# Allergic Respiratory Diseases: Causes, Symptoms and Treatment

# Allergic Respiratory Diseases: Causes, Symptoms and Treatment

Edited by Kim Geller

hayle
medical

New York

Hayle Medical,
750 Third Avenue, 9ᵗʰ Floor,
New York, NY 10017, USA

Visit us on the World Wide Web at:
www.haylemedical.com

ISBN: 978-1-63241-646-9

**Cataloging-in-Publication Data**

Allergic respiratory diseases : causes, symptoms and treatment / edited by Kim Geller.
    p. cm.
Includes bibliographical references and index.
ISBN 978-1-63241-646-9
1. Allergy. 2. Respiratory organs--Diseases. 3. Respiratory organs--Diseases--Etiology.
4. Symptoms. 5. Respiratory organs--Diseases--Treatment. 6. Immunology. I. Geller, Kim.
QR188 .A45 2019
616.97--dc23

# Table of Contents

# Preface

Respiratory diseases are the pathological conditions that affect the tissues and organs of the respiratory system such as the upper respiratory tract, pleura and pleural cavity, alveoli, bronchi, bronchioles, trachea, the nerves and muscles of breathing. Allergic respiratory diseases are caused due to exposure to an allergen. Asthma is a common allergic respiratory disease affecting nearly 300 million people worldwide. It is an inflammatory disease of the airways of the lungs, and is characterized by recurring symptoms like airway obstruction and bronchospasm. Avoiding exposures to allergens and irritants, inhaling corticosteroids and use of long-acting beta agonists are the chief strategies for the management of asthma. Sinusitis is another respiratory disease that can be caused by allergies. It is strongly correlated to asthma. The condition allergic fungal sinusitis occurs in people with nasal polyps and asthma. Allergic respiratory diseases are diagnosed by performing a blood test, chest X-ray, biopsy of the lung or pleura, bronchoscopy, etc. Several medications may be used to block allergic mediators and their actions, such as antihistamines, epinephrine, glucocorticoids, etc. This book brings forth some of the most innovative concepts and elucidates the unexplored aspects of allergic respiratory diseases. It includes some of the vital pieces of work being conducted across the world, on the causes, symptoms and treatments of such conditions. Those in search of information to further their knowledge will be greatly assisted by this book.

After months of intensive research and writing, this book is the end result of all who devoted their time and efforts in the initiation and progress of this book. It will surely be a source of reference in enhancing the required knowledge of the new developments in the area. During the course of developing this book, certain measures such as accuracy, authenticity and research focused analytical studies were given preference in order to produce a comprehensive book in the area of study.

This book would not have been possible without the efforts of the authors and the publisher. I extend my sincere thanks to them. Secondly, I express my gratitude to my family and well-wishers. And most importantly, I thank my students for constantly expressing their willingness and curiosity in enhancing their knowledge in the field, which encourages me to take up further research projects for the advancement of the area.

**Editor**

# The need for patient-focused therapy for children and teenagers with allergic rhinitis: a case-based review of current European practice

Alexandra F Santos[1,2,3], Luis Miguel Borrego[4,5], Giuseppina Rotiroti[6], Glenis Scadding[6] and Graham Roberts[7,8,9,10*]

## Abstract

Allergic rhinitis is a common problem in childhood and adolescence, with a negative impact on the quality of life of patients and their families. The treatment modalities for allergic rhinitis include allergen avoidance, anti-inflammatory symptomatic treatment and allergen specific immunotherapy. In this review, four cases of children with allergic rhinitis are presented to illustrate how the recently published EAACI Guidelines on Pediatric Allergic Rhinitis can be implemented in clinical practice.

**Keywords:** Allergy, Rhinitis, Pediatric rhinitis, Immunotherapy, Guidelines

## Introduction

Allergic rhinitis is a common problem in childhood and adolescence [1]. This is partly the reason why it is often under perceived by patients and families, under diagnosed and its impact underestimated. Allergic rhinitis causes chronic disturbing symptoms which have a negative effect on physical, social and psychological well-being, as well as on school performance of children and teenagers [2-4]. There are multiple associated co-morbidities [5], which further contribute to the direct and indirect costs of rhinitis [6]. Recently, a European Academy of Allergy and Clinical Immunology (EAACI) position paper on pediatric rhinitis was published to address the need for guidance on the management of this condition in the pediatric age group [7]. The main treatment modalities for pediatric allergic rhinitis include: avoidance of the relevant allergens, symptomatic treatment with H1-anti-histamines, intranasal corticosteroids and oral leukotriene-receptor antagonists, and allergen-specific immunotherapy (Figure 1). In this review article, we have used four pediatric cases to illustrate key aspects of the treatment of pediatric allergic rhinitis as an exercise to help implementing the aforementioned EAACI guidelines in clinical practice.

## Case 1

### *The importance of patient education and of a good nasal spray technique*

Six-year-old girl presented to clinic in June with troublesome hay fever symptoms. She had significant nasal obstruction and pruritus, sneezing and watery nasal discharge. The symptoms had started in early April and were progressively worsening. In previous years, she had had similar symptoms from April to July, but was asymptomatic during the rest of the year. Her doctor had prescribed oral cetirizine and intranasal mometasone furoate about 4 weeks after the symptoms started, but this treatment did not result in significant improvement. She stopped using the intranasal corticosteroid two weeks later because she was having frequent nose bleeds and had developed nasal crusting that she associated with the use of the nasal spray.

Skin prick testing was positive to grass pollens and negative to other common airborne allergens. After checking the patient's nasal spray technique, the allergy clinic team realised that she was not using it properly and spent some time providing appropriate training.

The patient was prescribed a very short course of rescue decongestant to open up her congested nasal airway and intranasal isotonic saline to minimise the formation of nasal crusting. She was advised to use daily intranasal

* Correspondence: g.c.roberts@soton.ac.uk
[7]David Hide Asthma and Allergy Research Centre, St Mary's Hospital, Isle of Wight, UK
[8]Human Development and Health and Clinical Experimental Sciences Academic Subunits, University of Southampton Faculty of Medicine, Southampton, UK
Full list of author information is available at the end of the article

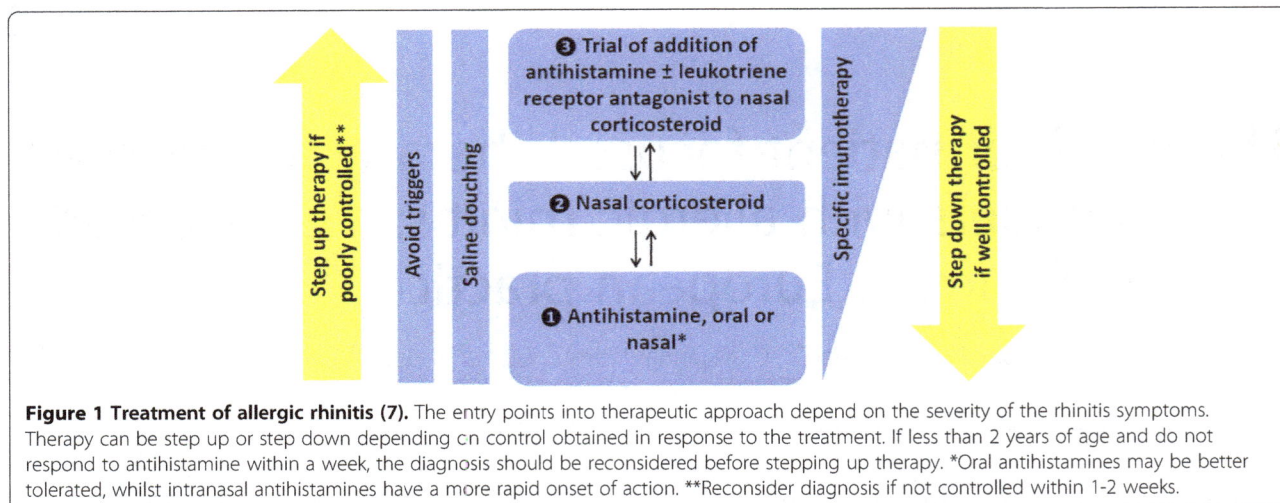

**Figure 1 Treatment of allergic rhinitis (7).** The entry points into therapeutic approach depend on the severity of the rhinitis symptoms. Therapy can be step up or step down depending on control obtained in response to the treatment. If less than 2 years of age and do not respond to antihistamine within a week, the diagnosis should be reconsidered before stepping up therapy. *Oral antihistamines may be better tolerated, whilst intranasal antihistamines have a more rapid onset of action. **Reconsider diagnosis if not controlled within 1-2 weeks.

mometasone furoate and cetirizine until the end of the pollen season, whilst attempting to minimise direct exposure to grass pollen. Her family was educated to start cetirizine and intranasal corticosteroids about 2 weeks before the beginning of the grass pollen season in the following years.

Case 1 highlights the importance of adherence to treatment and of a correct application technique of the nasal spray for maximum effect and for minimising side effects. Nasal drops and nasal sprays require different techniques (Figure 2) [8]. Poor technique is a common cause of treatment failure, so it is important to spend time in clinic explaining the appropriate use of these devices and providing hands-on training [9]. It is also important to explain the nature of the treatment, its safety profile and possible side effects. Patients should be given realistic expectations about the results of the treatment and should be informed that complete resolution does not usually occur in the treatment of chronic conditions such as allergic rhinitis. For example, in the case of intranasal corticosteroids, patients should be informed that they take a few days before any effects can be noticed. Appropriate information helps in ensuring concordance with therapy, which is critical for a good control of the nasal inflammation and for the improvement of the symptoms.

Minimising allergen exposure is also an important part of the management of this condition. Given her grass pollen allergy, she was advised to minimize early morning and evening activities outdoors, to avoid going out after thunderstorms or on windy days during the pollen season, to wear sunglasses when outside, to avoid mowing the grass or being near it when it is being mowed, to keep windows closed as much as possible and use air-conditioning and to wash her hair at the end of the day when she arrives home as well as to bathe her eyes and douche her nose frequently during the grass pollen season.

Finally, pollen levels rise slowly at the start of the pollen season with symptoms only presenting at a threshold level. Prior to this, exposure to small amounts of allergen will attract inflammatory cells into the nasal airway exacerbating symptoms when pollen levels rise further. Commencing hayfever treatment a few weeks prior to the expected start of the seasons, can be very helpful in delaying symptom onset and in achieving symptom control.

### Case 2
#### *The role of anti-leukotrienes in the treatment of allergic rhinitis*
An 8-year-old boy was referred to the Allergy clinic due to nasal symptoms consisting of rhinorrhoea, sneezing and nasal itching since he was 5. His parents reported that the symptoms usually persisted throughout the year, worsened during the winter, particularly with exposure to house dust, but had not disturbed his sleep or daily activities. While exercising, he usually developed wheeze and cough that subsided with rest. His physical examination was normal and skin prick tests were positive for house dust mite (HDM). Allergen avoidance and a once daily, non-sedative H1-antihistamine (desloratadine) resulted in improvement of the nasal symptoms but his exercise-induced complaints persisted. An anti-leukotriene (montelukast) was therefore added resulting in better control of the lower respiratory symptoms.

This patient had classic symptoms and signs of allergic rhinitis with rhinorrhoea, pruritus and sneezing. The presence of allergic sensitization to HDM suggests a diagnosis of allergic rhinitis.

According to the Allergic Rhinitis and its Impact on Asthma (ARIA) guidelines [10], his rhinitis would be classified as persistent based on the duration of symptoms and mild according to the impact of the disease

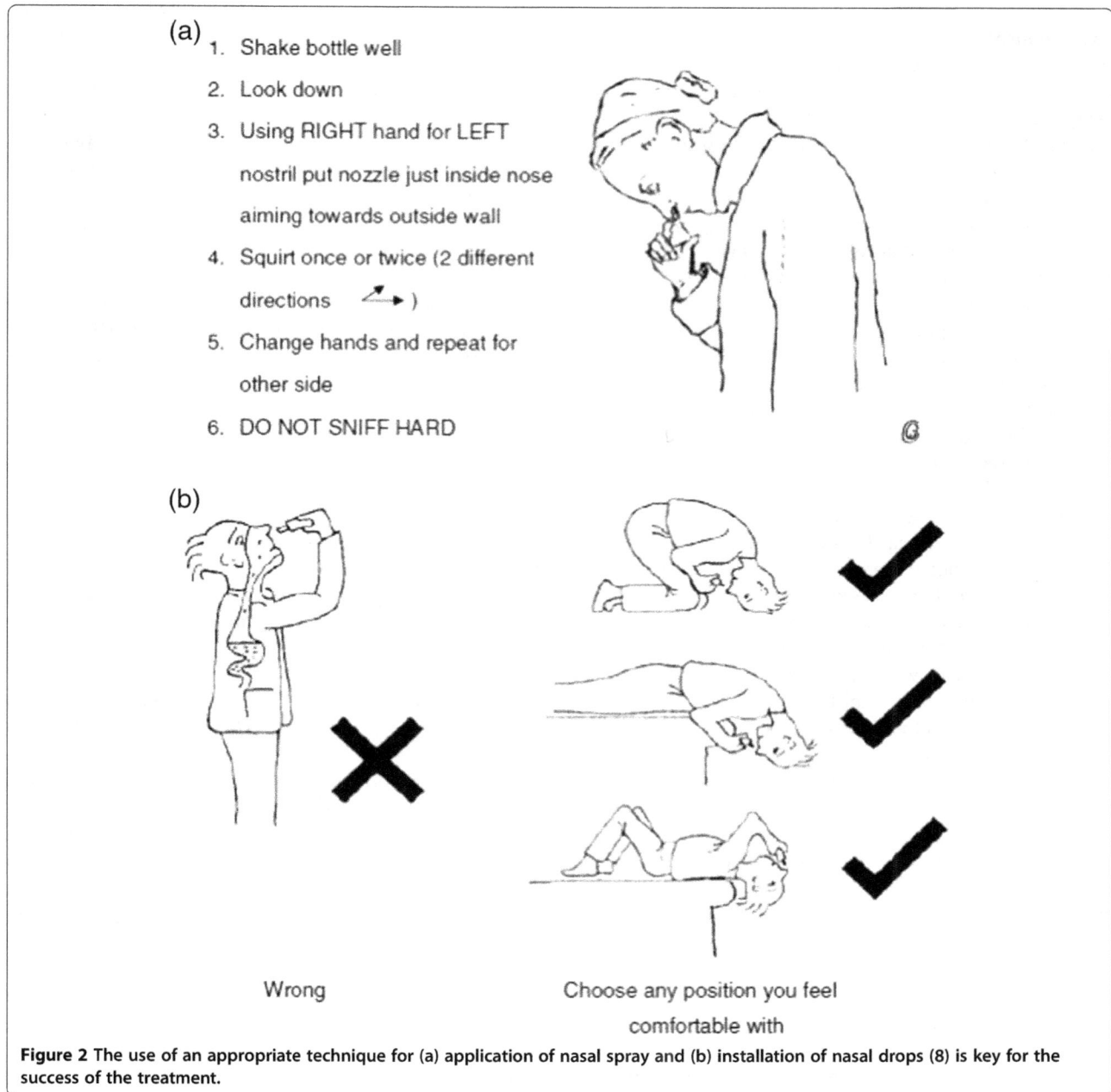

(a)
1. Shake bottle well
2. Look down
3. Using RIGHT hand for LEFT nostril put nozzle just inside nose aiming towards outside wall
4. Squirt once or twice (2 different directions ⤳ )
5. Change hands and repeat for other side
6. DO NOT SNIFF HARD

(b)

Wrong

Choose any position you feel comfortable with

**Figure 2** The use of an appropriate technique for (a) application of nasal spray and (b) installation of nasal drops (8) is key for the success of the treatment.

[10]. He also had wheeze in association with exercise. Various studies have shown that rhinitis and bronchial hyper-reactivity frequently co-exist in children [11-14] and that treatment of rhinitis can improve asthma control [15].

Allergen avoidance measures and anti-histamine therapy led to partial clinical improvement. It has been reported that allergen avoidance should be the first intervention for allergic rhinitis although interventional studies suggest that it is of limited value for allergens such as house dust mite. Regarding therapy, antihistamines can be used as first-line therapy, although nasal corticosteroids are more effective particularly in reducing mucosal oedema and may also have beneficial effects on asthma [13,15-19]. Nevertheless, antihistamines may be preferred in mild rhinitis, especially if there is no nasal obstruction, as in this case. Adding montelukast to the treatment improved symptom control. Anti-leukotriene receptor antagonists have been shown to be effective for controlling exercise-induced asthma and preventing the seasonal decrease in lung function parameters in patients with grass pollen allergy [20]. They may be used as add-on therapy to control rhinitis in patients with concomitant asthma [13,16-19].

## Case 3

### The treatment of coexisting conjunctivitis in allergic rhinitis

A 10 year-old girl was referred to the Allergy outpatient clinic for rhino-conjunctivitis of one year's duration. Her symptoms of rhinorrhoea, nasal blockage, sneezing and itching started when she was 7. She reported that her symptoms only occurred from March to June. They had now worsened with the addition of bilateral ocular *pruritus*, conjunctival *hyperaemia* and watering eyes. During these episodes she could not do her usual daily activities outdoors and did not sleep well. Physical examination was normal and skin prick tests were positive for grass pollen.

Considerable improvement occurred with allergen avoidance and oral levocetirizine once daily. After adding a nasal corticosteroid (mometasone furoate) once a day to the treatment, complete clinical remission occurred with good control of both ocular and nasal symptoms.

In the presence of rhinorrhoea, nasal obstruction, pruritus and sneezing [21] which develop seasonally and sensitization to pollen [10], a diagnosis of allergic rhinitis was made. According to the ARIA guidelines [10], it was classified as persistent rhinitis, since symptoms occurred more than 4 days a week and more than 4 weeks a year and as moderate/severe, since it affected her daily activities and sleep [10]. This case highlights that despite having only seasonal symptoms, patients can present with persistent moderate-severe rhinitis, which has implications for therapy.

This child also had allergic conjunctivitis, with bilateral ocular pruritus, hyperaemia and watery eyes, which is very common in patients with pollen-induced allergic rhinitis. Allergic conjunctivitis is the commonest co-morbidity associated with allergic rhinitis [22].

As described before, minimization of contact with the relevant allergens should be the first-line intervention. So, she was advised to avoid outdoor activities during the periods of high pollen count, to wear sunglasses when outside and to open the windows only during the evening and night.

Nasal corticosteroids were prescribed, ameliorating nasal and ocular symptoms. Nasal corticosteroids are considered to be the most effective treatment to control nasal inflammation in moderate to severe allergic rhinitis [13,16-18], especially in the presence of nasal obstruction [7,18]. Moreover, some studies have shown that fluticasone furoate and mometasone furoate improve conjunctivitis since some of the eye symptoms result from nasal inflammation and nasal-ocular reflex activation [23]. A recent systematic review and meta-analysis suggest that leukotriene receptor antagonists may also have a beneficial effect in ocular symptoms of seasonal allergic rhinitis [24].

Nasal corticosteroids are well tolerated, being recommended for children and adolescents with allergic rhinitis, from the age of two [23,25-27]. Newer nasal corticosteroids (e.g. fluticasone propionate [28], mometasone furoate [29])

are safe, and do not impair growth velocity [30], as opposed to older nasal corticosteroids, such as beclomethasone and budesonide. However, a recent study shows small impairment of growth with fluticasone furoate administered over a one-year period to prepubescent children with perennial allergic rhinitis [31]. Therefore, when prescribing nasal corticosteroids to children, one should balance the benefits and risks, prefer the ones with documented fewer adverse effects and explain to parents the safety and efficacy of this treatment in order to avoid loss of adherence to therapy and "steroid-phobia".

Finally, non-sedative antihistamines are useful as add-on therapy to nasal corticosteroids [7,10,16-18,32] and were prescribed for this patient with good results. First-generation antihistamines are not recommended for the treatment of allergic rhinitis as they cause sedation and may affect cognitive function and reduce academic and/or work performance [2,33].

## Case 4

### The role of allergen specific immunotherapy in the treatment of allergic rhinitis in children

Twelve-year-old boy presented with very disruptive symptoms of rhinitis with significant nasal obstruction as well as sneezing, rhinorrhoea and very disturbing nasal and ocular pruritus. These symptoms developed every year during the summer months and were persistent and severe, affecting his ability to sleep and his performance at school. His exam marks were lower in his summer examinations compared to those earlier in the year. He also felt that his nose problems were restricting his sport and social activities during the period when the weather was good; he liked playing outside. He was tested for different airborne allergens and both skin and specific IgE testing showed sensitization to grass pollen confirming grass pollen allergy. The previous years, he had been prescribed loratadine, intranasal mometasone furoate, montelukast and sodium cromoglicate eye drops, which he was taking. Despite good adherence, he continued to have poor disease control.

Given his continued symptoms, that were impacting on this quality of life, despite optimal pharmacotherapy, he was started on sublingual immunotherapy to grass pollen. He took the first dose in clinic and continued with the treatment at home. He initially had some local pruritus but this settled after a couple of weeks. One year into this treatment, he was already feeling some improvement and was able to reduce the medication he was taking to loratadine only.

Allergen-specific immunotherapy (IT) is the only disease-modifying treatment for allergic rhinitis. It is able to change the natural history of this condition and to provide long-term remission [34,35]. It is indicated in patients over 5 years old with demonstrable IgE to clinically relevant allergens, particularly in patients where pharmacological treatment has failed to control symptoms [36]. Since he was having troublesome symptoms despite maximum pharmacological therapy and the symptoms were due to grass pollen exposure to which he had detectable IgE, he was a good candidate for this treatment. There are standardized extracts to grass pollen commercially available to administer via the subcutaneous or the sublingual route [37,38]. Although there are very few head-to-head studies comparing subcutaneous immunotherapy (SCIT) and sublingual immunotherapy (SLIT), both forms are effective if appropriately used [39,40]. In terms of safety, SCIT more frequently causes systemic adverse events while SLIT tends to cause more local side effects, which are usually mild and resolve with continuation of treatment [41,42]. Severe adverse events are commonly associated with uncontrolled asthma, high allergen exposure during therapy, concomitant diseases such as severe infections and inexperienced health care staff. Premedication with an antihistamine may decrease the rate of adverse effects [43]. The decision on whether to do SLIT or SCIT depends on a variety of factors, including patient's preference about home-based versus hospital-based treatment, fear of injections, costs and concordance.[44]. In children, SLIT is more widely accepted but may have lower patient adherence [45]. Although SLIT is given at home, the first dose should be given at the doctor's office. This is also the opportunity to give detailed instructions about how to administer the treatment and about the precautions to be taken. Patients should be informed about possible adverse reactions and about the ways to treat them. Apart from the effectiveness in reducing symptoms and medication use, another potential advantage of allergen-specific immunotherapy is its preventative effects in reducing asthma and the development of further allergic sensitizations [46-50]. This is particularly important in the pediatric age groups. When clinically indicated, IT should be started early in the disease process, before significant remodelling and fixed airway obstruction has developed in the case of patients with asthma. As allergen-specific immunotherapy is the only disease-modifying treatment available for allergic rhinitis and respiratory allergy, it may be considered as a therapeutic option even before trying maximal therapy, depending on individual cases, clinical practice and finance.

## Conclusions

1. Patient education and appropriate nasal device training are very important for an effective and safe treatment of allergic rhinitis in children.
2. Allergen avoidance is part of the treatment of allergic rhinitis.
3. Symptomatic relief and reduction of nasal inflammation may be obtained with nasal corticosteroids, which are globally the most

effective therapy. Oral anti-histamines and anti-leukotrienes can also prove effective.
4. Allergen-specific immunotherapy is the only disease-modifying treatment for allergic rhinitis and has the potential to prevent the development of further allergic sensitization and asthma.

**Abbreviations**
ARIA: Allergic rhinitis and its impact on asthma; EAACI: European Academy of Allergy and Clinical Immunology; HDM: House dust mite; IT: Immunotherapy; SCIT: Subcutaneous immunotherapy; SLIT: Sublingual immunotherapy.

**Competing interests**
GS has received research grants from GSK, ALK; honoraria for articles, consulting, lectures/ chairing and/or advisory boards from ALK, Bausch & Lomb, Church & Dwight, Circassia, GSK, Groupo Uriach, Meda, Merck, Ono, Shionogi, Stallergenes.
The other authors declared no competing interests.

**Authors' contributions**
GR designed the manuscript, AFS and LMB wrote the first draft and all authors commented on the manuscript and accepted the final version. All authors read and approved the final manuscript.

**Author details**
[1]Department of Paediatric Allergy, Division of Asthma, Allergy & Lung Biology, King's College London, London, UK. [2]MRC & Asthma UK Centre in Allergic Mechanisms of Asthma, London, UK. [3]Immunoallergology Department, Coimbra University Hospital, Coimbra, Portugal. [4]CUF Descobertas Hospital, Lisbon, Portugal. [5]CEDOC, Nova Medical School, Universidade Nova de Lisboa, Lisbon, Portugal. [6]The Royal National Throat, Nose and Ear Hospital & University College London Hospitals, London, UK. [7]David Hide Asthma and Allergy Research Centre, St Mary's Hospital, Isle of Wight, UK. [8]Human Development and Health and Clinical Experimental Sciences Academic Subunits, University of Southampton Faculty of Medicine, Southampton, UK. [9]Respiratory Biomedical Research Unit, University Hospital Southampton NHS Foundation Trust, Southampton, UK. [10]Paediatric Allergy and Respiratory Medicine, University Child Health (MP803), University Hospital Southampton NHS Foundation Trust, Southampton, UK.

**References**
1. Asher MI, Montefort S, Bjorksten B, Lai CK, Strachan DP, Weiland SK, et al. Worldwide time trends in the prevalence of symptoms of asthma, allergic rhinoconjunctivitis, and eczema in childhood: ISAAC Phases one and three repeat multicountry cross-sectional surveys. Lancet. 2006;368(9537):733–43.
2. Walker S, Khan-Wasti S, Fletcher M, Cullinan P, Harris J, Sheikh A. Seasonal allergic rhinitis is associated with a detrimental effect on examination performance in United Kingdom teenagers: case-control study. J Allergy Clin Immunol. 2007;120(2):381–7.
3. Silva CH, Silva TE, Morales NM, Fernandes KP, Pinto RM. Quality of life in children and adolescents with allergic rhinitis. Braz J Otorhinolaryngol. 2009;75(5):642–9.
4. Roberts G, Hurley C, Lack G. Development of a quality-of-life assessment for the allergic child or teenager with multisystem allergic disease. J Allergy Clin Immunol. 2003;111(3):491–7.
5. Lack G. Pediatric allergic rhinitis and comorbid disorders. J Allergy Clin Immunol. 2001;108(1 Suppl):S9–15.
6. Bousquet J, Reid J, van Weel C, Baena Cagnani C, Canonica GW, Demoly P, et al. Allergic rhinitis management pocket reference 2008. Allergy. 2008;63(8):990–6.
7. Roberts G, Xatzipsalti M, Borrego LM, Custovic A, Halken S, Hellings PW, et al. Paediatric rhinitis: position paper of the European academy of allergy and clinical immunology. Allergy. 2013;68(9):1102–16.
8. Scadding GK, Durham SR, Mirakian R, Jones NS, Leech SC, Farooque S, et al. BSACI guidelines for the management of allergic and non-allergic rhinitis. Clin Exp Allergy. 2008;38(1):19–42.

9.   Gani F, Pozzi E, Crivellaro MA, Senna G, Landi M, Lombardi C, et al. The role of patient training in the management of seasonal rhinitis and asthma: clinical implications. Allergy. 2001;56(1):65–8.

10.  Bousquet J, Khaltaev N, Cruz AA, Denburg J, Fokkens WJ, Togias A, et al. Allergic Rhinitis and its Impact on Asthma (ARIA) 2008 update (in collaboration with the World Health Organization, GA 2) LEN and AllerGen). Allergy. 2008;63 Suppl 86:8–160.

11.  Kurukulaaratchy RJ, Raza A, Scott M, Williams P, Ewart S, Matthews S, et al. Characterisation of asthma that develops during adolescence; findings from the Isle of wight birth cohort. Respir Med. 2012;106(3):329–37.

12.  Hamouda S, Karila C, Connault T, Scheinmann P, de Blic J. Allergic rhinitis in children with asthma: a questionnaire-based study. Clin Exp Allergy. 2008;38 (5):761–6.

13.  Ballardini N, Kull I, Lind T, Hallner E, Almqvist C, Ostblom E, et al. Development and comorbidity of eczema, asthma and rhinitis to age 12: data from the BAMSE birth cohort. Allergy. 2012;67(4):537–44.

14.  Kurukulaaratchy RJ, Fenn M, Matthews S, Arshad SH. Characterisation of atopic and non-atopic wheeze in 10 year old children. Thorax. 2004;59(7):563–8.

15.  Lohia S, Schlosser RJ, Soler ZM. Impact of intranasal corticosteroids on asthma outcomes in allergic rhinitis: a meta-analysis. Allergy. 2013;68(5):569–79.

16.  Anolik R. Clinical benefits of combination treatment with mometasone furoate nasal spray and loratadine vs monotherapy with mometasone furoate in the treatment of seasonal allergic rhinitis. Ann Allergy Asthma Immunol. 2008;100(3):264–71.

17.  Martin BG, Andrews CP, van Bavel JH, Hampel FC, Klein KC, Prillaman BA, et al. Comparison of fluticasone propionate aqueous nasal spray and oral montelukast for the treatment of seasonal allergic rhinitis symptoms. Ann Allergy Asthma Immunol. 2006;96(6):851–7.

18.  Di Lorenzo G, Pacor ML, Pellitteri ME, Morici G, Di Gregoli A, Lo Bianco C, et al. Randomized placebo-controlled trial comparing fluticasone aqueous nasal spray in mono-therapy, fluticasone plus cetirizine, fluticasone plus montelukast and cetirizine plus montelukast for seasonal allergic rhinitis. Clin Exp Allergy. 2004;34(2):259–67.

19.  Simons FE, Simons KJ. Histamine and H1-antihistamines: celebrating a century of progress. J Allergy Clin Immunol. 2011;128(6):1139–50. e1134.

20.  Keskin O, Alyamac E, Tuncer A, Dogan C, Adalioglu G, Sekerel BE. Do the leukotriene receptor antagonists work in children with grass pollen-induced allergic rhinitis? Pediatr Allergy Immunol. 2006;17(4):259–68.

21.  Scadding GK, Durham SR, Mirakian R, Jones NS, Drake-Lee AB, Ryan D, et al. BSACI guidelines for the management of rhinosinusitis and nasal polyposis. Clin Exp Allergy. 2008;38(2):260–75.

22.  Bjorksten B, Clayton T, Ellwood P, Stewart A, Strachan D. Worldwide time trends for symptoms of rhinitis and conjunctivitis: phase III of the international study of asthma and allergies in childhood. Pediatr Allergy Immunol. 2008;19(2):110–24.

23.  Anolik R, Nathan RA, Schenkel E, Danzig MR, Gates D, Varghese S. Intranasal mometasone furoate alleviates the ocular symptoms associated with seasonal allergic rhinitis: results of a post hoc analysis. Int Arch Allergy Immunol. 2008;147 (4):323–30.

24.  Gane J, Buckley R. Leukotriene receptor antagonists in allergic eye disease: a systematic review and meta-analysis. J Allergy Clin Immunol Pract. 2013;1(1):65–74.

25.  Ratner PH, Meltzer EO, Teper A. Mometasone furoate nasal spray is safe and effective for 1-year treatment of children with perennial allergic rhinitis. Int J Pediatr Otorhinolaryngol. 2009;73(5):651–7.

26.  Wandalsen GF, Mendes AI, Sole D. Objective improvement in nasal congestion and nasal hyperreactivity with use of nasal steroids in persistent allergic rhinitis. Am J Rhinol Allergy. 2010;24(1):e32–6.

27.  Nathan RA, Berger W, Yang W, Cheema A, Silvey M, Wu W et al. Effect of once-daily fluticasone furoate nasal spray on nasal symptoms in adults and adolescents with perennial allergic rhinitis. Ann Allergy Asthma Immunol. 2008;100(5):497–505.

28.  Allen DB, Meltzer EO, Lemanske Jr RF, Philpot EE, Faris MA, Kral KM, et al. No growth suppression in children treated with the maximum recommended dose of fluticasone propionate aqueous nasal spray for one year. Allergy Asthma Proc. 2002;23(6):407–13.

29.  Daley-Yates PT, Kunka RL, Yin Y, Andrews SM, Callejas S, Ng C. Bioavailability of fluticasone propionate and mometasone furoate aqueous nasal sprays. Eur J Clin Pharmacol. 2004;60(4):265–8.

30.  Skoner DP, Rachelefsky GS, Meltzer EO, Chervinsky P, Morris RM, Seltzer JM, et al. Detection of growth suppression in children during treatment with intranasal beclomethasone dipropionate. Pediatrics. 2000;105(2):E23.

31.  Lee LA, Sterling R, Maspero J, Clements D, Ellsworth A, Pedersen S. Growth velocity reduced with once-daily fluticasone furoate nasal spray in prepubescent children with perennial allergic rhinitis. J Allergy Clin Immunol Pract. 2014;2(4):421–7.

32.  Benninger M, Farrar JR, Blaiss M, Chipps B, Ferguson B, Krouse J, et al. Evaluating approved medications to treat allergic rhinitis in the United States: an evidence-based review of efficacy for nasal symptoms by class. Ann Allergy Asthma Immunol. 2010;104(1):13–29.

33.  Vuurman EF, van Veggel LM, Uiterwijk MM, Leutner D, O'Hanlon JF. Seasonal allergic rhinitis and antihistamine effects on children's learning. Ann Allergy. 1993;71(2):121–6.

34.  Niggemann B, Jacobsen L, Dreborg S, Ferdousi HA, Halken S, Host A, et al. Five-year follow-up on the PAT study: specific immunotherapy and long-term prevention of asthma in children. Allergy. 2006;61(7):855–9.

35.  Calderon MA, GerthvanWijk R, Eichler I, Matricardi PM, Varga EM, Kopp MV, et al. Perspectives on allergen-specific immunotherapy in childhood: an EAACI position statement. Pediatr Allergy Immunol. 2012;23(4):300–6.

36.  Bufe A, Roberts G. Specific immunotherapy in children. Clin Exp Allergy. 2011;41(9):1256–62.

37.  Wahn U, Tabar A, Kuna P, Halken S, Montagut A, de Beaumont O, et al. Efficacy and safety of 5-grass-pollen sublingual immunotherapy tablets in pediatric allergic rhinoconjunctivitis. J Allergy Clin Immunol. 2009;123(1):160–6. e163.

38.  Bufe A, Eberle P, Franke-Beckmann E, Funck J, Kimmig M, Klimek L, et al. Safety and efficacy in children of an SQ-standardized grass allergen tablet for sublingual immunotherapy. J Allergy Clin Immunol. 2009;123(1):167–73. e167.

39.  Calderon MA, Alves B, Jacobson M, Hurwitz B, Sheikh A, Durham S. Allergen injection immunotherapy for seasonal allergic rhinitis. Cochrane Database Syst Rev. 2007;1, CD001936.

40.  Radulovic S, Wilson D, Calderon M, Durham S. Systematic reviews of sublingual immunotherapy (SLIT). Allergy. 2011;66(6):740–52.

41.  Vance GH, Goldring S, Warner JO, Cox H, Sihra B, Hughes S, et al. A national audit of pollen immunotherapy for children in the United Kingdom: patient selection and programme safety. Clin Exp Allergy. 2011;41(9):1313–23.

42.  Fiocchi A, Pajno G, La Grutta S, Pezzuto F, Incorvaia C, Sensi L, et al. Safety of sublingual-swallow immunotherapy in children aged 3 to 7 years. Ann Allergy Asthma Immunol. 2005;95(3):254–8.

43.  Portnoy J, Bagstad K, Kanarek H, Pacheco F, Hall B, Barnes C. Premedication reduces the incidence of systemic reactions during inhalant rush immunotherapy with mixtures of allergenic extracts. Ann Allergy. 1994;73(5):409–18.

44.  Zuberbier T, Bachert C, Bousquet PJ, Passalacqua G, Walter Canonica G, Merk H, et al. GA (2) LEN/EAACI pocket guide for allergen-specific immunotherapy for allergic rhinitis and asthma. Allergy. 2010;65(12):1525–30.

45.  Senna G, Lombardi C, Canonica GW, Passalacqua G. How adherent to sublingual immunotherapy prescriptions are patients? The manufacturers' viewpoint. J Allergy Clin Immunol. 2010;126(3):668–9.

46.  Jacobsen L, Niggemann B, Dreborg S, Ferdousi HA, Halken S, Host A, et al. Specific immunotherapy has long-term preventive effect of seasonal and perennial asthma: 10-year follow-up on the PAT study. Allergy. 2007;62(8):943–8.

47.  Inal A, Altintas DU, Yilmaz M, Karakoc GB, Kendirli SG, Sertdemir Y. Prevention of new sensitizations by specific immunotherapy in children with rhinitis and/or asthma monosensitized to house dust mite. J Investig Allergol Clin Immunol. 2007;17(2):85–91.

48.  Des Roches A, Paradis L, Menardo JL, Bouges S, Daures JP, Bousquet J. Immunotherapy with a standardized Dermatophagoides pteronyssinus extract. VI. Specific immunotherapy prevents the onset of new sensitizations in children. J Allergy Clin Immunol. 1997;99(4):450–3.

49.  Pajno GB, Barberio G, De Luca F, Morabito L, Parmiani S. Prevention of new sensitizations in asthmatic children monosensitized to house dust mite by specific immunotherapy. A six-year follow-up study. Clin Exp Allergy. 2001;31(9):1392–7.

50.  Purello-D'Ambrosio F, Gangemi S, Merendino RA, Isola S, Puccinelli P, Parmiani S, et al. Prevention of new sensitizations in monosensitized subjects submitted to specific immunotherapy or not. A retrospective study. Clin Exp Allergy. 2001;31(8):1295–302.

# 2

# Airborne protein concentration: a key metric for type 1 allergy risk assessment—in home measurement challenges and considerations

Liz Tulum[*], Zoë Deag, Matthew Brown, Annette Furniss, Lynn Meech, Anja Lalljie and Stella Cochrane[*]

## Abstract

**Background:** Exposure to airborne proteins can be associated with the development of immediate, IgE-mediated respiratory allergies, with genetic, epigenetic and environmental factors also playing a role in determining the likelihood that sensitisation will be induced. The main objective of this study was to determine whether airborne concentrations of selected common aeroallergens could be quantified in the air of homes using easily deployable, commercially available equipment and analytical methods, at low levels relevant to risk assessment of the potential to develop respiratory allergies. Additionally, air and dust sampling were compared and the influence of factors such as different filter types on allergen quantification explored.

**Methods:** Low volume air sampling pumps and DUSTREAM® dust samplers were used to sample 20 homes and allergen levels were quantified using a MARIA® immunoassay.

**Results:** It proved possible to detect a range of common aeroallergens in the home with sufficient sensitivity to quantify airborne concentrations in ranges relevant to risk assessment (Limits of Detection of 0.005–0.03 ng/m$^3$). The methodology discriminates between homes related to pet ownership and there were clear advantages to sampling air over dust which are described in this paper. Furthermore, in an adsorption–extraction study, PTFE (polytetrafluoroethylene) filters gave higher and more consistent recovery values than glass fibre (grade A) filters for the range of aeroallergens studied.

**Conclusions:** Very low airborne concentrations of allergenic proteins in home settings can be successfully quantified using commercially available pumps and immunoassays. Considering the greater relevance of air sampling to human exposure of the respiratory tract and its other advantages, wider use of standardised, sensitive techniques to measure low airborne protein concentrations and how they influence development of allergic sensitisation and symptoms could accelerate our understanding of human dose–response relationships and refine our knowledge of thresholds of allergic sensitisation and elicitation via the respiratory tract.

**Keywords:** Indoor aeroallergens, Dust, Air sampling, Respiratory allergy, Protein risk assessment

## Background

Exposure to airborne allergenic proteins can be associated with the development of immediate, IgE-mediated

*Correspondence: liz.tulum@unilever.com;
Stella.A.Cochrane@unilever.com
SEAC Unilever Colworth, Colworth Science Park, Sharnbrook, Bedfordshire
MK44 1LQ, UK

respiratory allergies such as hay fever or baker's asthma The focus of this paper is measurement of exposure and as such other risk factors (genetic, epigenetic and environmental) associated with development of allergic sensitisation are not covered in detail here. It is important to appreciate however that not all individuals exposed to airborne allergenic proteins, but rather a subset, are at risk of sensitisation. Whilst measurement of airborne protein concentrations has been widely undertaken in many occupational settings, for example wheat flour proteins in bakeries, to understand potential risks to worker health [1], this approach is less frequently applied in other settings. Thresholds of allergic sensitisation and elicitation to proteins via respiratory exposure remain poorly defined. A few studies have included measurement of airborne protein concentrations during use of products by consumers. Results have been used to define exposure benchmarks for consumer risk assessment [2–8], but the number of these studies in the published literature remains limited. In contrast, the most commonly used technique in studies of environmental allergen exposure in homes and schools is still measurement of allergen in dust samples [e.g. 9–12] as a 'surrogate' indicator of exposure. As recently highlighted by Custovic (2015), whilst exposure to allergen(s) is a prerequisite for sensitisation, we do not fully understand human dose–response relationships with regards to allergen exposure and subsequent sensitisation and/or elicitation [13]. Custovic 2015 called for the development of standardised, reliable and reproducible methods for measuring allergen exposure. To this suggestion could be added the need for a standardised, relevant metric, which we propose should be inhalable protein concentration, as is used in existing risk assessment and management approaches.

This paper describes work undertaken as a proof of principle study, to investigate the feasibility of using commercially available air sampling pumps, deployable by study participants, and allergen measurement techniques to quantify airborne protein concentrations (in this case of common environmental aeroallergens) in homes, at concentrations relevant to potential use in risk assessment and furthering our understanding of human-dose response relationships associated with the development of IgE mediated allergies.

The main objective of the study was to determine whether 11 common aeroallergens could be quantified, down to sub $ng/m^3$ concentrations, in the air of 20 homes using a low volume air sampler. Secondary objectives were to understand the challenges associated with taking such measurements, investigate the influences of different factors such as filter material on such measurements and establish general feasibility and acceptability in a domestic environment.

## Methods
### Demographics
The occupants of 20 homes in Bedfordshire (United Kingdom) and the surrounding counties agreed to take part (minimum inhabitants in home n = 2). Data was collected from urban and rural areas—50:50 distribution. Sampling occurred during 2 weeks in December 2014

(winter) in the UK in the lounge and a bedroom in each home.

Information about the environment in the lounge and bedroom used for sampling were collected through a questionnaire. The questionnaire requested each participant to provide information on their general cleaning routine, details about the layout of the lounge and bedroom, how often bed linen was changed and how often vacuuming was carried out. Information about the number of people in the household and details about soft furnishings in the rooms was also requested as part of the questionnaire.

The number of people and pets in the house and/or room being monitored and the proportion of time they spent in the room during the lounge run were recorded by questionnaire. The typical activities of the occupants of the room were also recorded during this run. At least one member of the household was at home all day during this study, as they needed to be present to do the sampling and all participants were asked to go about their daily activities in both rooms in which samples were taken. As stated they were asked to hoover the lounge and change the bed to release potential reservoirs of allergen into the air but they could also have been present in either room throughout the sampling period.

Some panellists recorded that they brought their Christmas trees and decorations down from their lofts at the time of the study, which could have introduced additional dust or airborne allergens into the indoor environment.

Participants were requested not to clean extensively the weekend before the study.

All subjects provided written Panellist Agreement and retained a copy of the Experimental Design and Procedures. An ethical review was not required as the study did not involve any intrusive procedures, sampling of human tissues, nor capturing of identifiable, personal data.

### Sampling and assays
#### Indoor air sampling
Subjects collected two air samples on two separate days using an air sampling pump (Casella TUFF™ 4+, Bedford, UK, 3.5 l/min), connected to an IOM (Institute of Occupational Medicine, SKC Inc. PA) sampling head, which is a simple filter holder. During the day the pump was located either in the lounge or the bedroom for a 10-h sampling period (thus sampling a total air volume of 2.1 $m^3$) in each location. Samples were collected onto glass fibre filters (grade A) (Casella Measurement; 25 mm diameter, 0.8 μm pore size) the most commonly used and typically recommended filter for the pumps. During the bedroom sampling, the bed linen was changed 30 min

into the sampling period. At the end of the study, the filters were refrigerated until they could be dispatched to Indoor Biotechnologies Ltd for analysis.

Details of the sampling sites were recorded in a questionnaire. The sampling head attached to the TUFF 4 PLUS AIR SAMPLER was situated in the lounge approximately 1 m above floor level, attached to a retort stand and clamp. The pump itself could be placed on the carpeted floor to dampen the noise from the device, if required.

In the bedroom, the IOM sampling head attached to the TUFF 4 PLUS AIR SAMPLER was situated in the bedroom on a bedside table at pillow height. If the room did not contain a bedside table the sampling head was clamped at approximately 1 m from the floor. The pump itself could be placed on the carpeted floor to dampen the noise from the device.

Participants were advised that 'the pump should not be situated near to the television due to possible electrostatic disturbance'.

### Indoor dust sampling

A sample of dust from the flooring of each lounge was also collected by vacuuming two A4 areas 30 min into the air sampling time using a DUSTREAM® Collector containing nylon collection filters (pore size 40 µm) (Indoor Biotechnologies Ltd, Cardiff) [6].

### MARIA® assay analysis

The GF/A filters and dust samples from the in home study were placed into separate centrifuge tubes and extracted using PBS-Tween (0.05%); 2 ml of PBS-Tween was added to each air filter and per 100 mg of dust. Each centrifuge tube was then placed in a rocker for 2 h at room temperature. The extracts were then analysed by Indoor Biotechnologies Ltd using their fluorescent **Mul**tiplex **AR**ray for Indoor Allergens (MARIA®) technology (Indoor Biotechnologies Ltd, Cardiff, UK) [14, 15]. The MARIA® technology is based on xMAP® technology (Luminex Corp. Austin TX) which uses polystyrene microspheres that are labelled to create distinct sets of microspheres. Separate bead sets are covalently coupled with allergen-specific monoclonal antibodies, enabling the simultaneous capture and detection of multiple allergens in a single sample. The MARIA® assay allowed simultaneous detection of: mite (Der p 1, Der f 1, Mite Group 2), cat (Fel d 1), dog (Can f 1), mouse (Mus m1), rat (Rat n 1), German Cockroach (Bla g 2), Birch pollen (Bet v 1), Alternaria rot fungus (Alt a 1) and peanut allergens (Ara h 6—for dust and air samples this assay was in process of validation, however for filter comparison it had been validated).

### Filter comparison

Separate and in parallel to the in-home study, allergen adsorption and extraction from two different filter types (37 mm GF/A and 47 mm PTFE filters) was compared to investigate how filter type could impact upon allergen quantification. To achieve this, solutions of purified allergens, containing the 11 allergens used in the MARIA assay, were prepared in PBS (phosphate buffered saline, pH 7.4). 75 µl of these solutions were then added to 2 ml of PBS-Tween (0.05% Tween) in separate tubes such that each tube contained a total of 1, 5 and 10 ng of each allergen. Clean PTFE or GF/A filters were then inserted into the tubes and placed on a rocker for 2 h. These 'adsorption–extraction' samples were prepared in triplicate. 'No filter' control samples were also prepared by simply omitting addition of a filter. Control solutions were also analysed immediately after preparation and before rotation, the results of this analysis (not shown) were not significantly different from the rotated solutions. Allergen concentrations in the solutions after 2 h on a rocker were determined by Indoor Biotechnologies Ltd using the MARIA® assay as described in the preceding text.

## Results
### Filter comparison

All samples were analysed at three dilutions: neat, 1:2 and 1:4. A high degree of reproducibility was observed between different dilutions with an average CV (coefficient of variation) of 5.06%. The average variability between replicates was 7.16% (data not shown). The amounts of allergen measured using the MARIA® assay are summarised in Fig. 1 for the two types of filters incubated with 1, 5 and 10 ng allergen respectively.

The results indicate that the PTFE and GF/A filters absorb and release allergens to different extents, which also varies depending on the allergen and the concentration of the allergen present in the solution. For the majority of allergens (7/11) there was little difference between filter types or PTFE gave a slightly better recovery and equivalent recovery across the allergen doses e.g. as for mus m1. For four allergens however GF/A filters gave poor recovery values compared to PTFE and for 3 allergens (mite group 2 allergens, Can f 1 and Bet v 1) with no recovery at the lowest allergen dose which then plateaus significantly below the PTFE values at the higher doses. For the 4th allergen—Ara h 6—there was no difference in recovery across all doses, although recovery from the GF/A filters was lower, as already noted.

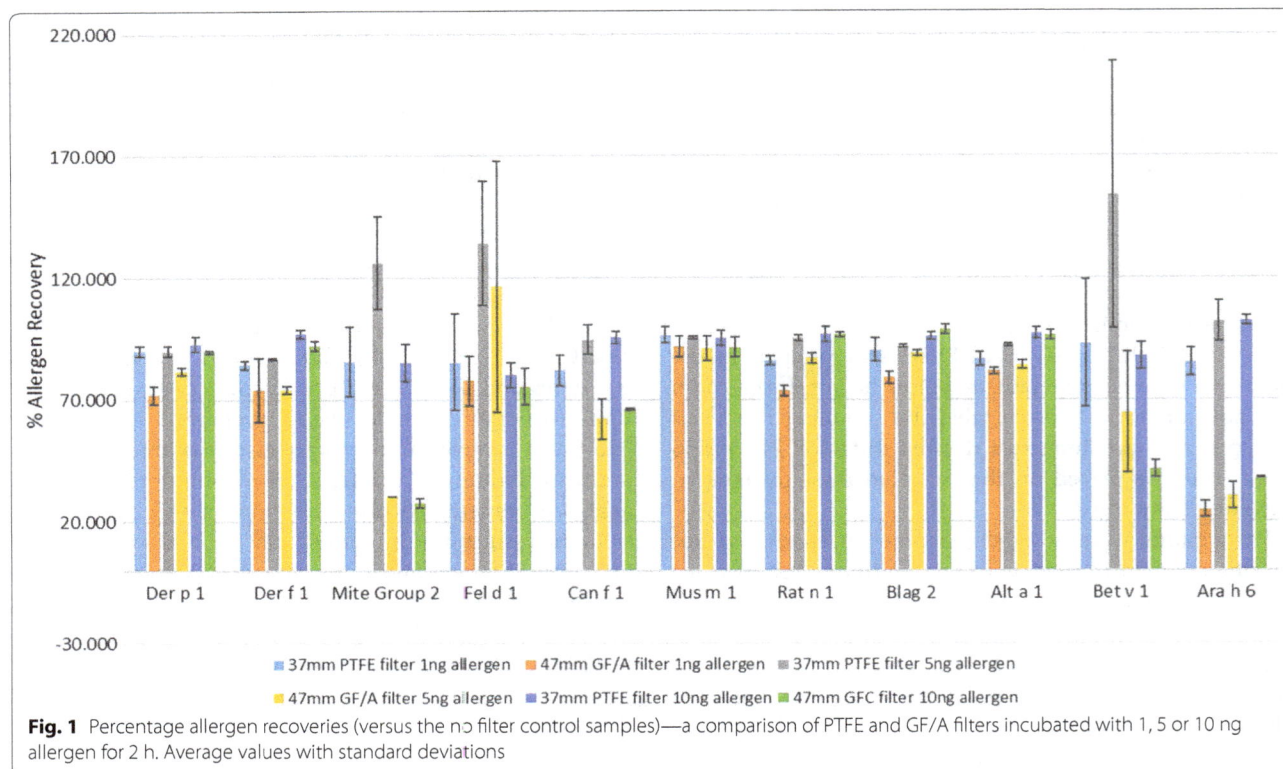

**Fig. 1** Percentage allergen recoveries (versus the no filter control samples)—a comparison of PTFE and GF/A filters incubated with 1, 5 or 10 ng allergen for 2 h. Average values with standard deviations

## In home study: demographics and study participant observations

The minimum and maximum number of inhabitants were 2 and 4 respectively. 7/20 homes had 2 inhabitants, 6/20 3 and 7/20 4.

Six households had a cat (one cat) and six had a dog (one which had two), none had both. One household had two guinea pigs and a cornsnake (fed mice).

Hoovering frequency was mostly weekly (12/20 homes) with the maximum and minimum frequencies being daily and every 2 weeks respectively. The duration of hoovering undertaken during the study ranged from 4 to 28 min.

The most typical frequency for bed linen changing was once every 2 weeks (13/20 homes) with the maximum and minimum frequencies being weekly and monthly respectively. The duration taken to change bed linen during the study was reported to be 6–20 min.

11 (55%) homes had carpet in the lounge versus 9 with laminate flooring and 18 (90%) had carpet in the bedroom versus 2 with laminate flooring.

Peanuts were consumed regularly in 8 of the 20 homes.

The majority of panellists found the sampling protocols easy to follow, however, there were a few instances of pumps either not starting properly, or (more rarely) switching themselves off mid-run, indicating that the TUFF 4 air sampler internal timers can sometimes be

unreliable, and that use should be carefully monitored and real-time study support provided for panellists to address and minimise the impact of such events upon any sampling (as was the case for this study). The pumps were relatively noisy to run but it was found that the noise could be dampened easily by placing the pumps on a carpeted surface. Panellists did quickly habituate to the noise throughout the 10-h run. It is possible to buy or make noise-cancelling boxes. In light of these findings the authors briefly investigated use of an alternative commercially available sampling pump, the SKC Leland Legacy, with a higher sampling rate of approximately 12 l/min. This was successfully used with a shorter (7 h) sampling period (data not shown).

### In home measurements: general observations

Common aeroallergens detected in the study were as follows: Der p1, Der f1 and mite group 2, cat, dog, rat, mouse, birch pollen, peanut (Ara h6). Mould (Alt a 1) and cockroach (Bla g 2) allergen were below the limit of detection (LoD) in all homes. Table 1 provides an overview of the maximum and minimum values recorded for each allergen across the homes, where they were detectable, along with the LoD. Overall allergen concentration ranges were 0.003–245 µg/g for dust and 0.005–18 ng/$m^3$ in air. The limit of detection ranges for the allergens

**Table 1** Minimum and maximum concentrations for all allergens measured above the LoD in air (lounge and bedroom) and dust (lounge only, where there was sufficient sample for extraction) across 20 homes

| Sample location | Der p 1 | Der f 1 | Mite group 2 | Fel d 1 | Can f 1 | Mus m 1 | Rat n 1 | Bet v 1 | Ara h 6 |
|---|---|---|---|---|---|---|---|---|---|
| Allergen concentration in ng/m³ air | | | | | | | | | |
| LOD ng/m³ air | 0.03 | 0.03 | 0.01 | 0.01 | 0.03 | 0.005 | 0.01 | 0.02 | 0.01 |
| Lounge air min | 0.05 | ND | ND | 0.2 | 0.07 | ND | ND | ND | ND |
| Lounge air max | 0.16 | ND | 0.04 | 14.1 | 9.74 | ND | ND | ND | 0.04 |
| Bedroom air min | ND | ND | ND | 0.13 | ND | ND | ND | ND | ND |
| Bedroom air max | 0.28 | 0.04 | 0.06 | 17.9 | 2.76 | 0.005 | ND | ND | ND |
| Allergen concentration in µg/g dust | | | | | | | | | |
| LOD µg/g dust | 0.012 | 0.012 | 0.004 | 0.004 | 0.012 | 0.002 | 0.004 | 0.01 | 0.004 |
| Lounge dust min | 0.014 | 0.028 | 0.009 | 0.006 | 0.014 | 0.003 | 0.02 | 0.02 | 0.005 |
| Lounge dust max | 17.80 | 9.042 | 10.010 | 42.01 | 244.89 | 0.005 | 0.06 | 0.07 | 3.73 |

*LOD* limit of detection, *ND* not detectable above LOD in any of the homes

were 0.002–0.012 µg/g for dust and 0.005–0.03 ng/m³ for air. These are extremely low detection ranges when compared to those achievable with conventional ELISA results.

As described in the filter comparison section GF/A filters, which were used for air sampling in the homes, gave poor recovery values compared to PTFE for 4 allergens (mite group 2 allergens, Can f 1, Bet v 1 and Ara h 6). Therefore, due to the uncertainty associated with the exposures measured for these allergens the absolute values in Table 1 should be treated with caution and whilst some observations associated with their detection are included in the following text, they were omitted from any statistical analyses.

A descriptive narrative is provided in the following text to give insights into the techniques used and where statistical analyses were possible the results are indicated in the text and relevant figure legends.

**Lounge (air and dust measured)**

If a home was cat or dog-free no corresponding allergens were detected in the air of the lounge however, specific allergen (Fel d 1 and/or Can f 1) was detected in the homes of people with either a cat or a dog. For example, for Fel d 1 airborne concentrations in lounges ranged from 0.24 to 14.1 ng/m³ (mean 3.25 ng/m³) in the 6/20 homes with cats, whereas no airborne Fel d 1 was measurable above the LoD in the 14/20 homes without cats. In contrast, dust levels did not reflect ownership—Fel d 1 was detected in dust even when animals were not present in the home, although there was a significant difference (P < 0.001) in the amount detected in homes with cats compared to those without when the data each group was compared by $T$ test (unpaired, 2-tailed). Fel d 1 dust levels in lounges from homes with cats ranged from 10.5

to 42.01 µg/g compared to < LoD-0.168 µg/g in homes without cats.

There was no significant difference in the levels of mite allergens (Der p 1 and Der f 1) found in rural homes when sampling dust, but some households didn't have enough dust sample for analysis. In contrast, the airborne concentrations of Der p 1 were significantly higher in urban homes as shown in Figs. 2 and 3.

When comparing homes containing carpet with those with solid flooring. As shown in Figs. 4 and 5 there were no significant differences in the concentrations of the 2 mite allergens in dust in homes with carpet compared to those with solid flooring, as was also the case when air was sampled. However, some homes, containing both

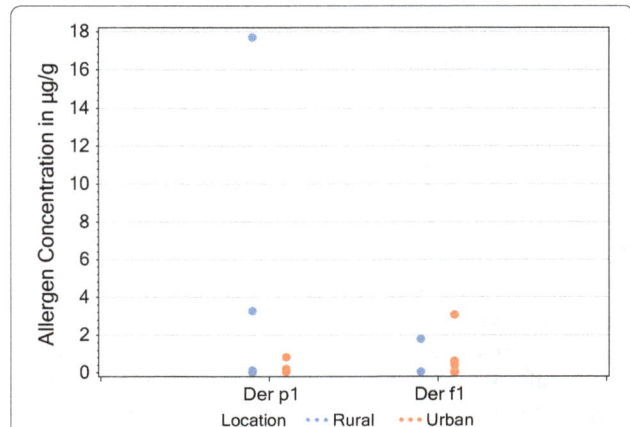

**Fig. 2** Comparison of measurable (above the LoD) mite allergen dust concentrations in the lounges of rural and urban homes (respective rural and urban sample sizes (n) were 5 and 8 for Der p1 and 2 and 5 for Der f1). Statistical analysis (T-test unpaired 2 t-tailed) comparing rural and urban measurable values gave P-values of 0.157 and 0.779 for Der p 1 and Der f 1 respectively

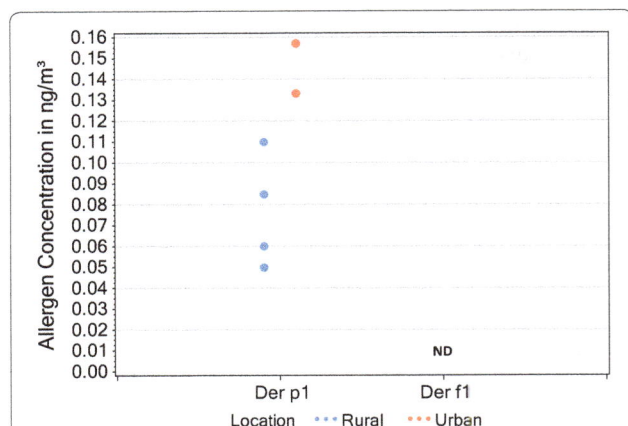

**Fig. 3** Comparison of measurable (above the LoD) mite allergen airborne concentrations in the lounges of rural and urban homes (Respective rural and urban sample sizes (n) were 4 and 2 for Der p1). Statistical analysis (T-test unpaired 2 t-tailed) comparing rural and urban measurable values P = 0.042. ND = not detected above the LOD

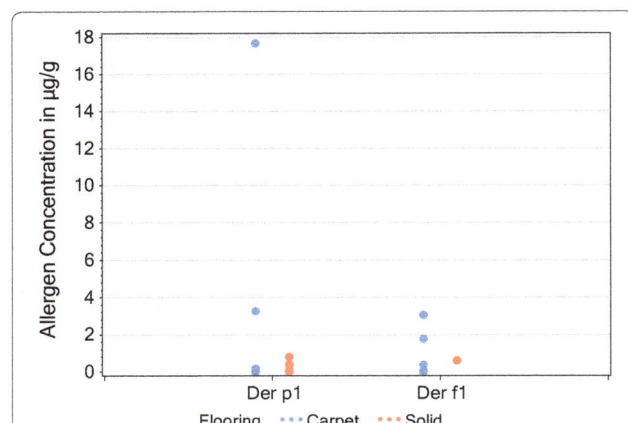

**Fig. 4** Comparison of measurable (above the LoD) mite allergen dust concentrations in lounges with carpets and those with solid flooring (Respective carpet and solid flooring sample sizes (n) were 9 and 4 for Der p1 and 6 and 1 for Der f1). Statistical analysis (T-test unpaired 2 t-tailed) comparing carpet and solid flooring measurable values gave a P-values of 0.569 for Der p 1. Analysis was not possible for Der f 1 due to the single solid flooring value

carpet and solid flooring, yielded insufficient dust during sampling to give accurate results.

Other aeroallergens found at detectable levels in the lounge air of some homes were: Ara h6 and Bet v 1, despite being 2 of the allergens more difficult to extract from GF/A filters. It was interesting to note that birch allergen was detectable in the air of the lounge of 2 homes in December, one of these was in a rural location with a birch tree in extremely close proximity.

## Bedroom (only air measured)

Ara h 6 was measurable in the bedroom air of only one home, but again this may reflect the difficulties associated with extracting this allergens from GF/A filters. Other aeroallergens found at detectable levels in the bedroom air of some homes were Der p1, Der f 1, Mite group 2, Fel d 1, mus m1 and Can f 1.

## Discussion

We demonstrate in this pilot study that it is possible to quantify very low airborne concentrations of a range of common aeroallergens, in homes using a commercially available Tuff 4 Plus pump sampling at low volumes (3.5 l/min) over long periods of time (10 h) coupled with analysis of GF/A filters using a MARIA® immunoassay.

The method used had enough sensitivity to quantify very low levels of allergen (0.005–18 ng/m³), encompassing values relevant to the risk assessment of exposure to proteins through use of consumer products (0.1–15 ng/m³) [1, 6]. It could also be of use in investigating and refining our understanding of human-dose response relationships and thresholds of allergic sensitisation and/or elicitation. However care should be taken when comparing data and benchmarking exposure values between studies to ensure all variables and potential confounding factors are considered, for example the use of high or low air volume sampling pumps and different filter types etc.

In terms of the filters used for detection of aeroallergens the data from the adsorption–extraction study suggests PTFE filters should be the preferred choice in the absence of any further information. However only a small number of allergens have been studied and validation studies should be undertaken to confirm the optimum filter type for allergen capture and subsequent extraction, which should optimized to prevent absorption to glassware and filter e.g. inclusion of Tween 20. As GF/A filters were used for the air sampling in the in home study the poor recovery noted for GF/A versus PTFE filters for mite group 2 allergens, Can f 1, Bet v 1 and Ara h 6 are such that we cannot rule out absorption to the filter as a confounding factor impacting upon detection and quantification of these allergens.

The study also showed clear advantages to air sampling compared to dust sampling. In some situations, there was simply insufficient (house) dust for extraction, whereas air can always be sampled. Additionally, the manner in which dust accumulates appears to blur the relationship between allergen levels in dust and relevant household characteristics such as pet ownership. Of course, it is air that is inhaled, not settled dust, and therefore an airborne concentration is most relevant to human respiratory tract exposure in a risk assessment context. Airborne measurements can provide insights into the patterns of exposure

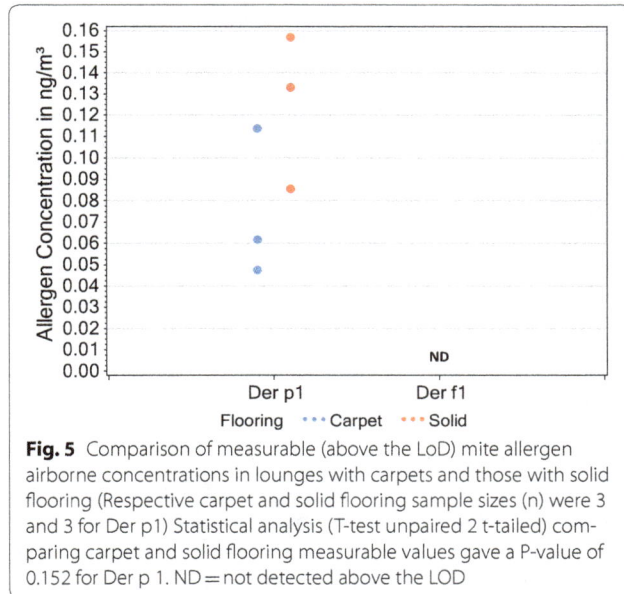

**Fig. 5** Comparison of measurable (above the LoD) mite allergen airborne concentrations in lounges with carpets and those with solid flooring (Respective carpet and solid flooring sample sizes (n) were 3 and 3 for Der p1) Statistical analysis (T-test unpaired 2 t-tailed) comparing carpet and solid flooring measurable values gave a P-value of 0.152 for Der p 1. ND = not detected above the LOD

whereas, at best, dust allergen content is more akin to a proxy for cumulative exposure.

Relationships were observed between homes in which peanut is eaten, the ownership of a cat/dog, pet free homes, and the presence of the applicable allergen in both air and dust.

Despite the reduced extraction efficiency observed with Ara h 6 and GF/A filters the peanut allergen Ara h 6 was detected in both air and dust samples from the lounges of 2 households and in the air sampled in the bedroom of one of these households. This is in contrast to the findings of Brough et al. [9] who failed to detect peanut in air samples from homes with high peanut levels in dust. Brough et al. used the same air sampling device as in this study and GF/A filters, but did not detect peanut allergen despite sampling for longer (22 h). However the limit of quantification of their analytical method was equivalent to 2.5 µg/m$^3$, compared to a limit of detection in this study of 0.01 ng/m$^3$, i.e. 5 orders of magnitude higher. Additionally, the assay used by Brough et al. [9], was the Neogen Veratox® peanut ELISA, designed primarily for use with foods, which according to Jayasena et al. [16] is most sensitive in the recognition of peanut allergens Ara h 3 and Ara h 1 and least sensitive in recognizing the more stable peanut allergens Ara h 2 and Ara h 6 [17]. Differences in stability may influence persistence in the home and therefore assays targeting a more stable allergenic protein could provide insight into exposure to allergenic proteins with the potential to persist and accumulate. Brough et al. [9] concluded 'Thus peanut protein is unlikely to cause either peanut sensitization or allergic

manifestations in patients with peanut allergy through inhalation unless the peanuts are deshelled in close proximity to them' a statement which cannot be substantiated in the light of our results. Birch pollen in air in December also suggests that in-home 'build up' can result in year-round exposure to allergens typically considered seasonal.

If homes were cat-free this was reflected by the lack of detectable Fel d 1 in air samples. However when dust was sampled Fel d 1 was detectable in almost all cat-free homes (though at lower levels than in homes with cats) illustrating that dust, as mentioned, is more akin to a proxy for cumulative exposure as opposed to air, which has the potential to provide data on patterns of exposure. Whilst absolute Fel d 1 values in air and dust samples were lower than reported in previous studies, reflecting the increased sensitivity (typically 10 × more sensitive) of the approach used and other variables such as a small number of homes, the magnitude of difference (2–3 orders of magnitude for dust) between cat-owning and cat-free homes was similar. For example, Custovic et al. [18] sampled dust from 75 British homes using a very similar approach, though coupled with a less sensitive immunoassay and reported an average Fel d 1 dust concentration of 237 µg/g in living rooms of homes with cats, whereas in this study the average concentration in lounge dust was 20 µg/g. In homes without cats, levels were ~ 260 × lower (mean of 0.9 µg/g) in the Custovic et al. study compared to ~ 500 × lower (mean of 0.04 µg/g) in this study. Custovic et al. [18] reported airborne Fel d 1 concentrations of 0.7–38 ng/m$^3$ in homes with cats and 0.24–1.78 ng/m$^3$ without cats (detectable in 22/75 i.e. 30% of such homes) compared to 0.24–14.1 ng/m$^3$ in the 6/20 homes with cats in our study and no detectable airborne Fel d 1 in any of the 14 homes without cats.

Using the same sampling pump as in this study but sampling variable volumes in *bedrooms* Custovic et al. [18] reported Fel d 1 airborne concentrations were 0.4–28 ng/m$^3$ in homes with cats and < 0.4 ng/m$^3$ in homes without cats. In comparison, in our study Fel d 1 airborne concentrations were 0.13–17.87 ng/m$^3$ in bedrooms of homes with cats and < 0.01 ng/m$^3$ in those without cats.

Custovic et al. [19] also investigated the relationship between dust and air measurements for Der p 1 and Can f 1 in addition to Fel d 1. Again using similar dust sampling, but for air sampling a higher volume air sampler (60 l/min) was used. Airborne Der p 1 was below the LoD of the assay used i.e. < 0.8 ng/m$^3$ in all homes, with Der p 1 levels in living room carpet dust ranging from 0.2 to 66 µg/g (mean 1.14 µg/g). In contrast, in our study, in lounges, airborne Der p 1 levels were detectable (> 0.03 ng/m$^3$) and measurable in 6 out of 20 homes. This illustrates that despite using a lower volume air sampler, when coupled with a sensitive immunoassay (MARIA®) airborne concentrations of Der p 1 could be quantified in homes with apparently lower Der p 1 dust reservoirs. Can f 1 data were not compared due to the aforementioned potential confounding factor associated with the use of GF/A filters and Can f 1 measurement in this study.

Custovic et al. [19] recognised the need for standardised methods to measure allergen exposure to enable robust assessment of the relationship between exposure, sensitisation and allergic symptoms. At the time of publication, it was concluded that the aerodynamics of each allergen should be considered and for 'larger/heavier' allergens such as dust mite allergens measuring levels in dust appeared to be best available index of exposure. However, whilst an index of exposure may be useful in understanding clinically relevant exposures for individuals, in order to further our understanding of the quantitative relationship between exposure and risk of sensitisation or development of allergic symptoms the quantity of inhaled allergen would be the ideal measure of personal exposure. We echo these thoughts and show in this publication that it is technically feasible with readily available and easy to use equipment and assays.

One aspect of airborne allergen exposure that is still poorly understood is the role of high peak airborne concentration exposure versus chronic low airborne exposure on sensitisation or elicitation. More extensive use of 'personal' exposure monitoring could provide insight regarding this issue. The pumps used in this study have successfully been used in a 'personal' monitoring study, with modifications so they could be carried and sampling timed over 24 h coupled with recording of participants' location and activity [20, 21]. One could envisage a similar study also incorporating a symptom diary to understand the relationship between exposure to an allergen and elicitation of symptoms in individuals with symptomatic allergy to that allergen.

In summary, whilst there have been some studies using air sampling to understand allergen exposure, the use of different combinations of high and low volume pumps sampling variable amounts of air, coupled with relatively insensitive immunoassays has led to variable success and a perception of the measurement of the allergen concentration of air being technically challenging and requiring specialist equipment. By contrast dust sampling is perceived as simpler and therefore still dominates as the technique used to obtain some 'index' of allergen exposure. This situation has hindered progress in our understanding of human dose–response relationships with regards to the development of immediate IgE mediated allergy to airborne proteins, which are essential to quantitative risk assessment. Now, with a variety

of pumps sampling at different rates being easily available and adaptable, improved protein capture filter materials and improvement in allergen detection and characterisation (e.g. stability and potential for persistence and home build up) we propose that it is time for a change and hopefully a step forward in research into human inhalational exposure to proteins. Finally, we would also suggest it is time to study exposure to a wider range of proteins, including those not associated with respiratory allergy, to further understand differences in allergenic 'potency'.

## Conclusions
Our study demonstrates that in-home measurements of low airborne allergen concentrations, at levels relevant for risk assessment of potential allergic sensitisation, are possible without bespoke specialist equipment. Such measurements can be achieved using equipment that can be easily deployed in homes by study participants. Wider use of such methodology should be pursued to further understanding of human dose–response relationships with regards to the development of immediate IgE mediated allergy to airborne proteins and refinement of current risk assessment data. This paper also highlights limitations of current approaches such as dust sampling compared to inhalable protein measurement.

**Authors' contributions**
All authors made substantial contributions to conception and design, or acquisition of data, or analysis and interpretation of data. More specifically: AL and SC were responsible for the formulation and evolution of overarching research goals. AL, LT, SC and ZD were responsible for study planning, coordination and management. LT, MB, AF and LM performed the experiments described, collected and curated the data. LT, ZD and SC analysed the study data. AL, LT, SC and ZD wrote the manuscript including the initial draft and subsequent revisions. All authors read and approved the final manuscript.

**Acknowledgements**
We appreciate the efforts of all participants in performing the collections and monitoring; thank you all. We would also like to thank James Hindley and Anna Kuklinska-Pijanka from Indoor Biotechnologies for their analytical expertise and support.

**Competing interests**
All authors are/were employees of Unilever.

**Funding**
This research was funded by Unilever.

## References

1. Baur X, Chen Z, Liebers V. Exposure-response relationships of occupational inhalative allergens. Clin Exp Allergy. 1998;28:537–44.
2. Johnston G, Innis JD, Mills KJ, Bielen F, Date RF, Weisgerber D, Sarlo K. Safety assessment for a leave-on personal care product containing a protease enzyme. Hum Exp Toxicol. 1999;8:527.
3. Kelling CK, Bartolo RG, Ertel KD, Smith LA, Watson DD, Sarlo K. Safety assessment of enzyme containing personal cleansing products: exposure characterization and development of IgE antibody to enzyme after a 6 month test. J Allergy Clin Immunol. 1998;101:179–87.
4. Sarlo K, Adamson GM, Hollis VL, Innis JD, Babcock LS, Kirchner DB. Development of allergic antibody to an enzyme in a body lotion: results of an 18-month clinical study. Immunotoxicology. 2004;1:71–7.
5. Sarlo K, Kirchner DB, Troyano E, Smith LA, Carr GJ, Rodriguez C. Assessing the risk of type 1 allergy to enzymes present in laundry and cleaning products: evidence from the clinical data. Toxicology. 2010;271:87–93.
6. Troyano E, McMillan D, Sarlo K, Li L, Wimalasena R. Approach to assessing consumer safety of botanical ingredients with emphasis to type I allergy. In: Dayan N, Kromidas L, editors. Formulating, packaging, and marketing of natural cosmetic products. Hoboken: Wiley; 2011 **(Chapter 9)**.
7. Pocalyko DJ, Chander P, Harding CR, Blaikie L, Watkinson A, Rawlings AV. The efficacy, stability and safety of topically applied protease in treating xerotic skin. In: Leyden JJ, Rawlings AV, editors. Skin moisturization. New York: Marcel Dekker; 2002. p. 365–84.
8. Blaikie L, Richold M, Whittle E, Lawrence RS, Keech S, Basketter DA. Airborne exposure from topically applied protein (proteolytic enzyme). Hum Exp Toxicol. 1999;18:528.
9. Brough HA, Makinson K, Penagos M, Maleki SJ, Cheng H, Douiri A, Stephens AC, Turcanu V, Lack G. Distribution of peanut protein in the home environment. J Allergy Clin Immunol. 2013;13:623–9.
10. Bertelsen RJ, Faeste CK, Granum B, Egaas E, London SJ, Carlsen KH, Lødrup Carlsen KC, Løvik M. Food allergens in mattress dust in Norwegian homes—a potentially important source of allergen exposure. Clin Exp Allergy. 2014;44:142–9.
11. Kanchongkittiphon W, Sheehan WJ, Friedlander J, Chapman MD, King EM, Martirosyan K, Baxi SN, Permaul P, Gaffin JM, Kopel L, Bailey A, Fu C, Petty CR, Gold DR, Phipatanakul W. Allergens on desktop surfaces in preschools and elementary schools of urban children with asthma. Allergy. 2014;69:960–3.
12. Krop EJ, Jacobs JH, Sander I, Raulf-Heimsoth M, Heederik J. Allergens and β-glucans in Dutch homes and schools: characterizing airborne levels. PLoS ONE. 2014;14(9):e88871.
13. Custovic A. To what extent is allergen exposure a risk factor for the development of allergic disease? Clin Exp Allergy. 2015;45:54–62.
14. King EM, Vailes LD, Tsay A, Satinover SM, Chapman MD. Simultaneous detection of total and allergen-specific IgE by using purified allergens in a fluorescent multiplex array. J Allergy Clin Immunol. 2007;120:1126–31.
15. King EM, Filep S, Smith B, Platts-Mills T, Hamilton RG, Schmechel D, Sordillo JE, Milton D, van Ree R, Krop EJ, Heederik DJ, Metwali N, Thorne PS, Zeldin DC, Sever ML, Calatroni A, Arbes SJ Jr, Mitchell HE, Chapman MD. A multi-center ring trial of allergen analysis using fluorescent multiplex array technology. J Immunol Methods. 2013;387:89–95.
16. Jayasena S, Smits M, Fiechter D, de Jong A, Nordlee J, Baumert J, Taylor SL, Pieters RH, Koppelman SJ. Comparison of six commercial ELISA kits for their specificity and sensitivity in detecting different major peanut allergens. J Agric Food Chem. 2015;63:1849–55.
17. Koppelman SJ, Hefle SL, Taylor SL, de Jong GA. Digestion of peanut allergens Ara h 1, Ara h 2, Ara h 3, and Ara h 6: a comparative in vitro study and partial characterization of digestion-resistant peptides. Mol Nutr Food Res. 2010;54:1711–21.
18. Custovic A, Simpson A, Pahdi H, Green RM, Chapman MD, Woodcock A. Distribution, aerodynamic characteristics, and removal of the major cat allergen Fel d 1 in British homes. Thorax. 1998;53:33–8.
19. Custovic A, Simpson B, Simpson A, Hallam C, Craven M, Woodcock A. Relationship between mite, cat, and dog allergens in reservoir dust and ambient air. Allergy. 1999;54:612–6.
20. Tovey ER, Willenborg CM, Crisafulli DA, Rimmer J, Marks GB. Most personal exposure to house dust mite aeroallergen occurs during the day. PLoS ONE. 2013;8:e69900.
21. Tovey ER, Liu-Brennan D, Garden FL, Oliver BG, Perzanowski MS, Marks GB. Time-based measurement of personal mite allergen bioaerosol exposure over 24 hour periods. PLoS ONE. 2016;18(11):e0153414.

# 3

# Quality indicators for the acute and long-term management of anaphylaxis: a systematic review

Sangeeta Dhami[1] ⓘ, Aadam Sheikh[2], Artonella Muraro[3], Graham Roberts[4,5], Susanne Halken[6], Monserat Fernandez Rivas[7], Margitta Worm[8] and Aziz Sheikh[9]*

## Abstract

**Background:** The quality of acute and long-term anaphylaxis management is variable and this contributes to the poor outcomes experienced by many patients. Clinical practice guidelines have the potential to improve outcomes, but implementing guideline recommendations in routine practice is challenging. Quality indicators have the potential to support guideline implementation efforts.

**Objective:** To identify quality indicators to support the acute and long-term management of anaphylaxis.

**Methods:** We conducted a systematic review of the literature that involved searching Medline, EMBASE and CINAHL databases for peer-reviewed published literature for the period 1 January 2005–31 December 2015. Additionally we searched Google for grey and unpublished literature. The identified indicators were descriptively summarized against the most recent international anaphylaxis guidelines (i.e. those produced by the European Academy of Allergy and Clinical Immunology) and critically evaluated using the Agency for Healthcare Research and Quality's criteria for indicator development.

**Results:** Our searches revealed 830 publications, from which we identified five sources for 54 indicators addressing both acute (n = 27) and long-term (n = 27) management of anaphylaxis. The majority of indicators were developed through expert consensus with relatively few of these having been formally piloted or tested to demonstrate that they could discriminate between variations in practice and/or that they were sensitive to change.

**Conclusions:** There is a need for a comprehensive set of quality indicators for anaphylaxis management. We have however identified some indicators for the acute and long-term management of anaphylaxis that could with relatively little additional work support efforts to translate guideline recommendations into clinical care.

**Keywords:** Allergy, Anaphylaxis, Guidelines, Implementation research, Indicators, Outcomes, Quality of care, Standards

## Background

Anaphylaxis is a "severe, life-threatening generalized or systemic hypersensitivity reaction" [1, 2] that is responsible for considerable morbidity and, in some cases, mortality. The quality of emergency and ongoing care for patients experiencing and/or with a history of anaphylaxis is variable and this contributes to the poor outcomes (e.g. high risk of recurrent episodes of anaphylaxis) seen [3]. In an attempt to standardize care, and thereby improve outcomes, a number of governments and professional bodies have developed clinical practice guidelines [4–7]. These aim to provide front-line clinicians with simple, concise, evidence-based recommendations for clinical care. Whilst undoubtedly a welcome development, there is a growing body of evidence demonstrating that guidelines often prove challenging to implement in routine clinical care [8]. To support this implementation process, attention is increasingly

*Correspondence: aziz.sheikh@ed.ac.uk
[9] Allergy and Respiratory Research Group, Asthma UK Centre for Applied Research, Usher Institute of Population Health Sciences and Informatics, The University of Edinburgh, Edinburgh, UK
Full list of author information is available at the end of the article

focusing on the need to develop tools that can help clinicians implement key recommendations and monitor progress with implementation efforts [9].

Quality standards and indicators are potentially important tools designed to help clinicians and healthcare organisations assess the quality of care being provided against agreed evidence-based recommendations [9]. These are now being used across a number of disease and clinical areas, but we are unaware of these currently being routinely used at scale in relation to anaphylaxis.

We are developing evidence-based tools to support translation of key anaphylaxis recommendations into clinical practice and in order to inform this process we undertook a systematic review to identify existing quality indicators for anaphylaxis and identify gaps where there is a need for further development.

## Methods

### Overview of methods, registration and reporting

We conducted a systematic review of the literature that involved searching for published and unpublished literature. It is registered in the PROSPERO database with registration number CRD42016035381. We reported findings using the principles advocated in the PRISMA guidelines [10] (Additional file 1).

### Search strategy

We developed a highly sensitive search strategy to identify papers on standards and/or quality indicators for anaphylaxis. This involved searching Medline, EMBASE and CINAHL databases for peer-reviewed published literature, and the Google database for searching grey literature published during the period 1 January 2005–31 December 2015. No language restrictions were employed. Our search terms are detailed in the Appendix.

### Inclusion criteria

We were interested in publications reporting on indicators for measuring the quality of acute and long-term care of anaphylaxis in patients of any age. We did not specify any criteria on how these were developed and there was therefore no study filter employed in selecting papers.

### Selection of indicators

Two reviewers independently selected manuscripts against the pre-specified inclusion criteria. Disagreements were resolved through discussion with arbitration by a third reviewer, where necessary.

### Data extraction

Two reviewers independently extracted indicator data onto a customized data extraction sheet. Disagreements were resolved through discussion; a third reviewer arbitrated in instances where agreement could not be reached. Where available, we also extracted data on how these indicators were developed, whether they had been tested and if they had been used in experimental contexts to demonstrate that they could capture improvements in the quality of care.

### Quality assessment of indicators

The quality of these indicators was then assessed against the criteria detailed using the four stage quality indicator process recommended by the Agency for Healthcare Research and Quality (AHRQ), namely:

1. Development: Identifying candidate indicators through a literature review and/or discussion with experts;
2. Implementation: Testing of candidate indicators, introducing them into software etc.;
3. Maintenance: Indicators need to be regularly checked and, if necessary, updated to keep abreast of latest developments; and
4. Retirement processes: Indicators need to be assessed at periodic intervals for relevance and in order to assess if they need to be discontinued [11].

We contacted the authors of these development tools for further clarification, if necessary.

### Data synthesis

We then mapped available indicators against the various recommendations in the most recent international anaphylaxis guidelines, namely those produced by the European Academy of Allergy and Clinical Immunology (EAACI) [12], identifying areas of overlap and gaps, and making an overall assessment of whether any particular indicator was considered appropriate for use in routine clinical practice. Available indicators were traffic-light color coded with green indicating that the indicators were suitable/nearly suitable for routine use as they had undergone the AHRQ process, amber indicating the need for some additional work, and red indicating the need for a substantial amount of additional underpinning work as most of the stages suggested by AHRQ had not been followed.

## Results

### Characteristics of included studies

Our searches identified 830 studies, of which five satisfied our inclusion criteria (see Fig. 1) [12–16]. The five sources of indicators are detailed in Table 1. In total, 54 individual indicators were identified: 27 for the acute management of anaphylaxis and the remaining 27 for

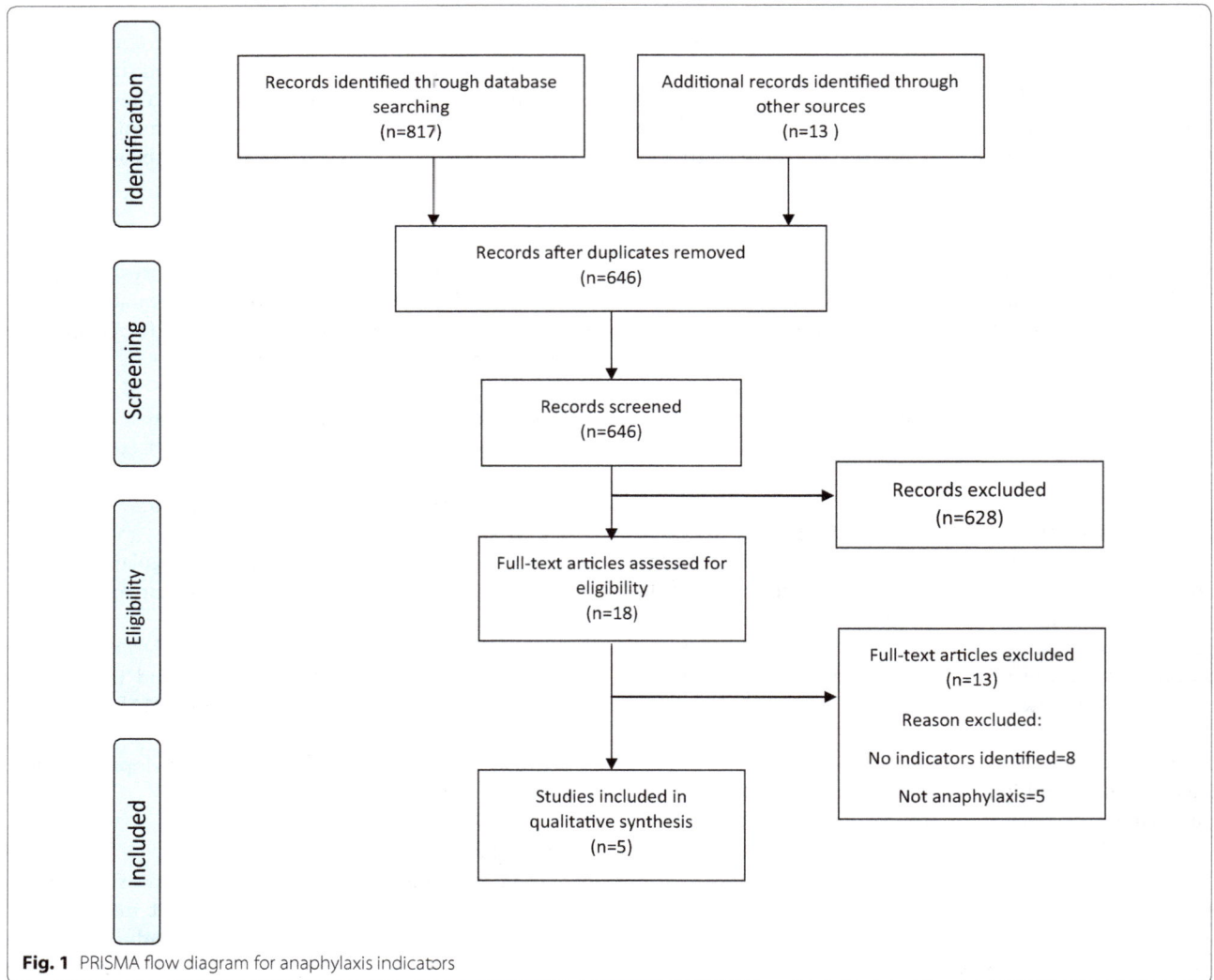

**Fig. 1** PRISMA flow diagram for anaphylaxis indicators

longer-term management. Indicators for the acute and longer-term management of anaphylaxis were identified by four of the five sources [12, 14–16]. Two sources of indicators only focused on children and young people [16, 17], and one focused solely on children attending Emergency Departments (ED) for the acute management of anaphylaxis [17].

Geographically, three sets of indicators were developed in the United Kingdom (UK) [14–16], the fourth was developed in Canada [17] and the fifth was pan-European in origin [12].

**Assessment of indicators against AHRQ criteria**

Table 2 summarizes our assessment of the quality of the indicators against each of the four criteria stipulated by AHRQ.

1. Measure development

The EAACI indicators [12] were derived from clinical guidelines in relation to key recommendations. The Levy indicators [14] were developed through expert consensus. The National Institute of Health and Clinical Excellence (NICE) indicators were derived from relevant guideline recommendations [15]. The Royal College of Paediatrics and Child Health (RCPCH) indicators were derived from a care pathway for children with suspected anaphylaxis [16]. The Stang indicators [17] were the only ones that had been developed through the stages suggested by AHRQ, namely formal processes to identify and assess indicators; furthermore, these were developed using National Quality Framework (NQF) measure evaluation criteria [19].

**Table 1 Source of indicators for the acute and long-term management of anaphylaxis**

| Author, year, country | Title | Indicators for the acute management of anaphylaxis | Indicators for the long-term management of anaphylaxis | No of indicators |
|---|---|---|---|---|
| European Academy of Allergy and Clinical Immunology (EAACI), 2014, Europe | Anaphylaxis: guidelines from the European Academy of Allergy and Clinical Immunology | Yes | Yes | 24 |
| Levy M, 2008, UK | Audit of self-administered injectable adrenaline prescription in primary care | Yes | Yes | 6 |
| National Institute for Health and Clinical Excellence (NICE), 2011, UK | Anaphylaxis clinical audit tool implementing NICE guidelines | Yes | Yes | 8 |
| Royal College of Paediatrics and Child Health (RCPCH), 2011, UK | RCPCH Allergy Care Pathways Project Audit criteria | Yes | Yes | 9 |
| Stang AS, et al., 2013, Canada | Quality indicators for high acuity pediatric conditions | Yes | No | 7 |

2. Implementation

The EAACI indicators [12] did not have any formal implementation assessment. The Levy indicators [14] are freely available for use from http://www.guideline-audit.com/adrenaline/audit_specification.php and had been successfully implemented in a number of UK general practices with the opportunity for benchmarking quality of care. NICE [15] had a generic implementation team and created a range of implementation tools, but it was unclear if the ability to implement these indicators in practice had been formally assessed. The RCPCH [16] give no mention of an implementation strategy. The Stang indicators were operationalized and tested in an ED setting [17].

3. Maintenance

None of the indicators had plans for formal maintenance checks.

4. Retirement

There were no plans for retirement of indicators, although EAACI [12], NICE [15] and the RCPCH [16] stated that they had established processes for the periodic review of their clinical guidelines/pathways.

**Mapping of indicators against guideline recommendations**

The EAACI Guidelines [12] made 16 recommendations on the acute management of anaphylaxis and indicators were developed by EAACI for all of these recommendations (Table 3). Six of these recommendations also had indicators identified from the other sources.

For the longer-term management of anaphylaxis, EAACI made eight recommendations and indicators were developed by EAACI for all of these (Table 4). Additional indicators from other sources were identified for five of these recommendations.

Tables 3 and 4 have been colour coded according to their compliance with the AHRQ criteria to show which

indicators are fit-for-purpose. Green identifies indicators that have been developed according to AHRQ principles and are ready to implement, red shows the indicators that need more developmental work before they can be implemented and amber falls between the two. These tables show that the Stang et al. [17] (coded green) and Levy [14] (coded amber) indicators could with relatively modest effort be rendered fit-for-purpose; gaps still however remained in relation to both acute and long-term management (coded red) where considerable development work is still required.

**Discussion**

**Statement of principal findings**

This study has demonstrated that there are now candidate quality indicators covering many aspects of the acute and long-term management of anaphylaxis. Only a few of these have however undergone the four stages of development recommended by AHRQ, namely implementation and maintenance and none of them have considered decisions on the maintenance or retirement of quality indicators [11]. Further work is therefore needed before any of these can be recommended for routine use in clinical practice [17]. That said, the indicators developed by Stang et al. [16] for acute management of anaphylaxis and those developed by Levy [14] for long-term management could be rendered fit-for-purpose with relatively modest additional effort. EAACI should therefore consider undertaking this work and adopting these indicators. Other areas in relation to both acute and long-term management require much more development work and evaluation.

**Strengths and limitations**

The key strengths of this work are that we used systematic review methods to identify relevant literature,

**Table 2 Assessment of indicators against AHRQ criteria**

| Reference | Identification of candidate indicators | | | Assessment of candidate indicators | | | | | Implementation | | | Mainte-nance | Retirement |
|---|---|---|---|---|---|---|---|---|---|---|---|---|---|
| | Literature review | Conceptual model | Expert engagement | Initial spec | Second literature review | Panel review | Risk adjust-ment | Empirical analysis | Coding | Testing | User docu-mentation | | |
| EAACI | No | Yes | Yes | No | No | No | No | No | No | No | No | No | No |
| Levy | No | Yes | Yes | Unclear | No | No | No | No | Yes | Yes | Yes | No | No |
| NICE | No | Yes | Yes | Yes | No | Unclear | Unclear | No | No | Unclear | Unclear | No | No |
| RCPCH | No | Yes | Yes | No | No | No | No | Unclear | No | Unclear | Unclear | No | No |
| Stang | Yes | Yes | Yes | Yes | Unclear | Yes | Yes | Yes | Yes | Yes | Yes | No | No |

**Table 3 Indicators for the acute management of anaphylaxis mapped to EAACI recommendations with assessment of indicator quality**

| Recommendation | Indicator | Source |
|---|---|---|
| Adrenaline is potentially life-saving and must therefore promptly be administered as the first-line treatment for the emergency management of anaphylaxis | % of children treated with an intramuscular adrenaline injection for an acute anaphylaxis reaction | Stang et al |
| | % of patients with anaphylaxis who received epinephrine in ED | Stang et al |
| | 100% of patients prescribed Adrenaline Auto-injectors should be for the correct dose | Levy |
| | % of patients at risk of anaphylaxis who have an unexpired adrenaline auto-injector | EAACI |
| | % of patients experiencing anaphylaxis who are promptly treated with adrenaline | EAACI |
| | The time of onset of the reaction should be recorded | NICE |
| Earlier administration of adrenaline should be considered on an individual basis when an allergic reaction is likely to develop into anaphylaxis | % of patients experiencing anaphylaxis who are promptly treated with adrenaline | EAACI |
| Adrenaline should be administered by intramuscular injection into the mid outer thigh | % of patients treated with epinephrine in ED treated by the appropriate route | Stang et al |
| | % of children treated with an intramuscular adrenaline injection for an acute anaphylaxis reaction | Stang et al |
| | % of patients who give the auto-injector into the mid-outer thigh | NICE |
| | Percentage of children treated with an intramuscular adrenaline injection for an acute anaphylaxis reaction | RCPCH |
| In patients requiring repeat doses of adrenaline, these should be administered at least 5 minutes apart | % of patients treated with >1 dose adrenaline, timing and who administered (parents, paramedics, self) | EAACI |

**Table 3  continued**

| Recommendation | Indicator | Source |
|---|---|---|
| With inadequate response to 2 or more doses of intramuscular adrenaline, adrenaline may be administered as an infusion by appropriately experienced intensive care, emergency department and critical care physicians, with appropriate cardiac monitoring | % of patients requiring intensive care support with anaphylaxis<br><br>Outcome if require ≥ 2 doses intramuscular adrenaline | EAACI |
| Trigger of the anaphylaxis episode should be removed | Time taken for removal of trigger among patients with anaphylaxis from medication or blood products<br><br>The circumstances immediately before the onset of symptoms should be recorded to help to identify the possible trigger | EAACI<br><br>NICE |
| Help should be called promptly and simultaneously with patient's assessment | Whether and when help is called | EAACI |
| Patients experiencing anaphylaxis should be positioned supine with elevated lower extremities if they have circulatory instability, sitting up if they have respiratory distress and in recovery position if unconscious | In patients with previous anaphylaxis, determine proportion of patients placed in the correct position whilst receiving treatment | EAACI |
| High flow oxygen should be administered by face mask to all patients with anaphylaxis | % of patients with anaphylaxis that were given high flow oxygen  in the community (ambulance) and in hospital | EAACI |
| Intravenous fluids (crystalloids) should be administered (boluses of 20 ml/kg) in patients experiencing cardiovascular instability | % of patients with anaphylaxis who received IV fluids (bolus and maintenance)<br><br>% of patients with blood pressure measurement as part of initial observations | EAACI<br><br>EAACI |
| Inhaled short-acting beta-2 agonists should additionally be given to relieve symptoms of bronchoconstriction | % of patients with  lower respiratory symptoms in the context of anaphylaxis given adrenaline<br><br>% of patients with  lower respiratory symptoms in the context of anaphylaxis inhaled beta-2-agonists but not adrenaline | EAACI<br><br>EAACI |

**Table 3  continued**

| Recommendation | Indicator | Source |
|---|---|---|
| Oral H1- (& H2)-antihistamines may relieve cutaneous symptoms of anaphylaxis | % of patients with anaphylaxis who self-administered antihistamines prior to adrenaline | EAACI |
| Systemic glucocorticosteroids may be used as they may reduce the risk of late phase respiratory symptoms. High dose nebulized glucocorticoids may be beneficial for upper airway obstruction | % of patients who received adrenaline treatment with and without glucocorticocosteroids | EAACI |
| Patients who presented with respiratory compromise should be closely monitored for at least 6-8 hours and patients who presented with circulatory instability require close monitoring for 12-24 hours | % of patients discharged within 6 hours compared to > 24 hours and outcome of reaction e.g. development of biphasic response, or need for repeat dose adrenaline<br><br>% of children with an acute episode of anaphylaxis transferred to hospital<br><br>% of children with an acute episode of anaphylaxis who are transferred to hospital are observed for a minimum of 4 hours<br><br>All children younger than 16 years given emergency treatment for suspected anaphylaxis should be admitted to hospital under the care of a paediatric medical team | EAACI<br><br>RCPHCP<br><br>RCPHCP<br><br>NICE |
| Before discharge, the risk of future reactions should be assessed and an adrenaline auto-injector should be prescribed to those at risk of recurrence | % of patients prescribed adrenaline auto-injector upon discharge following anaphylaxis<br><br>After emergency treatment for suspected anaphylaxis, people (or, as appropriate, their parent and/or carer) should be offered an appropriate adrenaline injector as an interim measure before the specialist allergy service appointment | EAACI<br><br>NICE |

formally considered the appropriateness of the methods to develop and deploy these indicators using the four stage process recommended by the AHRQ [11] and then systematically mapped these against the recent EAACI anaphylaxis guidelines [5].

The limitations of this work also need to be considered. This includes the possibility that we failed to identify relevant literature and indicators, although we tried to minimize this risk by not having any restriction of languages on our searches, searching grey literature and by

**Table 3  continued**

| Recommendation | Indicator | Source |
|---|---|---|
| Patients should be provided with a discharge advice sheet, including allergen avoidance measures (where possible) and instructions for the use of the adrenaline auto-injector. Specialist and food allergy specialist dietitian (in food anaphylaxis) follow-up should be organized. Contact information for patient support groups should also be provided | % of patients with discharge advice sheet and training on use of adrenaline auto-injector upon discharge following anaphylaxis | EAACI |
| | After emergency treatment for suspected anaphylaxis, people should be offered a referral to a specialist allergy service | NICE |
| | Before discharge a healthcare professional with the appropriate skills and competencies should offer people (or, as appropriate, their parent and/or carer) the following: • information about anaphylaxis, including the signs and symptoms of an anaphylactic reaction • information about the risk of a biphasic reaction • information on what to do if an anaphylactic reaction occurs (use the adrenaline injector and call emergency services) • a demonstration of the correct use of the adrenaline injector and when to use it • advice about how to avoid the suspected trigger (if known) • information about the need for referral to a specialist allergy service and the referral process • information about patient support groups | NICE |

contacting a panel of experts. There may also have been experiences of using these indicators that have not yet found their way into the peer-reviewed or grey literature. This issue could be further investigated through, for example, contacting electronic health record and software vendors to see which if any have been computed and with what results.

**Interpretation in the light of other published literature**
Anaphylaxis, in comparison to other disease areas, is relatively undeveloped in terms of quality indicators [18]. For example, NICE has developed indicators for a number of disorders—particularly long-term conditions—that have been used to incentivize improvements in care through the UK Quality and Outcomes Framework (QOF) [19, 20]. Examples of areas in which these have been used include asthma, atrial fibrillation, blood pressure and cancer care [21]. Similarly, in the US indicators

are in widespread use in hospital practice focusing, for example, on re-hospitalization of patients within 30 days of discharge, which can be used to penalize hospitals [22, 23]. By imposing financial penalties for those with the highest readmission rates and thus penalizing those with poor levels of care, the hope is to improve the quality of care delivered [24].

**Implications for policy, practice and research**
Indicator development, implementation testing, and maintenance and retirement considerations should be seen as integral to the process of producing guidelines as this will maximize the chances of translating guideline recommendations into routine clinical practice and thereby improve outcomes. Quality indicators can improve this translational process through associated financial incentives and penalties as noted above, but they can also be used in more subtle ways through, for

**Table 4 Indicators for the longer-term management of anaphylaxis mapped to EAACI recommendations with assessment of indicator quality**

| Recommendation | Indicator | Source |
|---|---|---|
| An anaphylaxis management plan should be used from the time of diagnosis to prevent future reactions, and aid recognition and treatment of any further reactions | 100% of patients with a recorded diagnosis of anaphylaxis have evidence of receiving a written self-management plan. | Levy |
| | At least 80% of patients with a recorded diagnosis of anaphylaxis have been reviewed in the past year? | Levy |
| | 100% of patients or their parents/ representatives with a prescription for self-administered adrenaline should have been taught to use device. | Levy |
| | At least 80% of patients or their parents/ representatives have demonstrated they can use their autoinjector, in the past 12 months | Levy |
| | At least 80% of patients with a prescription for self-administered adrenaline have a recorded diagnosis of anaphylaxis? | Levy |
| | % of patients attended the ED because of a further severe allergic reaction and length of ED stay | EAACI |

example, benchmarking efforts, supporting audit cycles and quality improvement initiatives. These comparative processes, particularly if they involve financial incentives and fines or reputational damage, need to be undertaken with care and with appropriate case mix adjustment, if appropriate [25].

Key next steps are for a multi-stakeholder group to formally consider these existing candidate indicators, chose between existing indicators, propose alternative indicators where considered necessary, develop additional indicators to fill the recommendation gaps, and then undertake formal field work to support implementation efforts. In due course, plans also need to be put into place to consider indicator maintenance and retirement related issues. The AHRQ framework can prove useful to guide this process [11].

**Conclusions**

Indicators were identified for all of the recommendations made in the EAACI Anaphylaxis Guidelines, though none of these satisfied all four criteria specified by AHRQ. There are some indicators, particularly in relation to

**Table 4 continued**

| Recommendation | Indicator | Source |
|---|---|---|
| | % of patients hospitalized because of a further severe allergic reaction and length of hospital stay EAACI | |
| | % of patients died because of a further severe allergic reaction | EAACI |
| | The acute clinical features should be documented | EAACI |
| | The circumstances immediately before the onset of symptoms should be recorded to help to identify the possible trigger | NICE |
| | After emergency treatment for suspected anaphylaxis, people should be offered a referral to a specialist allergy service | NICE |
| | | NICE |
| | After emergency treatment for suspected anaphylaxis, people (or, as appropriate, their parent and/or carer) should be offered an appropriate adrenaline injector as an interim measure before the specialist allergy service appointment | NICE |
| | Percentage of children with an acute episode of anaphylaxis who are investigated with specific allergy tests | RCPCH |
| | Percentage of children who carry an adrenaline injector who have been weighed for a review of their adrenaline dose | RCPCH |
| | Percentage of children (and their families) at risk of anaphylaxis educated to use an adrenaline injector at every health care visit for their acute severe allergies | RCPCH |

**Table 4  continued**

| Recommendation | Indicator | Source |
|---|---|---|
| | Percentage of children with anaphylaxis where the health professionals ensured that schools and early years settings are informed of how to deal with an acute event | RCPCH |
| | | RCPCH |
| Subcutaneous venom immunotherapy is recommended in venom allergic patients with a previous episode of anaphylaxis and adults with systemic cutaneous reactions | % of patients who have an increased quality of life compared to those without treatment | EAACI |
| Training in the recognition and management of anaphylaxis should be offered to all patients and caregivers of children at risk of anaphylaxis ideally from the time of diagnosis | 100% of patients or their parents/ representatives with a prescription for self-administered adrenaline should have been taught to use device. | Levy |
| | At least 80% of patients or their parents/ representatives have demonstrated they can use their autoinjector, in the past 12 months | Levy |
| | 100% of patients with a recorded diagnosis of anaphylaxis have evidence of receiving a written self-management plan | Levy |
| | Adrenaline auto-injector training devices should be available in physician offices or hospitals; if no time for training immediate referral to allergist | EAACI |

acute management, which would require relatively little effort to render them fit-for-purpose. We also identified some indicators, which may prove suitable in relation to assessing the quality of long-term anaphylaxis care. Other indicators, however, require much more developmental work. To progress this work, stakeholders now need to consider the findings from this review and then undertake additional formative work to ensure that there are a

**Table 4  continued**

| Recommendation | Indicator | Source |
|---|---|---|
| | The acute clinical features should be documented | NICE |
| | Percentage of children (and their families) at risk of anaphylaxis educated to use an adrenaline injector at every health care visit for their acute severe allergies | RCPCH |
| | Percentage of children with anaphylaxis where the health professionals ensured that schools and early years settings are informed of how to deal with an acute event | RCPCH |
| Training in the recognition and management of anaphylaxis, including use of adrenaline auto-injectors, should be offered to all professionals dealing with patients at risk of anaphylaxis | % of EDs with clinical guidelines for the treatment of anaphylaxis in children | Stang et al |
| | % of healthcare professionals who are trained in the recognition and management of anaphylaxis | EAACI |
| Training packages should be developed with the target groups | Number and quality of anaphylaxis training packages | EAACI |
| Training should cover allergen avoidance, symptoms of allergic reactions, when and how to use an adrenaline auto-injector and what other measures are needed within the context of an anaphylaxis management plan | 100% of patients or their parents/ representatives with a prescription for self-administered adrenaline should have been taught to use device. | Levy |
| | At least 80% of patients or their parents/ representatives have demonstrated they can use their autoinjector, in the past 12 months | Levy |
| | % of patients or caregivers who receive training | EAACI |

**Table 4 continued**

| Recommendation | Indicator | Source |
|---|---|---|
| Training may involve more than one session to allow revision, an interactive scenario-based approach, a standardized program with manual and educational material and simulation tools. Content and language should be tailored to be understood and memorized | At least 80% of patients with a recorded diagnosis of anaphylaxis have been reviewed in the past year? | Levy |
| | 100% of patients or their parents/ representatives with a prescription for self-administered adrenaline should have been taught to use device. | Levy |
| | % of patients or caregivers who receive training | EAACI |
| Educational interventions should ideally incorporate psychological principles and methods to address anxiety so that children and families may function well at home, at school/work, and socially despite their risk of future reactions and should ideally be part of their educational training. This can be done in a group format. Some patients, with severe anxiety of ongoing duration, may need more in-depth one to one psychological intervention | Optimization of adaptive anxiety levels in trained patients and caregivers | EAACI |

Green, amber and red show which indicators have been developed according to AHRQ criteria, green being the closest and red the furthest

range of suitable indicators that have been both appropriately developed and demonstrated to work in practice to achieve the desired outcome, namely helping to assess the quality of anaphylaxis care delivered to patients.

**Authors' contributions**
AS conceived this study, which was led by SD. AM, GR, SH, MFR and MW commented on an earlier draft of this manuscript. All authors read and approved the final manuscript.

**Author details**
[1] Evidence-Based Health Care Ltd, Edinburgh, UK. [2] UCL, London, UK. [3] Food Allergy Referral Centre Veneto Region, Department of Women and Child Health, Padua General University Hospital, Padua, Italy. [4] The David Hide Asthma and Allergy Research Centre, St Mary's Hospital, Newport Isle of Wight, NIHR Respiratory Biomedical Research Unit, University Hospital Southampton NHS Foundation Trust, Southampton, UK. [5] Faculty of Medicine, University

of Southampton, Southampton, UK. [6] Hans Christian Andersen Children's Hospital, Odense University Hospital, Odense, Denmark. [7] Hospital Clínico San Carlos - Jefe del Servicio de Alergia, Madrid, Spain. [8] Chartie-Universitats-medizin, Berlin, Germany. [9] Allergy and Respiratory Research Group, Asthma UK Centre for Applied Research, Usher Institute of Population Health Sciences and Informatics, The University of Edinburgh, Edinburgh, UK.

### Acknowledgements
We would like to thank U. Nurmatov for conducting searches and Zakariya Sheikh for technical support.

### Competing interests
AS, GR, AM, GR, SH, MFR and MW are all members of the EAACI Anaphylaxis Guidelines and contributed to the development of the EAACI indicators. AS also contributed to the RCPCH indicators.

### Funding
EAACI.

## Appendix
### Search strategy 1: MEDLINE and EMBASE
1. anaphylaxis/
2. anaphyl*.mp.
3. ((acute or severe or major or serious or life threatening or fatal*) and (allerg* or hypersensiti*)).mp.
4. hypersensitivity immediate/
5. exp food hypersensitivity/
6. respiratory hypersensitivity/
7. exp drug hypersensitivity/
8. ((food or egg? or nut? or peanut? or milk or wheat or drug? or respiratory or asthma* or sting* or venom*) adj3 (allerg* or hypersensiti*)).tw.
9. ((allerg* or hypersensiti*) adj5 reaction*).tw.
10. or/1–9
11. quality indicators.mp. or exp Quality Indicators, Health Care/
12. quality standard.mp.
13. "Process Assessment (Health Care)"/or clinical best practice.mp.
14. clinical audit.mp. or exp Clinical Audit/
15. patient experience.mp.
16. (quality and outcomes framework).mp.
17. or/11–16
18. 10 and 17

### Search strategy 2: CINAHL
(anaphylaxis or anaphylaxis management) AND (quality indicators or quality standard or clinical audit or patient experience).

### Search strategy 3: Google Scholar
Free key word search "anaphylaxis management and quality indicators 2005–2015.

### References
1. Johansson SGO, Bieber T, Dahl R, Friedmann PS, Lanier B, Lockey RF, et al. A revised nomenclature for allergy for global use: report of the Nomenclature Review Committee of World Allergy Organization. J Allergy Clin Immunol. 2004;113:832–6.
2. Muraro A, Roberts G, Clark A, Eigenmann PA, Halken S, Lack G, et al. The management of anaphylaxis in childhood: position paper of the European academy of allergology and clinical immunology. Allergy. 2007;62(8):857–71.
3. Mullins RJ. Anaphylaxis: risk factors for recurrence. Clin Exp Allergy. 2003;33(8):1033–40.
4. Soar J, Pumphrey R, Cant A, Clarke S, Corbett A, Dawson P, et al. Emergency treatment of anaphylactic reactions—guidelines for healthcare providers. Resuscitation. 2008;77(2):157–69. doi:10.1016/j.resuscitation.2008.02.001.
5. Muraro A, Roberts G, Worm M, Bilò MB, Brockow K, Fernández Rivas M, et al. Anaphylaxis: guidelines from the European Academy of Allergy and Clinical Immunology. Allergy. 2014;69(8):1026–45. doi:10.1111/all.12437.
6. Simons E, Ardusso L, Beatrice Bilò M, El-Gamal Y, Ledford D, Ring J, et al. World Allergy Organization guidelines for the assessment and management of anaphylaxis. World Allergy Organ J. 2010;4(2):13–37.
7. Vale S, Smith J, Said M, Mullins R, Loh R. ASCIA guidelines for prevention of anaphylaxis in schools, pre-schools and childcare: 2015 update. J Paediatr Child Health. 2015. doi:10.1111/jpc.12962.
8. Shuttleworth A. A practical approach to implementing guidelines. Nursing Times, 30 Nov 2007. http://www.nursingtimes.net/a-practical-approach-to-implementing-guidelines/304506.fullarticle.
9. NICE quality standards and indicators. https://www.nice.org.uk/standards-and-indicators.
10. PRISMA transparent reporting of systematic reviews and meta-analyses. http://www.prisma-statement.org/PRISMAStatement/Default.aspx.
11. AHRQ quality indicators: quality indicator measure development, implementation, maintenance, and retirement. http://www.qualityindicators.ahrq.gov/Downloads/Resources/Publications/2011/QI_Measure_Development_Implementation_Maintenance_Retirement_Full_5-3-11.pdf.
12. Muraro A, Roberts G, Worm M, Bilò MB, Brockow K, Fernández Rivas M, et al. Anaphylaxis: guidelines from the European Academy of Allergy and Clinical Immunology. Allergy. 2014. doi:10.1111/all.12437.
13. Levy M. Audit of self-administered injectable adrenaline prescription in primary care. http://www.guideline-audit.com/adrenaline/audit_specification.php.
14. National Institute for Health and Clinical Excellence (NICE). Anaphylaxis clinical audit tool implementing NICE guidelines. 2011. https://www.nice.org.uk/guidance/cg134/resources.
15. Royal College of Paediatrics and Child Health (RCPCH). RCPCH Allergy Care Pathways Project Audit criteria, Apr 2011. http://www.rcpch.ac.uk/system/files/protected/page/2011_RCPCH_Allergy_Audit_v5_0.pdf.
16. Stang AS, Straus SE, Crotts J, Johnson DW, Guttmann A. Quality indicators for high acuity pediatric conditions Pediatrics. 2013;132(4). http://pediatrics.aappublications.org/content/132/4/752.long.
17. Gill PJ, O'Neill B, Rose P, Mant D, Harnden A. Primary care quality indicators for children: measuring quality in UK general practice. Br J Gen Pract. 2014;64(629):e752–7. doi:10.3399/bjgp14X682813.
18. Lee S, Stachler RJ, Ferguson BJ. Defining quality metrics and improving safety and outcome in allergy care. Int Forum Allergy Rhinol. 2014;4(4):284–91. doi:10.1002/alr.21284.

19. Roland M. Linking physicians' pay to the quality of care—a major experiment in the United Kingdom. N Engl J Med. 2004;351:1448–54. doi:10.1056/NEJMhpr041294.

20. Roland M, Campbell S. Successes and failures of pay for performance in the United Kingdom. N Engl J Med. 2014;370:1944–9. doi:10.1056/NEJMhpr1316051.

21. The NICE Indicator Menu for the QOF National Institute for Health and Care Excellence. https://www.nice.org.uk/Standards-and-Indicators/QOFIndicators.

22. Joynt KE, Jha AK. Characteristics of hospitals receiving penalties under the Hospital Readmissions Reduction Program. JAMA. 2013;309(4):342–3. doi:10.1001/jama.2012.94856.

23. Joynt KE, Jha AK. A path forward on Medicare readmissions. N Engl J Med. 2013;368:1175–7. doi:10.1056/NEJMp1300122.

24. Desai AS, Stevenson LW. Rehospitilisation for heart failure: predict or prevent? Circulation. 2012. doi:10.1161/CIRCULATIONAHA.112.125435.

25. Millett C, Majeed A, Saxena S, Laverty A, Alshamsan R, Lee J, et al. Impact of the 2004 General Practitioner Contract on health improvement and inequalities in cardiovascular disease and diabetes: findings from a systematic review and national and local quantitative studies. NIHR Service Delivery and Organisation Programme. Published June 2011. http://www.nets.nihr.ac.uk/__data/assets/pdf_file/0007/82393/ES-08-1716-209.pdf.

# 4

# Peak nasal inspiratory flow as outcome for provocation studies in allergen exposure chambers: a GA²LEN study

Georg Boelke[1][*] ⓘ, Uwe Berger[2], Karl-Christian Bergmann[1], Carsten Bindslev-Jensen[3], Jean Bousquet[4], Julia Gildemeister[5], Marek Jutel[6,7], Oliver Pfaar[8,9], Torsten Sehlinger[10] and Torsten Zuberbier[1]

## Abstract

**Background:** The GA²LEN chamber has been developed as a novel mobile allergen exposure chamber (AEC) allowing standardized multicenter trials in allergy. Hitherto, subjective nasal symptom scores have been the most often used outcome parameter, but in standardized modern trials objective parameters are preferred. Despite its practicability, the objective parameter peak nasal inspiratory flow (PNIF) has been rarely used for allergy trials in the setting of allergen exposure chambers. This study aims to evaluate PNIF as an outcome parameter for provocation studies in AECs.

**Methods:** In a randomized controlled blinded setting subjects suffering from allergic rhinitis were exposed to grass pollen, birch pollen, house dust mite and/or placebo in the GA²LEN chamber. Different allergen concentrations were used to evaluate symptom severities. Patients had to perform PNIF before and every 30 min during a challenge using a portable PNIF meter.

**Results:** 86 subjects participated in 203 challenges, altogether. House dust mite provocations caused the greatest reduction in PNIF values, followed by grass pollen and birch pollen. Provocations with every allergen or pollen concentration led to a significant decrease ($p < 0.05$) in PNIF compared to baseline. Furthermore, positive correlations were obtained between PNIF and peak expiratory flow, height and weight, and inverse correlations between PNIF and total nasal symptom score, nasal congestion score and visual analog scale of overall subjective symptoms.

**Conclusion:** PNIF is a helpful and feasible tool for conducting provocation trials with allergens, especially grass pollen and house dust mite, in an AEC.

**Keywords:** Allergen exposure chamber (AEC), Allergy trial, GA²LEN chamber, Peak nasal inspiratory flow (PNIF), Provocation study

## Background

Depending on the geographic location and age of the patients, allergic rhinitis (AR) affects up to 10–40% of world's population [1–3]. The prevalence of sensitization to airborne or indoor allergens reaches even higher values [4, 5]. Clinically AR presents especially with nasal congestion, sneezing, nasal pruritus and nasal discharge [6]. In Europe, major causes for seasonal allergic rhinitis are pollen from grass species (e.g. *Phleum pratense*), birch trees (betula) for northern Europe and olive (olea) for the Mediterranean regions, respectively, and house dust mites (HDM) and animal dander as the most common reason for perennial allergic rhinitis [7, 8]. AR is known to result in a decreased quality of life, sleep disorders, missing days at work or school, decreased productivity, and eventually causing direct and indirect medical costs of billions [9–11]. Hence, there is a great need for developing new treatment options and conducting

---
*Correspondence: georg.boelke@charite.de
[1] Charité – Universitätsmedizin Berlin, corporate member of Freie Universität Berlin, Humboldt-Universität zu Berlin, and Berlin Institute of Health, Department of Dermatology and Allergy, Allergy-Center-Charité, Berlin, Germany
Full list of author information is available at the end of the article

clinical trials in the field of allergy. However, these trials are known to be time consuming due to their immanent demand on the pollen season. Furthermore, the amount of pollen each subject gets exposed to depends on several uncontrollable factors like climate, lifestyle and the actual pollen load in the air [12]. To overcome these difficulties, allergen exposure chambers (AEC) were developed and have been used for years in Europe, North America and Asia [13]. They provide a controlled, stable and reproducible environment regardless of the natural pollen season. Recently, the GA$^2$LEN chamber was introduced, a mobile exposition chamber using a unique technique of exposure that allows individual allergen exposure for each patient during a challenge [14]. Besides subjective scoring through the patient itself during allergen challenges, there is a need for objective parameters as well. Out of the three most common methods to objectify nasal symptoms, namely rhinomanometry, acoustic rhinometry and peak nasal inspiratory flow (PNIF), the PNIF has been rarely used in the allergen chamber setting. It is cheap, portable and provides highly reproducible results despite depending on the patients' cooperation [15]. Moreover, it correlates with subjective feeling of nasal obstruction, and is both easy and fast to learn [16–18]. PNIF measures the total nasal flow, therefore it is not dependent on the changing resistances between the left and right nostril during the nasal cycle. This study aims to evaluate PNIF as an outcome parameter for allergen provocations in an AEC. Moreover, associations between PNIF and biometric data (age, weight, height), PNIF and oral peak expiratory flow (PEF), and PNIF and subjective symptom scores and visual analog scales (VAS) are investigated.

## Methods
### Subjects
The study was conducted between January 2015 and May 2016 in Berlin, Germany. The majority of the trials were performed outside and only a few inside of the regional pollen season. Included were both male and female subjects between 18 and 75 years old with a history of AR caused by grass and/or birch pollen and/or house dust mite for at least two years, a positive skin prick test (SPT) (wheal diameter ≥3 mm than negative control) for grass mix, birch and/or house dust mite (*Dermatophagoides pteronyssinus* and/or *Dermatophagoides farinae*), and/or ImmunoCAP score ≥2 for the allergen they were exposed to. Both smokers and non-smokers were included in this study. Exclusion criteria were pregnancy, acute or chronic rhinosinusitis, severe asthma, prior immunotherapy, and treatment with a nasal decongestant, nasal glucocorticoid, oral antihistamine, oral chromone derivates (up to 7 days prior to exposure) or systemic glucocorticoids (up to 30 days prior to exposure). Every patient gave written informed consent

prior to exposure. The study was approved by the ethical committee of the Charité (No. EA1/193/14 for grass/birch and EA1/152/15 for HDM) and conducted following the guidelines from the Declaration of Helsinki.

## Methods and material
Subjects were included based on history and skin test independent of symptom severity during an exposure. The study was planned as modified double-blinded and placebo-controlled, patients did neither know if they were exposed to an allergen nor the amount of the allergen. Right before each provocation, patients were randomly assigned to a seat using a randomization software. Beforehand, particle disperse units above each seat had been prepared by a technician uninvolved in the interactions between investigators and patients. The investigators were sitting in a separated control room exposing the patients according to a preset randomized pattern only revealed at the start without any interactions during the exposure with the patients to ensure a completely blinded study. Patients were exposed for 90–240 min for grass/birch pollen and 60–90 min for HDM. To get comparable results, we focus on data from exposures for at least 120 min regarding grass/birch pollen and 90 min for HDM. Before the challenge began, patients had to sit on their designated seats for at least 15 min to get acclimated. Before and every 10 min during the challenge, patients had to evaluate their nasal symptoms (itching, sneezing, rhinorrhea, congested nose) on a symptom check card using a rating scale ranging from zero points (no symptoms present) to three points (severest symptoms present). All four symptoms were summed up to the total nasal symptom score (TNSS) with a highest possible score of 12 points. Moreover, before exposure started and every 30 min during exposure patients measured their PEF using a portable peak flow meter (PFM20, Omron Healthcare Europe, Hoofddorp, Netherlands) and their PNIF using a portable PNIF meter (In-check, Inspiratory flow meter, Clement Clarke International, Essex, UK). Before the baseline measurements were conducted, each patient was given a short training about how to perform the test correctly and to have some trials to avoid a training effect. Each measurement was taken in a seated position, the best of at least two successful measurements was noted. PNIF und PEF meter were kept in a closable bag next to the patient all throughout the exposure to protect them from contamination with allergen and were only taken out for the measurements. The patients evaluated their overall subjective symptoms being asked to assess their present general well-being using a 10 cm (cm) visual analog scale (VAS) ranging from very good (0 cm) to very bad (10 cm) directly before and every 30 min after the start of each challenge. Immediately before and after each

challenge participants underwent spirometry for safety. Patients could participate multiple times and if eligible for each allergen and their different concentrations. For this study, only their last visit for each allergen and its different concentrations was included to avoid duplicates.

**Allergen exposure chamber**

The GA$^2$LEN chamber consists of two standard 24 ft. containers (one for observation and storage, the other one for the exposition chamber itself), the outer dimensions are 7.43 × 5.10 × 2.86 m (length × width × height). It can contain up to nine patients per run. Each patient gets their individual allergen exposure. Due to strong laminar airflow on both sides of the exposition chamber and almost no airflow in the area where the subjects are seated, there is no mixture of air and the contained allergen between the subjects guaranteeing their individual exposure. Detailed information on the technical aspect has been published by Zuberbier et al. [14]. Climate conditions were permanently controlled all throughout the exposures [temperature was set at 20.5 °C (±0.5 K), humidity at 55% (±5%)]. Patients were exposed to 4000 and 8000 grains/m$^3$ *Phleum pratense*, 4000, 8000 and 16,000 grains/m$^3$ *Betula pendula* (both *Allergon AB, Ängelholm, Sweden*), and 250 μg/m$^3$ house dust mite raw material (computed value, consists of whole bodies, body parts and feces; GMP material, equivalent to 400 ng Der p 1/m$^3$).

**Statistics**

Data was analyzed and diagrams were created with the help of IBM SPSS Statistics Version 24.0 for Windows (Armonk, NY: IBM Corp.) and Microsoft Excel 2013 (Redmond, WA). The challenges were initially performed as validation trials for the chamber, thus no specific power analysis for differences in PNIF was calculated. To compare between the groups, the relative PNIF value in percent was computed (PNIF%). Therefore, the subject's baseline PNIF was determined as 100%. PNIF% is reported as medians with bias corrected and accelerated bootstrap 95% confidence intervals of the median (95% BCa CI), absolute PNIF values as mean ± standard deviation (SD). A p level of <0.05 was accepted as significant. Kruskal–Wallis test and Mann–Whitney-U test were used for comparisons between the different treatment groups, Friedman test was used when differences in-between a group were examined. Pairwise comparisons as post hoc tests were computed using the Dunn–Bonferroni approach. Spearman rank correlations were calculated to assess associations between PNIF and age, height, weight, PEF, nasal congestion score, TNSS and VAS. For correlations with baseline PNIF, each subject was only included once with their best PNIF baseline

value. For correlations between PNIF and subjective symptom scores and VAS, each challenge was included using its mean PNIF%, its mean TNSS and nasal congestion score from beginning to end of exposure, and its mean VAS during a provocation test minus baseline VAS, respectively. Area under the curve (AUC) was calculated using the trapezoid rule and is reported as medians and 95% BCa CI.

**Results**

86 patients were included, 47 of them were female (54.7%). Men had a mean PNIF at baseline of 174.2 (±SD 59.9 L/min) and women 126.3 (±SD 31.0 L/min). No differences were found for PNIF at baseline between in- and out-side the pollen season provocations in the chamber. Detailed demographics are described in Table 1.

**Grass**

34 subjects were tested with 4000 grains/m$^3$ of grass pollen, 22 subjects with 8000 grains/m$^3$ and 22 subjects with placebo. Mean reduction from baseline PNIF was 32.4 (±SD 20.9 L/min) in the 4000 grains/m$^3$ group, 45.3 (±SD 23.7 L/min) in the 8000 grains/m$^3$ group and 12.0 (±SD 14.9 L/min) in the placebo group (Table 2). The relative PNIF compared to baseline (PNIF%) reduction was 29.7%, 95% CI (20.1, 32.8) for 4000 grains/m$^3$, 36.8%, 95% CI (27.8, 43.8) for 8000 grains/m$^3$ and 8.9%, 95% CI (1.3, 15.7) for placebo (Additional file 1: Table S1). Kruskal–Wallis-test found significant differences between the PNIF% values of the groups after 30 min ($\chi^2 = 10.357$, p = 0.006), after 60 min ($\chi^2 = 22.390$, p < 0.001), after 90 min ($\chi^2 = 26.829$, p < 0.001) and after 120 min ($\chi^2 = 20.789$, p < 0.001). Post-hoc tests revealed significant differences for both 4000 and 8000 grains/m$^3$ compared to placebo at each time of measurement (Fig. 1). Furthermore, a significant difference between both active

**Table 1 Patient demographics**

| Parameter (n = 86) | Male, n = 39 (45.3%) | Female, n = 47 (54.7%) |
|---|---|---|
| Age in years, mean (range) | 29.3 (19–74) | 26.4 (19–47) |
| Height in m, mean (range) | 1.83 (1.72–1.96) | 1.69 (1.55–1.80) |
| Weight in kg, mean (range) | 78.5 (54–96) | 62.9 (47–88) |
| Active smokers (%) | 6 (15.4%) | 4 (8.5%) |
| Sensitization to grass (%) | 32 (82.1%) | 39 (83%) |
| Sensitization to birch (%) | 29 (74.4%) | 38 (80.9%) |
| Sensitization to house dust mite (%) | 23 (59%) | 32 (68.1%) |
| PNIF in L/min, mean (± SD) | 174.2 (±59.9) | 126.3 (±31.0) |
| PEF in L/min, mean (± SD) | 588.3 (±83.8) | 401.3 (±75.0) |
| FEV1% predicted, mean (± SD) | 92.2 (±11.5) | 89.6 (±12.0) |

*FEV1* forced expiratory volume in one second, *PNIF* peak nasal inspiratory flow, *PEF* peak expiratory flow, *SD* standard deviation

**Table 2  PNIF values (in L/min) for challenges with grass pollen, birch pollen and house dust mite (HDM)**

| Pollen | Concentration | PNIF baseline (±SD) | PNIF 30 min (±SD) | PNIF 60 min (±SD) | PNIF 90 min (±SD) | PNIF 120 min (±SD) |
|--------|--------------|---------------------|-------------------|-------------------|-------------------|--------------------|
| Grass | Placebo | 123.4 (±55.4) | 106.8 (±40.4) | 109.3 (±44.9) | 114.3 (±51.1) | 115.2 (±56.3) |
| | 4000 grains/m$^3$ | 130.7 (±54.8) | 102.7 (±50.9) | 99.3 (±52.7) | 95.7 (±52.5) | 95.6 (±50.7) |
| | 8000 grains/m$^3$ | 135.5 (±52.7) | 98.0 (±50.9) | 84.1 (±46.3) | 82.5 (±47.6) | 96.1 (±48.3) |
| Birch | Placebo | 132.5 (±63.1) | 118.6 (±58.8) | 116.4 (±56.9) | 112.7 (±51.2) | 117.5 (±56.9) |
| | 4000 grains/m$^3$ | 143.6 (±37.5) | 126.1 (±42.4) | 118.9 (±41.7) | 117.9 (±37.2) | 120.2 (±44.2) |
| | 8000 grains/m$^3$ | 140.8 (±43.3) | 122.7 (±44.7) | 115.6 (±45.6) | 119.9 (±40.5) | 118.9 (±39.5) |
| | 16,000 grains/m$^3$ | 143.6 (±47.2) | 118.6 (±47.8) | 110.0 (±43.6) | 108.6 (±53.5) | 114.6 (±50.3) |
| HDM | Placebo | 136.9 (±46.4) | 121.9 (±50.1) | 106.1 (±52.0) | 104.4 (±51.3) | X |
| | 250 µg/m$^3$ | 139.4 (±55.1) | 95.2 (±38.6) | 80.0 (±38.0) | 81.5 (±40.2) | X |

*PNIF* peak nasal inspiratory flow, *SD* standard deviation

groups could be detected for PNIF% values at 60 min ($z = 15.004$, $p = 0.046$). Friedman test showed significant differences in each of the both active groups for every PNIF% value compared to their baseline, whereas no significant difference could be computed in the placebo group at all. The AUC for PNIF% was significant lower for both active groups [4000 grains/m$^3$ 8957.6 (8433.0, 10,046.6); 8000 grains/m$^3$ 8241.7 (7278.1, 9055.6)]

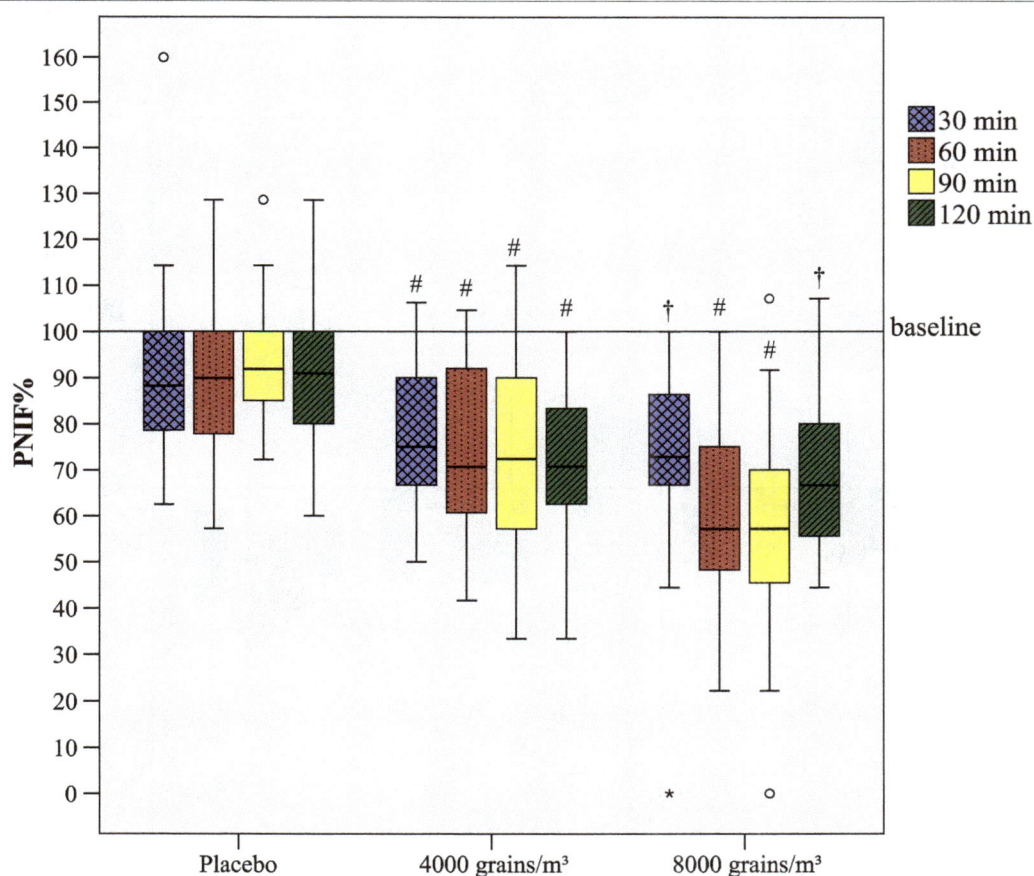

**Fig. 1** Reduction of PNIF during exposure with grass pollen in the GA$^2$LEN chamber. PNIF development during exposure with *Phleum pratense*. A hash marks a reduction compared to baseline $p < 0.001$, a dagger a reduction compared to baseline $p < 0.01$. Outliers are presented as degree sign, extreme outliers as asterisk. PNIF% from both actively exposed groups (4000 and 8000 grains/m$^3$) is significantly lower ($p < 0.05$) than in the placebo group at every associated time of measurement. PNIF% is displayed as medians and boxplots

compared to placebo [11,114.6 (10,331.8, 11,766.7)] (p < 0.001).

### Birch

28 subjects were challenged with 4000 grains/m$^3$ of birch pollen, 33 subjects with 8000 grains/m$^3$, 11 subjects with 16,000 grains/m$^3$ and 22 subjects with placebo. PNIF dropped from baseline during exposure 22.8 (±SD 25.3 L/min) for 4000 grains/m$^3$ concentration [PNIF% reduction 15.4%, 95% CI (8.8, 20.5)], 21.5 (±SD 23.6 L/min) for 8000 grains/m$^3$ [12.0%, 95% CI (9.4, 21.7)], 30.7 (±SD 21.9 L/min) for 16,000 grains/m$^3$ [19.6%, 95% CI (12.5, 28.4)], and 16.2 (±SD 22.6 L/min) for placebo [8.5%, (1.3, 17.1)] (Table 2; Additional file 1: Table S1). Friedman test found significant differences for every actively exposed group compared to their baseline value in PNIF%. In detail, at challenges with 8000 grains/m$^3$ each point of measurement differed significantly from the baseline, whereas at challenges with 4000 and 16,000 grains/m$^3$ each point of measurement from minute 60 and further on did. In the placebo group, only at point of measurement at

minute 90 a significant difference compared to baseline could be found (Fig. 2). However, PNIF% showed no significant difference between the challenge groups, even though a trend was clearly recognizable. Hence, the three groups that got actively exposed to birch pollen were summarized into one active group. In addition, only those tests runs were included where test subjects reached a TNSS greater than two points on at least two symptom check cards. Eventually, 38 challenges were included into the active group, the placebo group remained the same. Mean reduction from baseline for absolute PNIF values in the active group was 31.2 (±SD 24.8 L/min) and 20.4%, 95% CI (15.8, 25.0) for relative values (Additional files 2, 3: Tables S2, S3). Values in the placebo group stayed the same as reported earlier. Mann–Whitney-U test found significant differences when comparing the PNIF% values between active and placebo group after 60 min (z = −2.809, p = 0.005), after 90 min (z = −2.380, p = 0.017) and after 120 min (z = −2.133, p = 0.033) (Additional file 4: Fig. S1). Moreover, the AUC of PNIF% was significantly lower in the active group [9878.6 (9115.4, 10,250.0)]

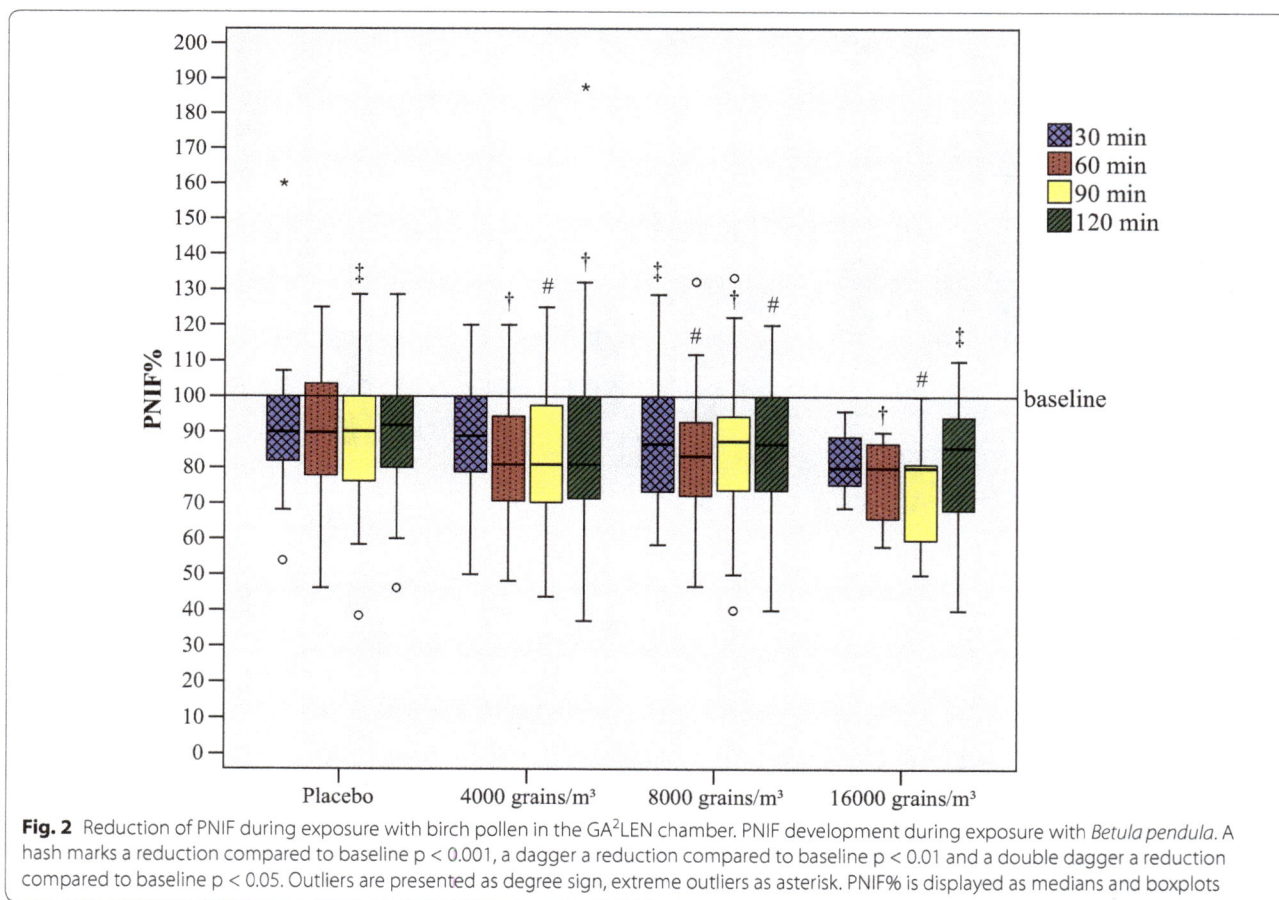

**Fig. 2** Reduction of PNIF during exposure with birch pollen in the GA$^2$LEN chamber. PNIF development during exposure with *Betula pendula*. A hash marks a reduction compared to baseline p < 0.001, a dagger a reduction compared to baseline p < 0.01 and a double dagger a reduction compared to baseline p < 0.05. Outliers are presented as degree sign, extreme outliers as asterisk. PNIF% is displayed as medians and boxplots

than in the placebo group [11,092.9 (10,105.3, 11,921.1)] (z = −2.754, p = 0.006).

## House dust mite
24 patients were exposed to 250 µg/m³ HDM material, 18 patients participated in a placebo run. Mean change from baseline was 53.8 (±SD 33.9 L/min) in the active group and 26.1 (±SD 28.7 L/min) in the placebo group for absolute values (Table 2; Additional file 5: Fig. S2), 40.1%, 95% CI (25.8, 44.4) and 20.7%, 95% CI (6.1, 33.3) for relative values, respectively (Additional file 1: Table S1). Mann–Whitney-U test found significant differences between both groups regarding their PNIF% values after 30 min (z = −2.975, p = 0.003), after 60 min (z = −2.328, p = 0.020) and after 90 min (z = −2.327, p = 0.020)

(Fig. 3). Similar to the other conducted challenges with grass and birch, comparisons of absolute PNIF values found no significant difference due to the unequal baselines. AUC for PNIF% was significant lower in the active group [6156.4 (5666.7, 7100.0)] than in the placebo group [7440.0 (6458.8, 8727.3)] (z = −2.872, p = 0.004). Furthermore, Friedman test showed a significant difference at each point of measurement during exposure compared to baseline in the active group. Though, the placebo group differed also significantly from their baseline value at points of measurement after 60 min and after 90 min.

## Comparison between the allergens
Please find these results in the Additional file 6: Appendix S1 and Additional file 7: Figure S3.

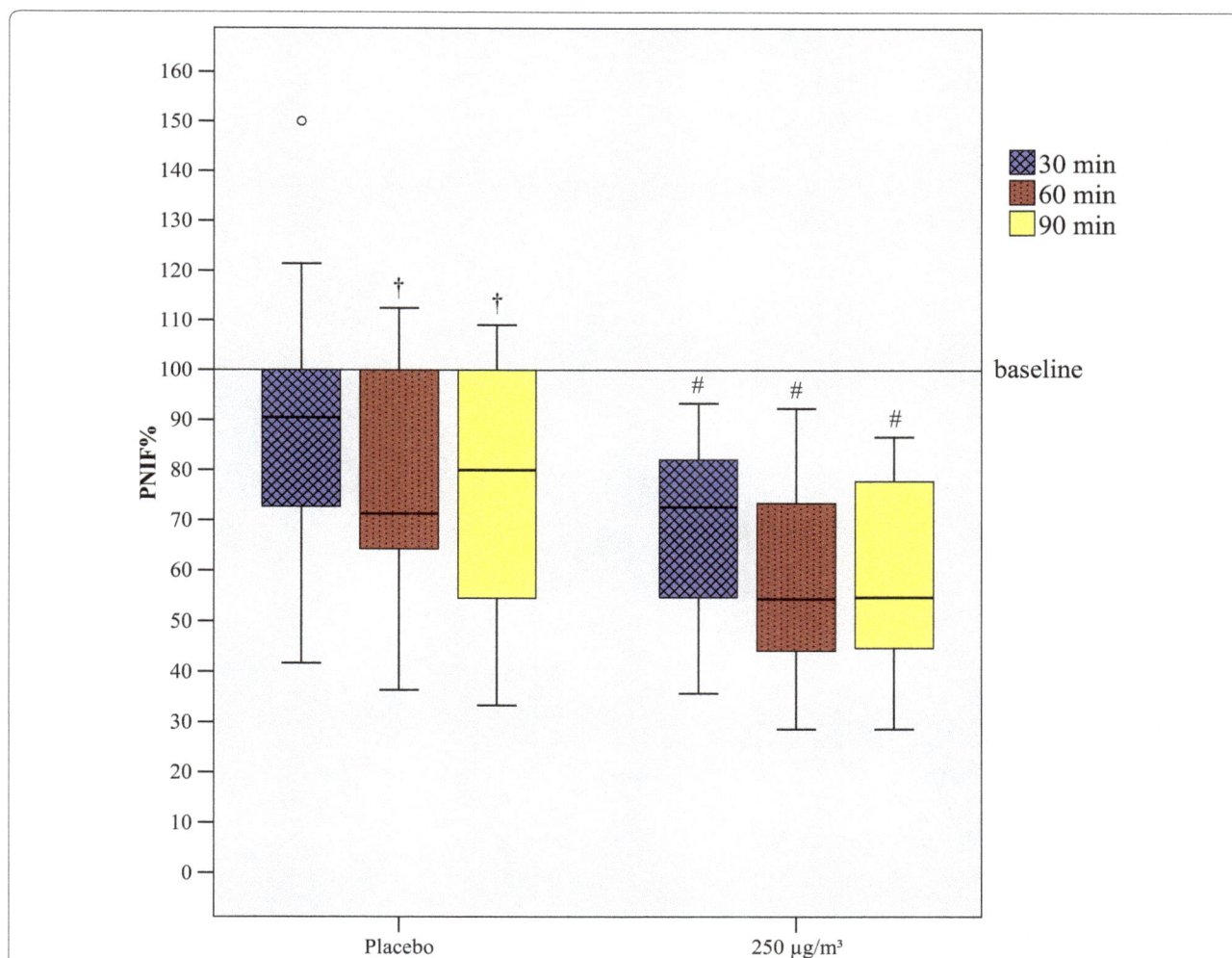

**Fig. 3** Reduction of PNIF during exposure with house dust mite (Der p 1) in the GA²LEN chamber. PNIF development during exposure with house dust mite material. A hash marks a reduction compared to baseline p < 0.001, a dagger a reduction compared to baseline p < 0.01. Outliers are presented as degree sign. PNIF% from the actively exposed group (250 µg/m³) is significantly lower (p < 0.05) than in the placebo group at every associated time of measurement. PNIF% is displayed as medians and boxplots

## Correlations

Positive weak to moderate correlations could be found between PNIF and PEF ($r_s$ = .499, p < 0.001), PNIF and height ($r_s$ = .404, p < 0.001) and PNIF and weight ($r_s$ = .308, p < 0.001). A correlation between PNIF and age was not visible ($r_s$ = .005, p = 0.96). Furthermore, an inverse moderate to strong correlation could be computed between PNIF% and TNSS ($r_s$ = −.585, p < 0.001), as well as inverse weak to moderate correlations between PNIF% and nasal congestion score ($r_s$ = −.415, p < 0.001), and PNIF% and VAS of overall subjective symptoms ($r_s$ = −.361, p < 0.001) (Fig. 4).

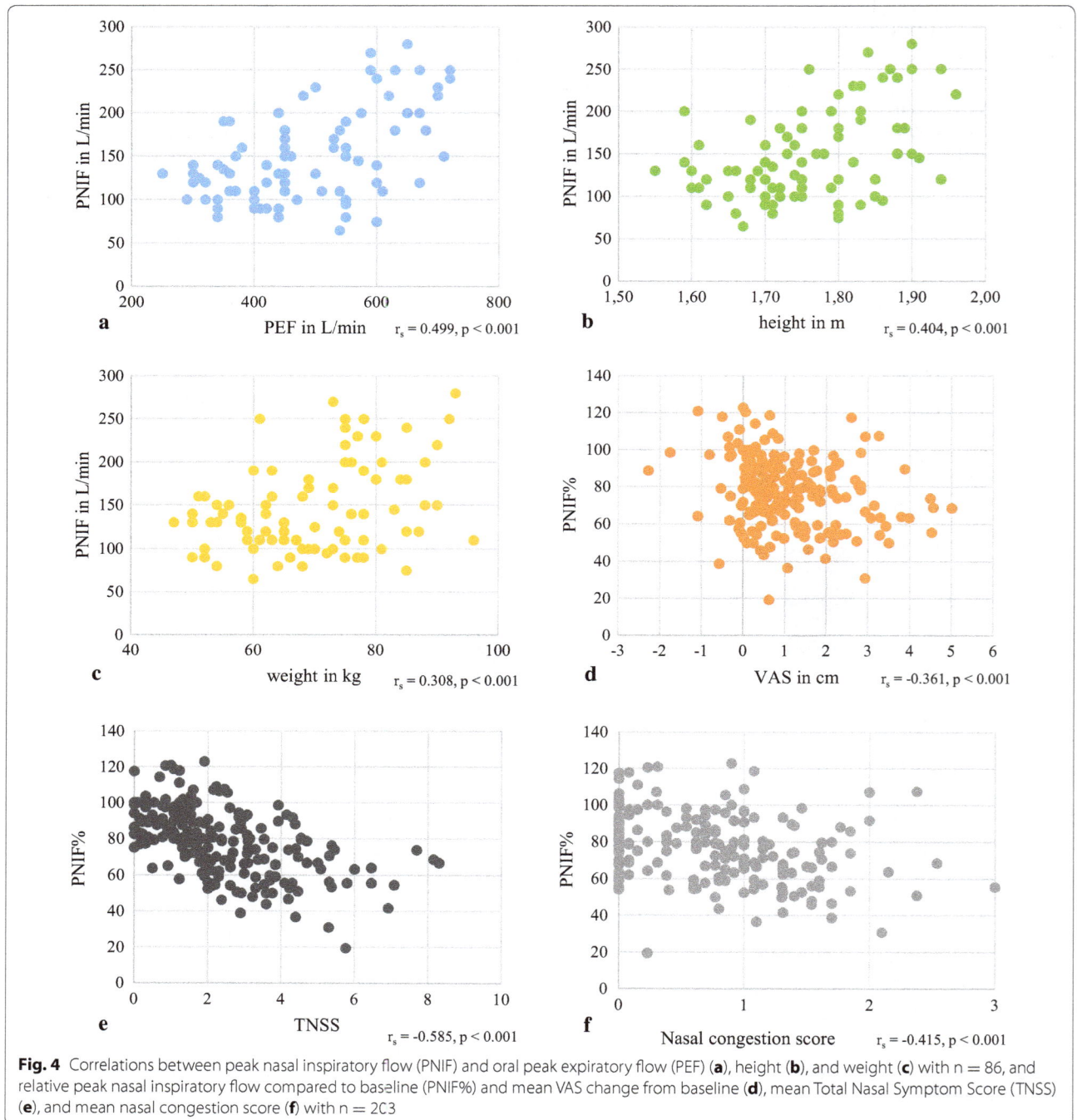

**Fig. 4** Correlations between peak nasal inspiratory flow (PNIF) and oral peak expiratory flow (PEF) (**a**), height (**b**), and weight (**c**) with n = 86, and relative peak nasal inspiratory flow compared to baseline (PNIF%) and mean VAS change from baseline (**d**), mean Total Nasal Symptom Score (TNSS) (**e**), and mean nasal congestion score (**f**) with n = 2C3

## Discussion

PNIF has been recommended and been used as an outcome parameter in allergen immunotherapy trials [19, 20], pharmacological trials [21, 22], nasal allergen challenges [23, 24], before surgical interventions [25, 26], and is also a feasible tool in assessing nasal patency in both children [27] and adults [28, 29]. This was the first study to evaluate peak nasal inspiratory flow as an outcome parameter in an allergen exposure chamber. Overall, 86 subjects participated in 203 individual challenges with either grass pollen, birch pollen, house dust mite material or placebo. At baseline, male subjects reached a PNIF of 174.2 ± 59.9 L/min and female subjects of 126.3 ± 31.0 L/min. Measurements were taken in a seated position, as there exists no significant difference to standing position [30], and the best of at least two successful measurements was noted due to no additional benefit in a third trial [15]. Reproducibility and no demand for priming exposures were previously reported [14]. Our results confirm a study by Denguezli Bouzgarou et al. who found almost exact same values in a healthy North African population with a mean PNIF in male subjects of 174 ± 54 and 126 ± 33 L/min in female subjects [31]. Looking at data for a European population our values were lower than data obtained by Åkerlund et al. [32], but comparable to findings from Ottaviano et al. with a PNIF of 143 ± 48.6 L/min for male and 121.9 ± 36 L/min for female [33]. A study by Klossek et al. in a French population found clearly lower normal ranges in PNIF though. Even when only reporting the values obtained from the subjects, who reported no nasal discomfort at all, men had a mean PNIF of 100.3 ± 43.6 L/min and women of 79.3 ± 32.2 L/min [34]. However, an explanation for these low values was not found. The greatest reduction in PNIF was elicited by HDM in our study, followed by grass pollen and birch pollen. PNIF also decreased mildly in the placebo group, even when no patient in the chamber was exposed to an allergen. Whether the decline results apart from the placebo effect itself, from decreasing patients' effort during the exposure, increased osmolarity of nasal mucus due to increased ventilation from the measurements, or despite 55% humidity too dry air, needs to be further investigated. Standard deviation of some results for absolute PNIF values exceeded the mean value caused by the unequal distribution. Hence, it is of utmost importance to compare the relative reductions. Decreased PNIF is known in HDM allergy as allergic subjects usually present with nasal obstruction [35]. However, little is known about the differences in nasal symptoms elicited by different airborne pollen. In our challenges PNIF decreased in subjects exposed to grass pollen much greater in both absolute and relative values than in subjects exposed to birch pollen. Nonetheless, both kinds of pollen had in common that

the more the pollen concentration increased the more PNIF reduction was induced. These results imitate the conditions in nature as described by Caillaud et al. who described a linear relationship between birch pollen concentration and symptoms elicited until symptom severity reaches a plateau when a certain threshold concentration is exceeded [36]. As demanded by a recently published position paper from the European Academy of Allergy and Clinical Immunology (EAACI) it is important to compare the obtained results between the existing exposure chambers [37]. To the authors knowledge only two studies conducted in an Environmental Exposure Unit (EEU) in Kingston, Ontario have used PNIF as an outcome parameter in clinical trials [38, 39]. Both studies were clinical evaluations of the EEU for birch pollen and grass pollen exposure, respectively. Focusing just on the reported PNIF data for provocations with grass pollen, the mean reduction of PNIF after 180 min of exposure compared to baseline to either 2500 or 3500 grains/m$^3$ grass pollen (*Lolium perenne*) was 29.8 and 42.9 L/min, respectively, resulting in a relative reduction of 30.4 and 34.2%, respectively. These results match our findings with a PNIF reduction of 35.2 L/min (relative reduction 29.3%) after 120 min exposure to 4000 grains/m$^3$ of grass pollen compared to baseline. However, allergic patients were not provoked to placebo in the EEU, thus the effect of the chamber itself to allergic subjects is unknown. Furthermore, the technology of pollen distribution is totally different in both chambers. Whereas in the EEU and most of the other existing chambers pollen gets distributed via fans all over the exposition room, the GA$^2$LEN chamber provides an individual exposure to every subject giving an exact knowledge of the concentration every test subject got exposed to. Hence, even when using the same allergen concentration the results might not be directly comparable. Both chambers provoked less reduction in PNIF during challenges with birch pollen. That is why it can be suspected that birch allergy elicit less nasal congestion and other symptoms are more present. This needs to be further evaluated. In our study, we found moderate positive correlations between PNIF and weight, height and oral peak inspiratory flow. Even though some publications denied a correlation between PNIF and weight [32] or PNIF and height [40], other studies confirmed these associations, especially for PNIF and PEF [41–43]. In our study PNIF and subjective nasal symptoms were found to correlate inversely with a Spearman's rank correlation coefficient $r_s = -0.59$ between PNIF and TNSS, and $r_s = -0.42$ between PNIF and nasal congestion score. Other studies, that were using exactly the same TNSS as we did, computed correlations from $-0.50$ to $-0.62$ between PNIF and TNSS, confirming our analysis and thus consolidate the usefulness of PNIF as an objective control parameter for subjective symptoms [44, 45]. Furthermore, the publication from Ellis et al. reported a weak to moderate negative correlation from −0.32 to −0.37 between PNIF and subjective scoring of nasal congestion, which can be validated and even enhanced with data obtained in the GA²LEN chamber [38]. The correlation between PNIF and VAS of overall subjective symptoms was found to be at −0.36 in the GA²LEN chamber, thus being in the range of already published correlations of −0.39 to −0.48 between PNIF and VAS [17, 28, 29]. However, these studies focused only on the VAS of nasal obstruction in particular. Hence, our findings provide additional information about the relation of PNIF and the actual patient's perception of their overall symptom severity, which possibly represents real-life conditions more accurately.

## Conclusions

In conclusion, due to its portability, simple application and good correlation to subjective symptoms, PNIF is a valuable tool for provocation trials in AECs. However, more clinical trials comparing this outcome in different AECs facilities would be advisable.

## Additional files

**Additional file 1: Table S1.** PNIF% values for challenges with grass pollen, birch pollen and house dust mite

**Additional file 2: Table S2.** PNIF values for birch challenges (in L/min). Patients in active group were only included when they experienced a Total Nasal Symptom Score (TNSS) greater than 2 points on at least two symptom check cards.

**Additional file 3: Table S3.** PNIF% values for birch challenges. Patients in active group were only included when they experienced a Total Nasal Symptom Score (TNSS) greater than 2 points on at least two symptom check cards.

**Additional file 4: Figure S1.** Reduction of PNIF during exposure with birch pollen in the GA²LEN chamber. PNIF development during exposure with *Betula pendula*. Every challenge to birch pollen got pooled into one active group and only those runs were included where a TNSS greater than 2 points was reported on at least two symptom check cards throughout the whole challenge. A hash marks a reduction compared to baseline p < 0.001, a dagger a reduction compared to baseline p < 0.01, a double dagger a reduction compared to baseline p < 0.05. Outliers are presented as degree sign, extreme outliers as asterisk. FNIF% in the active group differed significantly (p < 0.05) from the placebo group at 60, 90 and 120 min. PNIF% is displayed as medians and boxplots.

**Additional file 5: Figure S2.** Example of individual PNIF development (in L/min) for every subject when exposed to house dust mite (**a** placebo, **b** 250 μg/m³).

**Additional file 6: Appendix S1.** Comparison between the different allergens.

**Additional file 7: Figure S3.** Comparison of different allergens and their PNIF outcome. PNIF development compared between the different allergens and placebo. Both grass pollen and house dust mite (HDM) elicited significantly greater PNIF% reductions at each associated time of measurement than placebo (p < 0.001) and birch pollen (p < 0.01). PNIF% is displayed as medians and boxplots. Outliers are presented as degree sign, extreme outliers as asterisk.

**Abbreviations**
AEC: allergen exposure chamber; AR: allergic rhinitis; AUC: area under the curve; cm: centimeter; FEV1: forced expiratory volume in one second; GA²LEN: Global Asthma and Allergy European Network; HDM: house dust mite; min: minutes; PEF: oral peak expiratory flow; PNIF: peak nasal inspiratory flow; SD: standard deviation; SPT: skin prick test; TNSS: total nasal symptom score; VAS: visual analog scale; 95% BCa CI: bias corrected and accelerated bootstrap 95% confidence interval of the median.

**Authors' contributions**
GB recruited patients, conducted the provocation trials, managed data, performed statistical analysis and drafted the manuscript. UB contributed to conception and design of the study, statistical analysis and draft of the manuscript. KCB contributed to conception and design of the study, conducted the provocation trials, supervised the study, and helped draft the manuscript. CBJ contributed to interpretation of the obtained data and draft of the manuscript. JB helped with statistical analysis, and discussion and contributed to draft of the manuscript. JG recruited patients, conducted the provocations, helped managing the databank, and contributed to draft of the manuscript. MJ contributed to conception and design of the study, and draft of the manuscript. OP contributed to conception and design of the study, helped with interpretation of the data and draft of the manuscript. TS designed the allergen exposure chamber, contributed to design of the study, supervised the technological aspect of the provocation trials, and helped drafting the manuscript. TZ designed, conceived and supervised the study, contributed to discussion of the results and draft of the manuscript. All authors read and approved the final manuscript.

**Author details**
[1] Charité – Universitätsmedizin Berlin, corporate member of Freie Universität Berlin, Humboldt-Universität zu Berlin, and Berlin Institute of Health, Department of Dermatology and Allergy, Allergy-Center-Charité, Berlin, Germany. [2] Department of Otorhinolaryngology, Aerobiology and Pollen Information Research Unit, Medical University of Vienna, Vienna, Austria. [3] Department of Dermatology and Allergy Centre, Odense University Hospital, Odense, Denmark. [4] CHRU, Montpellier University Hospital Center, Montpellier, France. [5] Mobile Chamber Experts GmbH, Berlin, Germany. [6] ALL-MED Medical Research Institute, Wrocław, Poland. [7] Department of Clinical Immunology, Wroclaw Medical University, Wrocław, Poland. [8] Department of Otorhinolaryngology, Head and Neck Surgery, Universitätsmedizin Mannheim, Medical Faculty Mannheim, Heidelberg University, Mannheim, Germany. [9] Center for Rhinology and Allergology, Wiesbaden, Germany. [10] Bluestone Technology GmbH, Woerrstadt, Germany.

**Acknowledgements**
None.

**Competing interests**
GB reports grants from ALK Abelló ("ALK Förderpreis Allergologie 2015") under consideration for publication, and employment and travel expenses by Mobile Chamber Experts GmbH outside the submitted work. KCB reports employment by Mobile Chamber Experts GmbH outside the submitted work. CBJ reports grants and payment for lectures from Hal Allergy, grants from Anergis, grants from Aimmune, outside the submitted work. JG reports employment by Mobile Chamber Experts GmbH outside the submitted work. OP reports grants and personal fees from ALK-Abelló, grants and personal fees from Allergopharma, grants and personal fees from Stallergenes Greer, grants and personal fees from HAL Allergy Holding B.V./HAL Allergie GmbH, grants and personal fees from Bencard Allergie GmbH/Allergy Therapeutics, grants and personal fees from Lofarma, grants from Biomay, grants from Nuvo, grants from Circassia, grants and personal fees from Biotech Tools S.A., grants and personal fees from Laboratorios LETI/LETI Pharma, personal fees from Novartis Pharma, personal fees from MEDA Pharma, grants and personal fees from Anergis S.A., personal fees from Sanofi US Services, personal fees from Mobile Chamber Experts (a GA2LEN Partner), personal fees from Pohl-Boskamp, outside the submitted work. TS has received payment to his institution for work under consideration from Mobile Chamber Expects GmbH and consultancy fees paid to his institution from Mobile Chamber Experts GmbH. TZ has received institutional funding for research and/or honoria for lectures and/

or consulting from AstraZeneca, AbbVie, ALK, Almirall, Astellas, Bayer Health Care, Bencard, Berlin Chemie, FAES, HAL, Henkel, Kryolan, Leti, L'Oreal, Meda, Menarini, Merck, MSD, Novartis, Pfizer, Sanofi, Stallergenes, Takeda, Teva and UCB. In addition, he is a member of ARIA/WHO, DGAKI, ECARF, GA$^2$LEN and WAO. GA$^2$LEN is a shareholder of Mobile Chamber Experts GmbH. The remaining authors declare that they have no competing interests.

## Funding
This study was supported by Mobile Chamber Experts GmbH. GB was supported by "ALK Förderpreis Allergologie 2015".

## References

1. Pefura-Yone EW, Kengne AP, Balkissou AD, Boulleys-Nana JR, Efe-de-Melingui NR, Ndjeutcheu-Moualeu PI, Mbele-Onana CL, Kenmegne-Noumsi EC, Kolontchang-Yomi BL, Theubo-Kamgang BJ, et al. Prevalence of asthma and allergic rhinitis among adults in Yaounde, Cameroon. PLoS ONE. 2015;10:e0123099.

2. Pols DH, Wartna JB, Moed H, van Alphen EI, Bohnen AM, Bindels PJ. Atopic dermatitis, asthma and allergic rhinitis in general practice and the open population: a systematic review. Scand J Prim Health Care. 2016;34:143–50.

3. Bauchau V, Durham SR. Prevalence and rate of diagnosis of allergic rhinitis in Europe. Eur Respir J. 2004;24:758–64.

4. Salo PM, Arbes SJ, Jaramillo R, Calatroni A, Weir CH, Sever ML, Hoppin JA, Rose KM, Liu AH, Gergen PJ, et al. Prevalence of allergic sensitization in the United States: results from the National Health and Nutrition Examination Survey (NHANES) 2005–2006. J Allergy Clin Immunol. 2014;134:350–9.

5. Bergmann KC, Heinrich J, Niemann H. Current status of allergy prevalence in Germany: position paper of the Environmental Medicine Commission of the Robert Koch Institute. Allergo J Int. 2016;25:6–10.

6. Wheatley LM, Togias A. Clinical practice. Allergic rhinitis. N Engl J Med. 2015;372:456–63.

7. D'Amato G, Cecchi L, Bonini S, Nunes C, Annesi-Maesano I, Behrendt H, Liccardi G, Popov T, van Cauwenberge P. Allergenic pollen and pollen allergy in Europe. Allergy. 2007;62:976–90.

8. Bousquet J, Khaltaev N, Cruz AA, Denburg J, Fokkens WJ, Togias A, Zuberbier T, Baena-Cagnani CE, Canonica GW, van Weel C, et al. Allergic Rhinitis and its Impact on Asthma (ARIA) 2008 update (in collaboration with the World Health Organization, GA(2)LEN and AllerGen). Allergy. 2008;63(Suppl 86):8–160.

9. McCrory DC, Williams JW, Dolor RJ, Gray RN, Kolimaga JT, Reed S, Sundy J, Witsell DL. Management of allergic rhinitis in the working-age population. Evid Rep Technol Assess (Summ). 2003;67:1–4.

10. Meltzer EO, Bukstein DA. The economic impact of allergic rhinitis and current guidelines for treatment. Ann Allergy Asthma Immunol. 2011;106:S12–6.

11. Small M, Piercy J, Demoly P, Marsden H. Burden of illness and quality of life in patients being treated for seasonal allergic rhinitis: a cohort survey. Clin Transl Allergy. 2013;3:33.

12. Day JH, Horak F, Briscoe MP, Canonica GW, Fineman SM, Krug N, Leynadier F, Lieberman P, Quirce S, Takenaka H, Cauwenberge P. The role of allergen challenge chambers in the evaluation of anti-allergic medication an international consensus paper. Clin Exp Allergy Rev. 2006;6(2):31–59.

13. Rosner-Friese K, Kaul S, Vieths S, Pfaar O. Environmental exposure chambers in allergen immunotherapy trials: current status and clinical validation needs. J Allergy Clin Immunol. 2015;135:636–43.

14. Zuberbier T, Abelson MB, Akdis CA, Bachert C, Berger U, Bindslev-Jensen C, Boelke G, Bousquet J, Canonica GW, Casale TB, et al. Validation of the Global Allergy and Asthma European Network (GA(2)LEN) chamber for trials in allergy: innovation of a mobile allergen exposure chamber. J Allergy Clin Immunol. 2017;139:1158–66.

15. Starling-Schwanz R, Peake HL, Salome CM, Toelle BG, Ng KW, Marks GB, Lean ML, Rimmer SJ. Repeatability of peak nasal inspiratory flow measurements and utility for assessing the severity of rhinitis. Allergy. 2005;60:795–800.

16. Nathan RA, Eccles R, Howarth PH, Steinsvåg SK, Togias A. Objective monitoring of nasal patency and nasal physiology in rhinitis. J Allergy Clin Immunol. 2005;115:S442–59.

17. Tsounis M, Swart KM, Georgalas C, Markou K, Menger DJ. The clinical value of peak nasal inspiratory flow, peak oral inspiratory flow, and the nasal patency index. Laryngoscope. 2014;124:2665–9.

18. Ottaviano G, Fokkens WJ. Measurements of nasal airflow and patency: a critical review with emphasis on the use of peak nasal inspiratory flow in daily practice. Allergy. 2016;71:162–74.

19. Scadding GW, Eifan AO, Lao-Araya M, Penagos M, Poon SY, Steveling E, Yan R, Switzer A, Phippard D, Togias A, et al. Effect of grass pollen immunotherapy on clinical and local immune response to nasal allergen challenge. Allergy. 2015;70:689–96.

20. Pfaar O, Demoly P, Gerth van Wijk R, Bonini S, Bousquet J, Canonica GW, Durham SR, Jacobsen L, Malling HJ, Mösges R, et al. Recommendations for the standardization of clinical outcomes used in allergen immunotherapy trials for allergic rhinoconjunctivitis: an EAACI Position Paper. Allergy. 2014;69:854–67.

21. Stjärne P, Mösges R, Jorissen M, Passàli D, Bellussi L, Staudinger H, Danzig M. A randomized controlled trial of mometasone furoate nasal spray for the treatment of nasal polyposis. Arch Otolaryngol Head Neck Surg. 2006;132:179–85.

22. Bachert C, Mannent L, Naclerio RM, Mullol J, Ferguson BJ, Gevaert P, Hellings P, Jiao L, Wang L, Evans RR, et al. Effect of subcutaneous dupilumab on nasal polyp burden in patients with chronic sinusitis and nasal polyposis: a randomized clinical trial. JAMA. 2016;315:469–79.

23. Nizankowska-Mogilnicka E, Bochenek G, Mastalerz L, Swierczyńska M, Picado C, Scadding G, Kowalski ML, Setkowicz M, Ring J, Brockow K, et al. EAACI/GA2LEN guideline: aspirin provocation tests for diagnosis of aspirin hypersensitivity. Allergy. 2007;62:1111–8.

24. Benichou AC, Armanet M, Bussière A, Chevreau N, Cardot JM, Tétard J. A proprietary blend of quail egg for the attenuation of nasal provocation with a standardized allergenic challenge: a randomized, double-blind, placebo-controlled study. Food Sci Nutr. 2014;2:655–63.

25. Bermüller C, Kirsche H, Rettinger G, Riechelmann H. Diagnostic accuracy of peak nasal inspiratory flow and rhinomanometry in functional rhinosurgery. Laryngoscope. 2008;118:605–10.

26. Menger DJ, Swart KM, Nolst Trenité GJ, Georgalas C, Grolman W. Surgery of the external nasal valve: the correlation between subjective and objective measurements. Clin Otolaryngol. 2014;39:150–5.

27. de Souza-Campos-Fernandes S, Ribeiro de Andrade C, da Cunha Ibiapina C. Application of Peak Nasal Inspiratory Flow reference values in the treatment of allergic rhinitis. Rhinology. 2014;52:133–6.

28. Hox V, Bobic S, Callebaux I, Jorissen M, Hellings PW. Nasal obstruction and smell impairment in nasal polyp disease: correlation between objective and subjective parameters. Rhinology. 2010;48:426–32.

29. Teixeira RU, Zappelini CE, Alves FS, da Costa EA. Peak nasal inspiratory flow evaluation as an objective method of measuring nasal airflow. Braz J Otorhinolaryngol. 2011;77:473–80.

30. Ottaviano G, Scadding GK, Iacono V, Scarpa B, Martini A, Lund VJ. Peak nasal inspiratory flow and peak expiratory flow. Upright and sitting values in an adult population. Rhinology. 2016;54:160–3.

31. Bouzgarou MD, Ben Saad H, Chouchane A, Cheikh IB, Zbidi A, Dessanges JF, Tabka Z. North African reference equation for peak nasal inspiratory flow. J Laryngol Otol. 2011;125:595–602.

32. Akerlund A, Millqvist E, Oberg D, Bende M. Prevalence of upper and lower airway symptoms: the Skövde population-based study. Acta Otolaryngol. 2006;126:483–8.

33. Ottaviano G, Scadding GK, Coles S, Lund VJ. Peak nasal inspiratory flow; normal range in adult population. Rhinology. 2006;44:32–5.

34. Klossek JM, Lebreton JP, Delagranda A, Dufour X. PNIF measurement in a healthy French population. A prospective study about 234 patients. Rhinology. 2009;47:389–92.

35. Potter PC, Group S. Levocetirizine is effective for symptom relief including nasal congestion in adolescent and adult (PAR) sensitized to house dust mites. Allergy. 2003;58:893–9.

36. Caillaud D, Martin S, Segala C, Besancenot JP, Clot B, Thibaudon M, Network FA. Effects of airborne birch pollen levels on clinical symptoms of seasonal allergic rhinoconjunctivitis. Int Arch Allergy Immunol. 2014;163:43–50.

37. Pfaar O, Calderon MA, Andrews CP, Angjeli E, Bergmann KC, Bønløkke JH, de Blay F, Devillier P, Ellis AK, Gerth van Wijk R, et al. Allergen exposure chambers: harmonizing current concepts and projecting the needs for the future—an EAACI Position Paper. Allergy. 2017;72:1035–42.

38. Ellis AK, Steacy LM, Hobsbawn B, Conway CE, Walker TJ. Clinical validation

of controlled grass pollen challenge in the Environmental Exposure Unit (EEU). Allergy Asthma Clin Immunol. 2015;11:5.

39. Ellis AK, Soliman M, Steacy LM, Adams DE, Hobsbawn B, Walker TJ. Clinical validation of controlled exposure to birch pollen in the Environmental Exposure Unit (EEU). Allergy Asthma Clin Immunol. 2016;12:53.

40. Blomgren K, Simola M, Hytönen M, Pitkäranta A. Peak nasal inspiratory and expiratory flow measurements-practical tools in primary care? Rhinology. 2003;41:206–10.

41. Phagoo SB, Watson RA, Pride NB. Use of nasal peak flow to assess nasal patency. Allergy. 1997;52:901–8.

42. Ottaviano G, Lund VJ, Coles S, Staffieri A, Scadding GK. Does peak nasal inspiratory flow relate to peak expiratory flow? Rhinology. 2008;46:200–3.

43. Ibiapina CC, de Andrade CR, Godinho R, Alvim CG, Cruz Á. Correlation between peak nasal inspiratory flow and peak expiratory flow in children and adolescents. Rhinology. 2012;50:381–5.

44. Wilson AM, Sims EJ, Orr LC, Coutie WJ, White PS, Gardiner Q, Lipworth BJ. Effects of topical corticosteroid and combined mediator blockade on domiciliary and laboratory measurements of nasal function in seasonal allergic rhinitis. Ann Allergy Asthma Immunol. 2001;87:344–9.

45. Scadding GW, Calderon MA, Bellido V, Koed GK, Nielsen NC, Lund K, Togias A, Phippard D, Turka LA, Hansel TT, et al. Optimisation of grass pollen nasal allergen challenge for assessment of clinical and immunological outcomes. J Immunol Methods. 2012;384:25–32.

# 5

# European Summit on the Prevention and Self-Management of Chronic Respiratory Diseases: report of the European Union Parliament Summit

Peter W. Hellings[1,2], David Borrelli[3], Sirpa Pietikainen[4], Ioana Agache[5], Cezmi Akdis[6,7], Claus Bachert[8], Michael Bewick[9], Erna Botjes[10], Jannis Constantinidis[11], Wytske Fokkens[2], Tari Haahtela[12], Claire Hopkins[13], Maddalena Illario[14], Guy Joos[15], Valerie Lund[16], Antonella Muraro[17], Benoit Pugin[18], Sven Seys[18,19], David Somekh[20], Pär Stjärne[21], Arunas Valiulis[22,23], Erkka Valovirta[24] and Jean Bousquet[25,26,27*]

## Abstract

A European Summit on the Prevention and Self-Management of Chronic Respiratory Diseases (CRD) was organized by the European Forum for Research and Education in Allergy and Airway Diseases. The event took place in the European Parliament of Brussels and was hosted by MEP David Borrelli and MEP Sirpa Pietikainen. The aim of the Summit was to correspond to the needs of the European Commission and of patients suffering from CRD to join forces in Europe for the prevention and self-management. Delegates of the European Rhinologic Society, European Respiratory Society, European Academy of Allergy and Clinical Immunology, European Academy of Paedi-atrics, and European Patients Organization EFA all lectured on their vision and action plan to join forces in achieving adequate prevention and self-management of CRD in the context of Precision Medicine. Recent data highlight the preventive capacity of education on optimal care pathways for CRD. Self-management and patient empowerment can be achieved by novel educational on-line materials and by novel mobile health tools enabling patients and doc-tors to monitor and optimally treat CRDs based on the level of control. This report summarizes the contributions of the representatives of different European academic stakeholders in the field of CRD.

**Keywords:** Advocacy, EUFOREA, Asthma, Mobile health technology, Allergy

## Background

The World Health Organization (WHO) rates Chronic Respiratory Diseases (CRD) as one of the 4 major chronic diseases of mankind (Fig. 1) [1]. CRD often start in early childhood and persist throughout the life cycle. They are a major cause of economic burden and largely impact on the general society. CRD represent a major global health problem leading to gender and social inequalities within and between countries [2]. CRD including allergies and chronic rhinosinusitis (CRS) are complex diseases intertwined with ageing. Asthma, CRS and allergic rhinitis (AR) are the most common non-communicable diseases in children and adults, and their prevalence and burden have increased in recent decades, reaching epidemic proportions [3–5]. The Polish Presidency of the Council of the European Union (EU) has therefore made prevention, early diagnosis and treatment of CRD a priority for the EU's public health policy [6] to prepare the Conclusions of the Council, December 2, 2011 [7]. This was reinforced by the Cyprus Presidency of the EU Council [8]. In October 2015, a symposium on Precision Medicine in Allergy and Airway diseases was organized in the EU parliament with active participation of the Commissioner of Health Vytenis Andriukaitis [9]. An innovative

*Correspondence: jean.bousquet@orange.fr
27 EUFOREA aisbl, 132, Ave. Brand Whitlock, 1200 Brussels, Belgium
Full list of author information is available at the end of the article

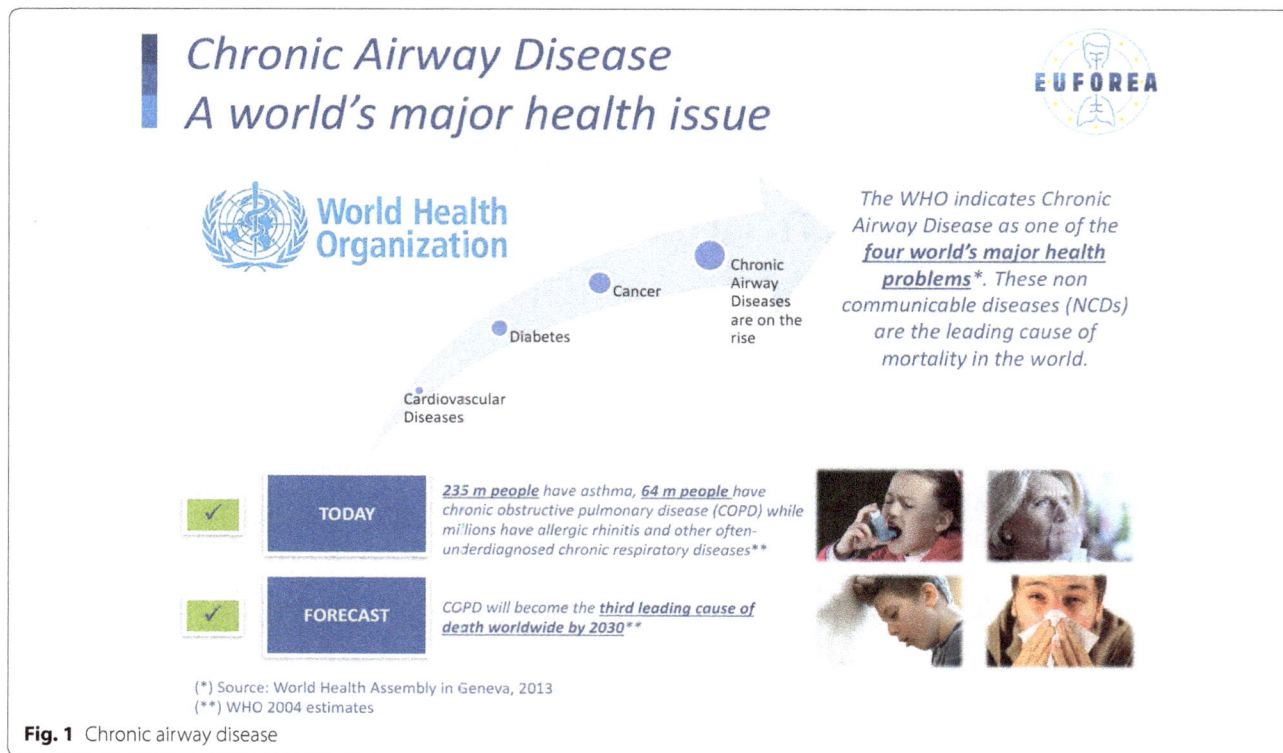

**Fig. 1** Chronic airway disease

integrated health system, built around systems and Precision Medicine and strategic partnerships, was proposed to combat CRD [10–13]:

- To better understand genetic determinants, environmental factors, molecular and cellular mechanisms underlying CRDs.
- To investigate social and economic factors leading to the onset, persistence and severity of CRDs.
- To phenotype and endotype patients, allowing implementation of the key pillars of Precision Medicine, i.e. personalized care, participation of the patient, prediction of success of treatment and prevention of disease.
- To develop unbiased and accurate biomarkers for multimorbidities, severity and follow-up of patients.
- To propose novel care pathways including multimorbidity and self-management strategies.
- To implement the principles of Precision Medicine into daily practice, in particular in primary care.
- To coach self-empowered patients through novel mobile health tools.
- To implement integrated care pathways with uniform information and treatment strategies provided by different care providers seen by patients.

A multidisciplinary practical platform with all stakeholders involved in CRD is currently missing. A symposium at the EU Parliament in October 2015 [9] proposed that the implementation of Precision Medicine into clinical practice may help to achieve the arrest of the epidemic of allergies and CRD. Participants underscored the need for optimal patient care in Europe, supporting joint action plans for disease prevention, patient empowerment, and cost-effective treatment strategies [9]. In the meantime, EUFOREA elaborated a European consensus report on the guidance of clinicians into the implementation of the principles of PM in daily practise [13].

The European Union Parliament Summit on March 29, 2017 aimed at providing practical approaches on the prevention and self-management of CRD, proposing care pathways implementing emerging technologies for predictive medicine centred around the patient (Figs. 2, 3). The Summit involved the active contribution of the scientific societies and patients' organisations, allowing a discussion on the innovative EUFOREA approaches to move forward on the prevention and self-management of CRD.

### The vision, mission and objectives of EUFOREA

EUFOREA is an international non-profit organisation forming an alliance of all stakeholders from national and international organizations, institutions, and agencies

European Summit on the Prevention and Self-Management of Chronic Respiratory Diseases: report...

45

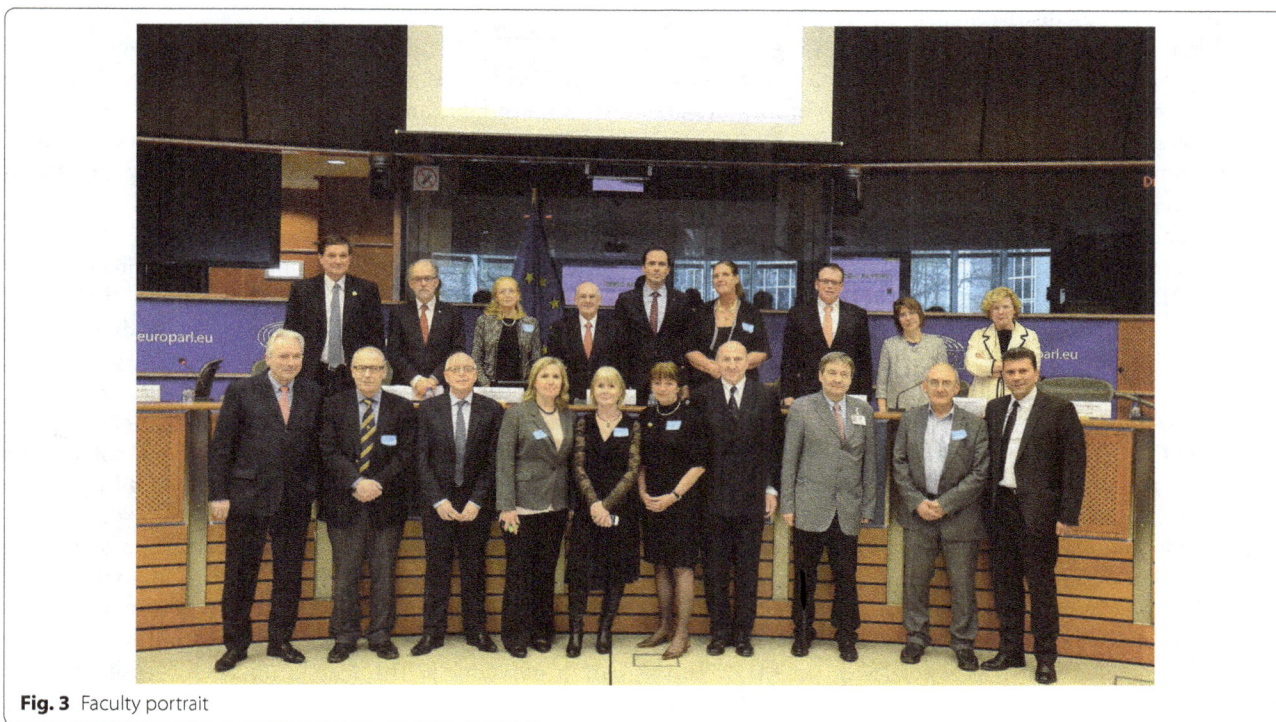

**Fig. 2** Programme announcement of EU Summit

**Fig. 3** Faculty portrait

working towards the common vision of preventing and improving the burden of asthma, allergic airway diseases and CRS. EUFOREA proposes to reduce the preventable and avoidable burden of morbidity and disability due to CRD by means of a multidisciplinary practical approach with all stakeholders at national, regional and global levels. Its aim is for populations to reach the highest attainable standards of health and productivity at every age and for CRD to no longer present as a barrier to well-being or socio-economic development. Given the novel scientific data on the prediction and prevention of allergic and airway diseases, the cost of inaction is unacceptable and there is an urgent need to undertake integrated actions in Europe, joining forces in a multi-specialty way with all stakeholders.

The main objective of EUFOREA is to initiate a comprehensive approach to prevent and fight CRD in upper and lower airways via the following strategies:

- To better educate the patients, the (para)medical community and the public
- To develop innovative care pathways including the key principles of Precision Medicine, i.e. prevention, personalized care, prediction and participation
- To empower the patients at the centre of the strategy, and to promote self-management and primary care
- To educate patients and health care providers on the optimal care pathways for CRD, taking into account 4 approaches: prevention, prediction, participation and personalized care
- To make recommendations of simple strategies for chronic airway disease management using emerging technologies for predictive medicine
- To promote active and healthy ageing
- To improve the work productivity of chronic airway disease sufferers
- To improve the well-being of chronic airway disease sufferers
- To reduce health and social inequities
- To support academic research in Europe in the field of CRD through a unique research support platform.

The added value of EUFOREA is to develop a unique strategic partnership for the prevention and control of CRD in order to tackle all components of prevention and to combat CRD from basic science to policies. EUFOREA provides a network through which collaborating parties can combine their strengths, thereby achieving major results that no one single partner could obtain alone. EUFOREA is meeting the need for a *pan-European multi-stakeholder platform* for the development of optimal and integrated care pathways for CRD, through a coordinated research and education activity portfolio. The EUFOREA platform unites educational and research initiatives of

all relevant stakeholders dealing with CRD through representatives of their official organizations: Primary Care physicians, Paediatricians and Allergologists via EAACI (European Academy of Allergy and Clinical Immunology), Respiratory physicians via ERS (European Respiratory Society), ENT doctors via ERS (European Rhinology Society), Allergy specialists of the ARIA (Allergic Rhinitis and its Impact on Asthma) expert group, Rhinologists of the EPOS expert committee, Patient organizations via EFA (European Federation of Allergy and Asthma Patient Organization), and Pharmacists via PGEU (Pharmaceutical Group at the European Parliament). The EUFOREA platform is unique given the multi-specialty nature and high academic profile of the multi-specialty advisory board taking part in the educational and clinical research activities of EUFOREA.

EUFOREA attempts to improve coordination between existing EU, governmental and non-governmental programmes to avoid duplication of efforts and wasting of resources.

### Action plan of EUFOREA

1. *ARIA* Care pathways implementing emerging technologies for predictive medicine in rhinitis and asthma across the life cycle

The Allergic Rhinitis and its Impact on Asthma (ARIA) initiative commenced during a WHO workshop in 1999 and was developed and implemented by the WHO Collaborating Centre on Asthma and Rhinitis [14, 15]. The initial goals were:

- To propose a new AR classification,
- To promote the concept of multi-morbidity in asthma and rhinitis, and
- To develop guidelines with all stakeholders that could be used globally for all countries and populations, in particular developing countries.

ARIA—disseminated and implemented in over 70 countries globally [16]—is now focusing on the implementation of emerging technologies for individualized and predictive medicine. MASK (MACVIA (*Contre les MAladies Chroniques pour un VIeillissement Actif*) [17]—ARIA Sentinel NetworK) [18] uses mobile technology to develop care pathways for the management of rhinitis and asthma by a multi-disciplinary group and by patients themselves. An App (Android and iOS) is available in 21 countries and 16 languages. It uses a visual analogue scale to assess symptom control and work productivity as well as a clinical decision support system. It is associated with an inter-operable tablet for physicians and other health care professionals. The scaling up strategy uses the recommendations of the European Innovation Partnership on Active and Healthy Ageing. The aim of the novel ARIA approach is to provide well-being and an active and healthy life to rhinitis sufferers, whatever their age, sex or socio-economic status, in order to reduce health and social inequalities incurred by the disease [19].

2. *EUFOREA mobile application 'mySinusitisCoach' CRS as a model for optimal patient coaching and empowerment*

CRS is a common disease but a stratification strategy is needed to provide a satisfactory management and to avoid unnecessary surgical interventions. MySinusitisCoach is being developed by EUFOREA, following a unique strategy with the following phases of development:

1. European CRS patient days to explore the needs and obstacles in current CRS care, including feedback on the mySinusitisCoach prototype using emerging technologies and the proposal of CRS interactive educational materials.

2. European meeting to align the patients' needs and KOL vision on the mySinusitisCoach prototype (Fig. 4), with feedback on the unique educational and coaching strategy of the CRS patients by mySinusitisCoach.

3. Preparation of the implementation of mySinusitisCoach in several regions in Europe with the support of local governmental authorities.

4. Analyses of the data generated by mySinusitisCoach, showing socio-economic value, secondary and tertiary prevention of CRD

5. Deployment of mySinusitisCoach in Europe, with data on real-life burden and cost of disease, (in)effective current treatment strategies, and demonstration of the major benefit of the instalment of mySinusitisCoach for the patient and the society.

3. EUFOREA Educational Platform: a practical approach

Patient education is the process by which health professionals and others impart information to patients and their caregivers that will alter their health behaviour or

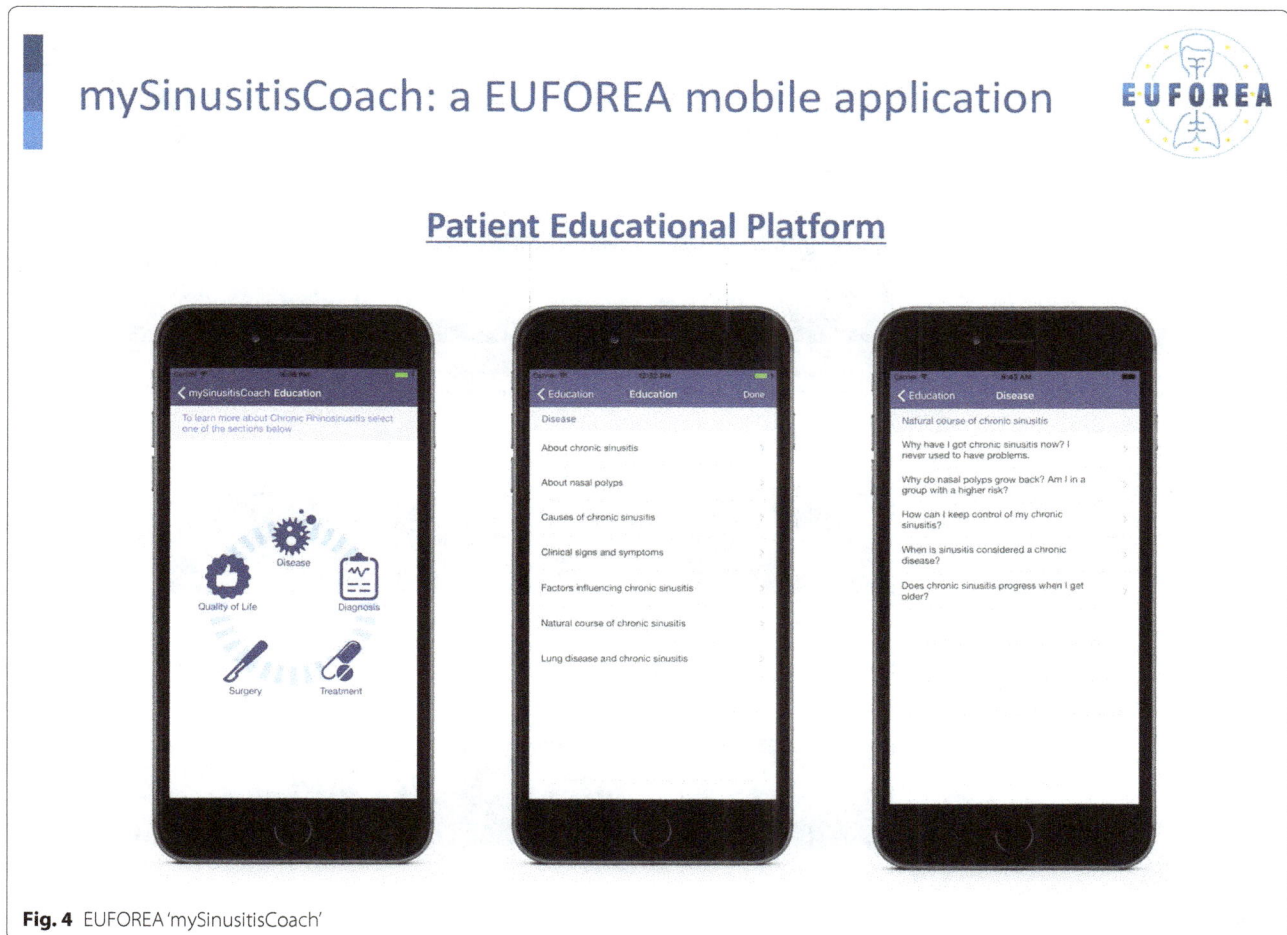

**Fig. 4** EUFOREA 'mySinusitisCoach'

improve their health status. Patient education for patients with chronic upper airway disease is one of the mainstays of EUFOREA (Fig. 5). European experts made a list of questions asked in their daily practice. Subsequently, interviews with small group of patients, individually and in groups, about their information needs were organized for understanding the patients' needs. A large web-based interview about information needs was then elaborated. Patients indicated that they needed more information at all stages of their disease and that they were not satisfied with the information available on the internet or from other sources. Patients were mostly interested to receive their information by means of a website or an App. Furthermore, they were very enthusiastic about the possibility of consulting a sinusitis coach (trained healthcare professional) by mail, chat or telephone. The EUFOREA website already contains the first series of patient information.

4.   EUFOREA Respiratory Research Platform for defining the RESEARCH NEEDS AND PRIORITIES in Europe

In November 2016, brainstorming sessions were held during the European Rhinology Research Forum (ERRF) on the research needs and priorities in the field of CRD with active participants from all over Europe. The major unmet needs and research priorities in the field of allergic rhinitis and Chronic Respiratory Diseases were highlighted from the perspectives of the patients and clinicians. This meeting resulted in the definition of the research priorities in the field of CRD and the joint action plan to meet these priorities [20]. A follow-up meeting is planned in the Royal Academy of Medicine of Belgium in Brussels on November 9 and 10, 2017, involving basic researchers, clinicians, representatives of patient organizations, and representatives of the industry and health authorities.

**The role of scientific societies**

European scientific societies are crucial in the management of CRD. They provide evidence-based, state-of-the art guidance for health practitioners by means of publishing research and knowledge including clinical practice guidelines, statements and technical standards as well as by providing continuing medical education (CME). In

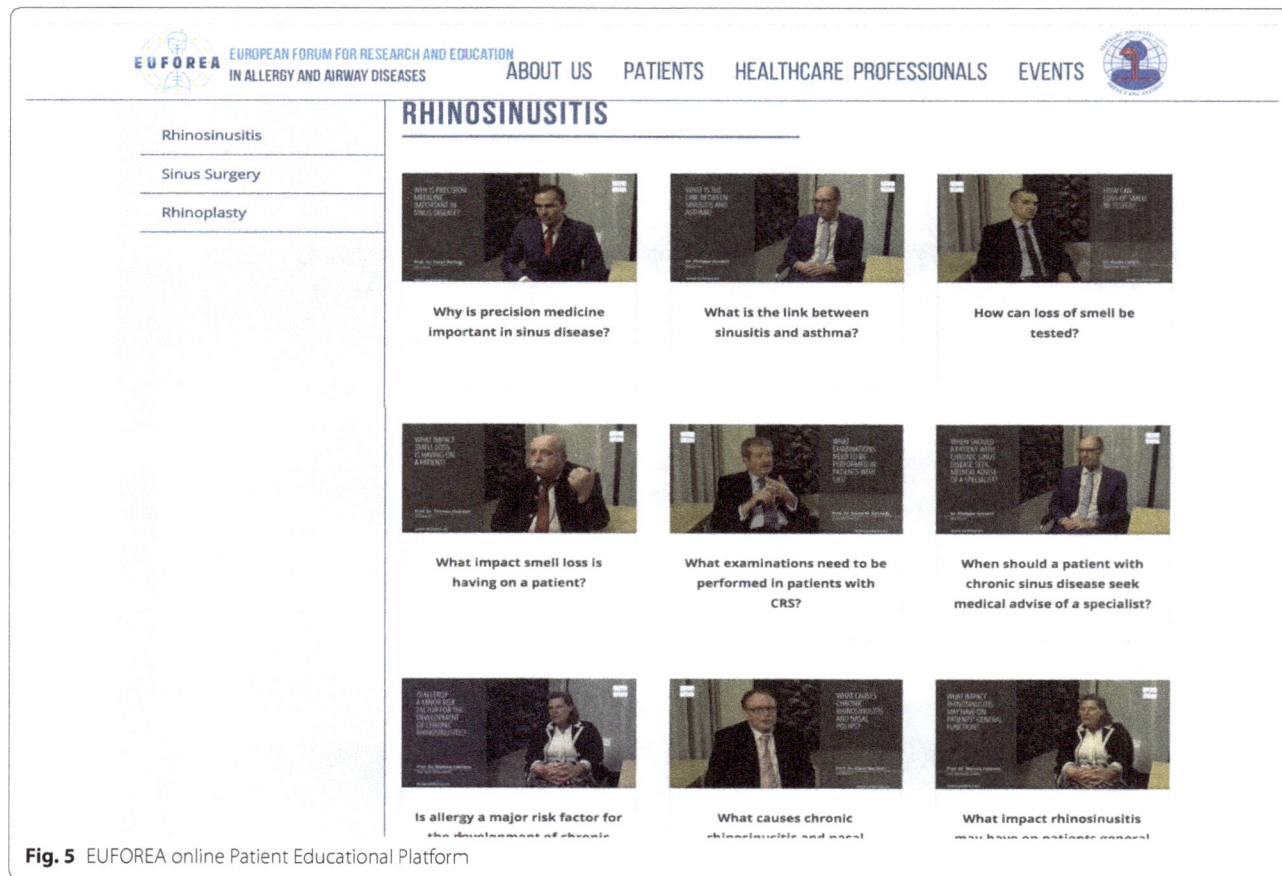

**Fig. 5** EUFOREA online Patient Educational Platform

addition, the large-scale annual or bi-annual congresses aim at transferring the latest scientific data to the clinicians. They bridge the gap between science and policy and advocate for policies committed to protecting public health. Scientific societies need to provide evidence-based input to ensure that airway diseases and their management is at the centre of policy decisions including air quality, European medical research, tobacco control and other preventative approaches such as occupational health issues. In conjunction with EFA, EAACI is currently launching a political Call to Action on Allergy and Asthma, with the support of the Interest Group on Allergy and Asthma of the European Parliament, led by the Finnish MEP Sirpa Pietikainen.

## Prevention of allergy and asthma in Finland
In the early 1990s, the new paradigm of asthma as an inflammatory disease was implemented into practice by the *Finnish Asthma Programme 1994–2004*. This improved care and cut costs both for individual patients and society [21]. New information of immune development in modern, urban societies has challenged the conventional thinking of allergy prevention. *The Finnish Allergy Programme 2008–2018* was initiated to turn avoidance strategy into tolerance strategy, and to take a step from treatment to prevention [22, 23]. Focusing on severe allergies and emphasizing allergy health rather than mild problems also targeted the use of health-care resources more efficiently. Revisiting of the asthma and allergy paradigms has led to actions relevant to society and health-care as a whole. In the Finnish society, burden of these conditions has started to decline [24]. The experience encourages medical communities and societies to lessen disability and costs caused by allergy and asthma and to improve public health.

## Therapeutic strategies to prevent asthma
Asthma often starts early in life and tends to persist across the life cycle [2, 25]. Thus, asthma prevention is a continuum from conception (or even before) to old age, integrating the complex network of risk factors (genome, exposome and disease endotypes and phenotypes) into a detailed roadmap for action [26]. Today the projection of children's diseases in adulthood is the key target for research and prerequisite of effective prevention as well as healthy ageing [27]. Wheezing is the major problem in both developed and developing countries affecting up to 50% of children under the age of 6 years. Even transient early wheeze is not only characterized by lower lung function but is also associated with chronic obstructive pulmonary disease in late adulthood [28]. An important work point is to protect children from active and passive smoking. Speed networking and new technologies based

e-research allow different projects to be integrated as well as the building of roads to modern paediatric respiratory medicine in EU countries [29].

A step-wise pathway is proposed: the tomorrow action plan relies on the multi-strategy approach focused on primary prevention and including the targeted hygiene concept. The 5-year programme relies on the wide use of health information technology translating vast amounts of "real-world" data unbiased by any pre-selection criteria into real-time clinical decision support at the point of care and harmonised disease management based on quality criteria [30]. The 10-year strategy integrates the multi-strategy approach with big data into personalised prevention plans [31]. Global, multi-discipline partnerships, rethinking healthcare, agreeing and implementing a fair balance between research and political priorities are all key points for an efficient asthma prevention strategy [32].

## Immunologic rationale for prevention of CRD
Dysregulated immune system, exposure to pollutants, irritants and allergens at home or to professional irritants in the work environment [33, 34], schools and workplace, genetic factors, and respiratory infections all play a role in the increased prevalence of CRD [35, 36]. Tobacco smoke is a key factor in the development and progression of CRD. Activation of the immune system cells and their interaction with tissue cells followed by chronic inflammation is a key mechanism in their pathogenesis. A defect in allergen tolerance is the cause of allergic diseases and is based on immunologic mechanisms. Recently, leakiness in the epithelial barrier is a major finding in all Chronic Respiratory Diseases such as asthma, AR and CRS [37, 38]. Several strategies are being developed to prevent respiratory diseases, including the restoration of barrier deficiency. Identification of risk groups and early intervention to restore the barrier function are essential for successful prevention strategies [39–41].

## A specific novel promising asthma prevention strategy resulted from the national survey in the United Kingdom
A prospective audit including more than 3 000 UK CRS surgical patients and assessing outcomes over a 5 year period showed significant improvement in the vast majority of patients [42]. Patients were then stratified by onset of symptoms to surgery into early (< 1 years), mid (1–5 years) and late (> 5 years) cohorts. This showed that the percentage change from baseline of CRS outcomes (SNOT22 scores) was greater in the early than in the late cohort at all time points ($p < 0.005$ at 1 years) when other demographic factors and extent of surgery were controlled [43]. Asthma prevalence was significantly higher

in the late group, suggesting that earlier sinus surgery is associated with better outcomes in both the upper and lower respiratory tract, altering natural history and preventing co-morbidities.

## Strategies for broad implementation of effective self-care

PROSTEP (Promotion of self-care in chronic diseases in the EU) is a tender designed to explore the added value of self-management in chronic diseases. It benefits from a thorough analysis of patient empowerment, including the relationship between self-management, joint decision-making and health literacy. PROSTEP stemmed from the EMPATHiE project (Empowering patients in the management of chronic diseases http://www.eu-patient.eu/whatwedo/Projects/EMPATHiE/), the first of two previous tenders, and from the experience of a platform of experts addressing the issues around the promotion of self-care in minor and self-limiting conditions (the PiSCE project). The overall requirements of this tender were (1) to conduct a study (consisting of a literature review and cost–benefit analysis) and (2) to set up a platform of experts in self-care in the field of chronic diseases to explore and propose possible methods of promotion of self-care for chronic diseases, taking into account previous and on-going policy work in this field such as the work of the CHRODIS JA. The 2-year project kicked off in January 2016.

## Patient's empowerment

The European Federation for Allergy and Airways Diseases Patients' Associations (EFA) has launched different projects at EU level to empower patients. They are built on three pillars: education, self-management and advocacy. One of the projects, Hey Ya, aims at improving health literacy in adolescent patients via raising self-awareness, confidence and attitude. This is particularly important in teenagers in whom poor adherence due to reduced health literacy is one of the major contributors to uncontrolled allergic airway disease. Secondly, the My Air Coach project was launched by the help of the Horizon 2020 Research and Innovation framework programme with the aim to develop a patient-friendly, sensor-based tool to collect clinical, environmental and behavioural data relating to the patient. Via self-management, it is a powerful tool for the prevention of complications. mHealth technology, jointly with patients' personal experience, are important for raising self-efficiency. Both Hey Ya and My Air Coach are important tools for improving teenagers' approach toward the diseases. Lastly, EFA supports and actively participates in advocacy campaigns at EU level. Recently, the Written Declaration on Chronic Respiratory Diseases was closed and signed by 115 MEPs. A new 'United Action for Allergy

and Asthma' was launched in the EU parliament in April 2017 to improve public policies. It addresses allergy and asthma and supports patients' rights.

## Technology transfer in rhinitis and asthma

The European Innovation Partnership on Active and Healthy Ageing (EIP on AHA) includes 74 Reference Sites. Scaling up is an essential component of the Action Plan B3 of the EIP on AHA (chronic diseases and remote monitoring) [27, 44]. A transfer innovation from an App developed by the MACVIA-France EIP on AHA reference site (Allergy Diary) to other reference sites will compare the phenotypic characteristics of rhinitis and asthma in adults and old age people using validated ICT tools (Allergy Diary [19] and CARAT: Control of Allergic Rhinitis and Asthma Test [45]) in 25 Reference Sites or regions across Europe. The aim is to better understand, assess the burden, diagnose and manage rhinitis and asthma in old age people.

## Conclusions

The high prevalence and major socio-economic impact of CRD require an inter-academic and multi-stakeholder approach for the successful implementation of prevention strategies leading to cost savings and reduction of burden. EUFOREA will continue its' mission to call for action by all stakeholders to implement Precision Medicine as the tool to arrest the epidemic of CRD. In Europe, there is an urgent need to join forces in the education of patients and medical care providers on prevention strategies, and to call for political action supported by all European academic stakeholders involved in the care of CRD.

## Authors' contributions
All authors participated to the European Parliament meeting and to the writing of the paper. They all agreed on the contents of the paper. All authors read and approved the final manuscript.

## Author details
[1] Department of Otorhinolaryngology, University Hospitals Leuven, KU Leuven, Louvain, Belgium. [2] Department of Otorhinolaryngology, Academic Medical Center, Amsterdam, The Netherlands. [3] Italian Member of the European Parliament, EFDD Group, Brussels, Belgium. [4] Finnish Member of the European Parliament, Brussels, Belgium. [5] Faculty of Medicine, Transylvania University, Brasov, Romania. [6] Swiss Institute of Allergy and Asthma Research (SIAF), University of Zurich, Davos, Switzerland. [7] Christine Kühne - Center for Allergy Research and Education (CK-CARE), Davos, Switzerland. [8] Upper Airways Research Laboratory, ENT Department, Ghent University Hospital, Ghent, Belgium. [9] Q4U Consultants Ltd, London, UK. [10] EFA - European Federation of Allergy and Airways Diseases Patients' Associations, Brussels, Belgium. [11] 1st Department of ORL, Head and Neck Surgery, Aristotle University, Thessaloníki, Greece. [12] Skin and Allergy Hospital, Helsinki University Hospital, Helsinki, Finland. [13] ENT Department, Guy's and St Thomas' Hospitals, London, UK. [14] Division for Health Innovation, Campania Region and Federico II University Hospital Naples (R&D and DISMET), Naples, Italy. [15] Department of Respiratory Medicine, Ghent University Hospital, Ghent, Belgium. [16] Royal National

Throat, Nose and Ear Hospital, University College London Hospitals, London, UK. [17] Food Allergy Referral Centre Veneto Region, Department of Women and Child Health, Padua General University Hospital, Padua, Italy. [18] European Forum for Research and Education in Allergy and Airway Diseases (EUFOREA), Brussels, Belgium. [19] Lab of Clinical Immunology, Department of Immunology and Microbiology, KU Leuven, Brussels, Belgium. [20] European Health Futures Forum (EHFF), Isle of Wright, UK. [21] Rhinology Department of Otorhinolaryngology, Karolinska University Hospital, Stockholm, Sweden. [22] Vilnius University Clinic of Children's Diseases and Public Health Institute, Vilnius, Lithuania. [23] European Academy of Paediatrics (EAP/UEMS-SP), Brussels, Belgium. [24] Department of Lung Diseases and Clinical Allergology, Univ. of Turku, and Allergy Clinic, Terveystalo, Turku, Finland. [25] MACVIA-France, Contre les MAladies Chroniques pour un VIeillissement Actif en France European Innovation Partnership on Active and Healthy Ageing Reference Site, Montpellier, France. [26] INSERM U 1168, VIMA: Ageing and Chronic Diseases Epidemiological and Public Health Approaches, UMR-S 1168, Université Versailles St-Quentin-en-Yvelines, Villejuif, Montigny le Bretonneux, France. [27] EUFOREA aisbl, 132, Ave. Brand Whitlock, 1200 Brussels, Belgium.

**Competing interests**
Pr Bousquet reports personal fees and other from Chiesi, Cipla, Hikma, Menarini, Mundipharma, Mylan, Novartis, Sanofi-Aventis, Takeda, Teva, Uriach, other from Kyomed, outside the submitted work. Dr Joos reports grants, personal fees and non-financial support from AstraZeneca; grants and personal fees from Boehringer Ingelheim, Chiesi, GlaxoSmithKline, Novartis ; personal fees from Sandoz, Teva, Mundipharma outside the submitted work. Dr Hopkins reports non-financial support from Fiagon, personal fees from GSK, Entellus, Medtronic, Optinose, outside the submitted work. Dr. Seys reports personal fees from Mylan, outside the submitted work. The remaning authors declare that they have no conflicts of interests.

**Funding**
Funding was provided by Euforea.

**References**
1. 2008–2013 Action plan for the global strategy for the prevention and control of non communicable diseases. Prevent and control cardiovascular diseases, cancers, Chronic Respiratory Diseases, diabetes. 2008. http://www.who.int/nmh/Actionplan-PC-NCD-2008.pdf.
2. Bousquet J, Anto JM, Berkouk K, Gergen P, Antunes JP, Augé P, et al. Developmental determinants in non-communicable chronic diseases and ageing. Thorax. 2015;70(6):595–7.
3. Samoliński B, Fronczak A, Włodarczyk A, Bousquet J. Council of the European Union conclusions on Chronic Respiratory Diseases in children. Lancet. 2012;379(9822):e45–6.
4. Hastan D, Fokkens WJ, Bachert C, Newson RB, Bislimovska J, Bockelbrink A, et al. Chronic rhinosinusitis in Europe-an underestimated disease. A GA²LEN study. Allergy. 2011;66(9):1216–23.
5. Jarvis D, Newson R, Lotvall J, Hastan D, Tomassen P, Keil T, et al. Asthma in adults and its association with chronic rhinosinusitis: the GA2LEN survey in Europe. Allergy. 2012;67(1):91–8.
6. Samoliński B, Fronczak A, Kuna P, Akdis CA, Anto JM, Bialoszewski AZ, et al. Prevention and control of childhood asthma and allergy in the EU from the public health point of view: Polish Presidency of the European Union. Allergy. 2012;67(6):726–31.
7. Council conclusions on prevention, early diagnosis and treatment of Chronic Respiratory Diseases in children: 31st EMPLOYMENT, SOCIAL POLICY, HEALTH and CONSUMER AFFAIRS Council meeting Brussels, 1 and 2 December 2011. Council of the European Union. 2011. http://www.consilium.europa.eu/.
8. Bousquet J, Tanasescu CC, Camuzat T, Anto JM, Blasi F, Neou A, et al. Impact of early diagnosis and control of Chronic Respiratory Diseases on active and healthy ageing. A debate at the European Union Parliament. Allergy. 2013;68(5):555–61.
9. Muraro A, Fokkens WJ, Pietikainen S, Borrelli D, Agache I, Bousquet J, et al. European symposium on precision medicine in allergy and airways diseases: report of the European Union parliament symposium (October 14, 2015). Allergy. 2016;71(5):583–7.
10. Bousquet J, Dahl R, Khaltaev N. Global alliance against Chronic Respiratory Diseases. Allergy. 2007;62(3):216–23.
11. Bousquet J, Jorgensen C, Dauzat M, Cesario A, Camuzat T, Bourret R, et al. Systems medicine approaches for the definition of complex phenotypes in chronic diseases and ageing. From concept to implementation and policies. Curr Pharm Des. 2014;20(38):5928–44.
12. Hellings PW, Fokkens WJ, Akdis C, Bachert C, Cingi C, Dietz de Loos D, et al. Uncontrolled allergic rhinitis and chronic rhinosinusitis: where do we stand today? Allergy. 2013;68(1):1–7.
13. Hellings PW, Fokkens WJ, Bachert C, Akdis CA, Bieber T, Agache I, et al. Positioning the principles of precision medicine in care pathways for allergic rhinitis and chronic rhinosinusitis: an EUFOREA-ARIA-EPOS-AIRWAYS ICP statement. Allergy. 2017. https://doi.org/10.1111/all.13162.
14. Bousquet J, Van Cauwenberge P, Khaltaev N, Aria Workshop Group, World Health Organization. Allergic rhinitis and its impact on asthma. J Allergy Clin Immunol. 2001;108(5 Suppl):147–334.
15. Bousquet J, Khaltaev N, Cruz AA, Denburg J, Fokkens WJ, Togias A, et al. Allergic Rhinitis and its Impact on Asthma (ARIA) 2008 update (in collaboration with the World Health Organization, GA(2)LEN and AllerGen). Allergy. 2008;63(Suppl 86):8–160.
16. Bousquet J, Schünemann HJ, Samolinski B, Demoly P, Baena-Cagnani CE, Bachert C, et al. Allergic Rhinitis and its Impact on Asthma (ARIA): achievements in 10 years and future needs. J Allergy Clin Immunol. 2012;130(5):1049–62.
17. Bousquet J, Mercier J, Avignon A, Bourret R, Camuzat T. MACVIA-LR (France) case study. Report EUR 27150 EN. In: Strategic intelligence monitor on personal health systems Phase 3 (SIMPHS3) JRC94487 Luxembourg: Publications Office of the European Union: JRC (Joint Research Centre) Science and policy report. Abadie F, editor. 2015. https://ec.europa.eu/jrc.
18. Bousquet J, Schunemann HJ, Fonseca J, Samolinski B, Bachert C, Canonica GW, et al. MACVIA-ARIA Sentinel NetworK for allergic rhinitis (MASK-rhinitis): the new generation guideline implementation. Allergy. 2015;70(11):1372–92.
19. Bousquet J, Hellings PW, Agache I, Bedbrook A, Bachert C, Bergmann KC, et al. ARIA 2016: care pathways implementing emerging technologies for predictive medicine in rhinitis and asthma across the life cycle. Clin Transl Allergy. 2016;6:47.
20. Hellings P, Akdis C, Bachert C, Bousquet J, Pugin B. EUFOREA Rhinology Research Forum 2016: report of the brainstorming sessions on needs and priorities in rhinitis and rhinosinusitis. Rhinology. 2017;55:202.
21. Haahtela T, Herse F, Karjalainen J, Klaukka T, Linna M, Leskelä R-L, et al. The Finnish experience to save asthma costs by improving care in 1987–2013. J Allergy Clin Immunol. 2017;139(2):408–14.
22. Haahtela T, von Hertzen L, Mäkelä M, Hannuksela M, Allergy Programme Working Group. Finnish Allergy Programme 2008–2018–time to act and change the course. Allergy. 2008;63(6):634–45.
23. von Hertzen LC, Savolainen J, Hannuksela M, Klaukka T, Lauerma A, Mäkelä MJ, et al. Scientific rationale for the Finnish Allergy Programme 2008–2018: emphasis on prevention and endorsing tolerance. Allergy. 2009;64(5):678–701.
24. Haahtela T, Valovirta E, Bousquet J, Mäkelä M, Allergy Programme Steering Group. The Finnish Allergy Programme 2008–2018 works. Eur Respir J. 2017. https://doi.org/10.1183/13993003.00470-2017.
25. Duijts L, Reiss IK, Brusselle G, de Jongste JC. Early origins of chronic obstructive lung diseases across the life course. Eur J Epidemiol. 2014;29(12):871–85.
26. Bloomfield SF, Rook GA, Scott EA, Shanahan F, Stanwell-Smith R, Turner P. Time to abandon the hygiene hypothesis: new perspectives on allergic disease, the human microbiome, infectious disease prevention and the role of targeted hygiene. Perspect Public Health. 2016;136(4):213–24.
27. Bousquet J, Barbara C, Bateman E, Bel E, Bewick M, Chavannes NH, et al. AIRWAYS-ICPs (European Innovation Partnership on Active

and Healthy Ageing) from concept to implementation. Eur Respir J. 2016;47(4):1028–33.

28. Kerkhof M, Boezen HM, Granell R, Wijga AH, Brunekreef B, Smit HA, et al. Transient early wheeze and lung function in early childhood associated with chronic obstructive pulmonary disease genes. J Allergy Clin Immunol. 2014;133(1):68–76.

29. Hadjipanayis A, Stiris T, Del Torso S, Mercier J-C, Valiul s A, Ludvigsson J. Europe needs to protect children and youths against secondhand smoke. Eur J Pediatr. 2017;176(1):145–6.

30. Blumenthal D. Stimulating the adoption of health information technology. N Engl J Med. 2009;360(15):1477–9.

31. Agache I, Akdis CA. Endotypes of allergic diseases and asthma: An important step in building blocks for the future of precision medicine. Allergol Int. 2016;65(3):243–52.

32. Guilleminault L, Ouksel H, Belleguic C, Le Guen Y, Germaud P, Desfleurs E, et al. Personalised medicine in asthma: from curative to preventive medicine. Eur Respir Rev. 2017;26(143):160010.

33. Hox V, Steelant B, Fokkens W, Nemery B, Hellings PW. Occupational upper airway disease: how work affects the nose. Allergy. 2014;69(3):282–91.

34. Hox V, Delrue S, Scheers H, Adams E, Keirsbilck S, Jorissen M, et al. Negative impact of occupational exposure on surgical outcome in patients with rhinosinusitis. Allergy. 2012;67(4):560–5.

35. European Academy of Allergy and Clinical Immunology. Global atlas of asthma. Zurich: European Academy of Allergy and Clinical Immunology; 2013.

36. European Academy of Allergy and Clinical Immunology. Global atlas of allergic rhinitis and chronic rhinosinusitis. Zurich: European Academy of Allergy and Clinical Immunology; 2014.

37. Steelant B, Farré R, Wawrzyniak P, Belmans J, Dekimpe E, Vanheel H, et al. Impaired barrier function in patients with house dust mite–induced allergic rhinitis is accompanied by decreased occludin and zonula occludens-1 expression. J Allergy Clin Immunol. 2016;137(4):1043–53.

38. Soyka MB, Wawrzyniak P, Eiwegger T, Holzmann D, Treis A, Wanke K, et al. Defective epithelial barrier in chronic rhinosinusitis: the regulation of tight junctions by IFN-γ and IL-4. J Allergy Clin Immunol. 2012;130(5):1087–96.

39. Muraro A, Lemanske RF, Hellings PW, Akdis CA, Bieber T, Casale TB, et al. Precision medicine in patients with allergic diseases: Airway diseases and atopic dermatitis-PRACTALL document of the European Academy of Allergy and Clinical Immunology and the American Academy of Allergy, Asthma and Immunology. J Allergy Clin Immunol. 2016;137(5):1347–58.

40. Canonica GW, Bachert C, Hellings P, Ryan D, Valovirta E, Wickman M, et al. Allergen Immunotherapy (AIT): a prototype of precision medicine. World Allergy Organ J. 2015;8(1):31.

41. Galli SJ. Toward precision medicine and health: opportunities and challenges in allergic diseases. J Allergy Clin Immunol. 2016;137(5):1289–300.

42. Browne JP, Hopkins C, Slack R, Topham J, Reeves B, Lund V, et al. Health-related quality of life after polypectomy with and without additional surgery. Laryngoscope. 2006;116(2):297–302.

43. Hopkins C, Rimmer J, Lund VJ. Does time to endoscopic sinus surgery impact outcomes in chronic rhinosinusitis? Prospective findings from the National Comparative Audit of Surgery for Nasal Polyposis and Chronic Rhinosinusitis. Rhinology. 2015;53(1):10–7.

44. Bousquet J, Farrell J, Crooks G, Hellings P, Bel EH, Bewick M, et al. Scaling up strategies of the chronic respiratory disease programme of the European Innovation Partnership on Active and Healthy Ageing (Action Plan B3: Area 5). Clin Transl Allergy. 2016;6:29.

45. Fonseca JA, Nogueira-Silva L, Morais-Almeida M, Azevedo L, Sa-Sousa A, Branco-Ferreira M, et al. Validation of a questionnaire (CARAT10) to assess rhinitis and asthma in patients with asthma. Allergy. 2010;65(8):1042–8.

# 6

# The hidden burden of adult allergic rhinitis: UK healthcare resource utilisation survey

David Price[1*], Glenis Scadding[2], Dermot Ryan[3,4], Claus Bachert[5], G. Walter Canonica[6], Joaquim Mullol[7], Ludger Klimek[8], Richard Pitman[9], Sarah Acaster[10], Ruth Murray[11] and Jean Bousquet[12,13,14,15]

## Abstract

**Background:** The affliction of allergic rhinitis (AR) has been trivialised in the past. Recent initiatives by the European Academy of Allergy & Clinical Immunology and by the EU parliament seek to rectify that situation. The aim of this study was to provide a comprehensive picture of the burden and unmet need of AR patients.

**Methods:** This was a cross-sectional, online, questionnaire-based study (June–July 2011) including symptomatic seasonal AR (SAR) patients ($\geq$18 years) from a panel. SAR episode pattern, severity, medication/co-medication usage, residual symptoms on treatment, number of healthcare visits, absenteeism and presenteeism were collected.

**Results:** One thousand patients were recruited (mild: n = 254; moderate/severe: n = 746). Patients with moderate/severe disease had significantly more symptomatic episodes/year (8.0 vs 6.0/year; p = 0.025) with longer episode-duration (12.5 vs 9.8 days; p = 0.0041) and more commonly used $\geq$2 AR therapies (70.5 vs 56.1 %; OR 1.87; p = 0.0001), looking for better and faster nasal and ocular symptom relief. The reported symptom burden was high irrespective of treatment, and significantly (p < 0.0001) higher in the moderate/severe group. Patients with moderate/severe AR were more likely to visit their GP (1.61 vs 1.19 times/year; OR: 1.49; p = 0.0061); due to dissatisfaction with therapy in 35.4 % of cases. Patients reported SAR-related absenteeism from work on 4.1 days/year (total cost to UK: £1.25 billion/year) and noted presenteeism for a mean of 37.7 days/year (vs 21.0 days/year; OR 1.71; p = 0.0048). Asthma co-morbid patients reported the need to increase their reliever- (1 in 2 patients) and controller-medication (1 in 5 patients) if they did not take their rhinitis medication.

**Conclusions:** This study differentiated between patients with mild and moderate/severe AR, demonstrating a burden of poorly controlled symptoms and high co-medication use. The deficiency in obtaining symptom control with what are currently considered firstline treatments suggests the need for a novel therapeutic approach.

**Keywords:** Allergic rhinitis, UK, Symptom episode, Co-medication, Absenteeism, Presenteeism

## Background

Allergic rhinitis (AR) has been trivialized over the years, despite its prevalence, chronicity and the burden it imposes on individuals and society [1–7]. Fortunately, the burden of AR is now being recognised both by the European Academy of Allergy & Clinical Immunology (EAACI) as well as at the EU parliament level, in order to highlight the profound impact this prevalent condition has on the quality of life (QoL) of AR sufferers and their families [8, 9]. Furthermore, the Polish presidency of the EU has highlighted the importance of early diagnosis and management of allergic diseases to promote active and healthy ageing [10], and made this an EU priority [11, 12]. All of these initiatives represent a fundamental shift in the perception of AR.

Reports in the literature already tell us that the daily burden of AR symptoms can be intrusive and debilitating, negatively impacting patients' QoL [4, 5], normal

*Correspondence: david@respiratoryresearch.org
[1] University of Aberdeen, Aberdeen, UK
Full list of author information is available at the end of the article

activities [6, 13], well-being, cognitive functioning [14] even mood [15] and sleep [16]. Most AR patients attending their healthcare provider have persistent disease, with many using multiple therapies [17]. AR imposes a high socioeconomic burden, particularly in terms of indirect costs, including absenteeism and presenteeism (i.e. productivity loss or under-performance at work and school) [18–21]. It has also been associated with poor asthma control; patients reporting severe rhinitis exhibit poorer asthma control than those with mild disease, with a negative impact equivalent to that of smoking [22].

Most AR patients visiting their physician have moderate/severe disease with persistent symptoms [2, 17, 23–25]. Insufficient symptom control by currently considered firstline therapies has been identified as a major concern [2, 4, 17], a situation which has not improved over time [6, 7]. Co-medication is common; patients self-medicate and doctors co-prescribe (antihistamines and intransal corticosteroids (INS) predominantly) [2, 3, 23, 26, 27] despite lack of evidence for this strategy in the literature [28–30]. AR patients have high expectations from their treatment [31], but most are dissatisfied with the results [32, 33]. Up to 40 % of patients have residual moderate/severe symptoms even after specialized treatment [17]. Management is often complicated by polysensitization [13, 34], the presence of allergic and non-allergic disease in the same patient (i.e. mixed rhinitis) [35] and confounded by phenotypes such as severe chronic upper airway disease (SCUAD) [36].

Clinical trials assess patients with the most severe symptoms with insufficient information from observational studies to understand the differences in burden between mild and moderate/severe rhinitis. To date, many surveys on the burden of AR have been conducted in Europe [2–5, 25] and in the US [6, 23, 37] but no cross-sectional questionnaire-based study, has assessed seasonal AR (SAR) episode pattern and duration, medication and co-medication usage (and the reasons for co-medicating), characterized residual symptoms on treatment nor provided information on healthcare visits, impact on asthma medication usage, absenteeism and presenteeism in a single study, stratified by disease severity (i.e. mild and moderate/severe).

The aim of this study was to describe the burden and unmet need of AR in one study, stratified by disease severity. AR patients have been included in hundreds of clinical trials without a true understanding of the real burden of this disease, the way patients experience their symptoms and how they and their health care provider manage their disease in real-life. A secondary aim was to use the data obtained to inform future AR clinical trial design and result relevancy.

## Methods
### Study design

This was a cross-sectional, online, questionnaire-based study designed to collect representative views of people diagnosed with SAR. It was carried out in the UK between June and July 2011. The survey content was informed by experts (see Additional file 1). Experts contributed to all aspects of the survey from item and response level development and provision of key concepts to explore to provision of full UK AR medication listings. Ethics approval was obtained from Independent Investigational Review Board Inc., (Florida, USA). Concept elicitation interviews with five patients were conducted prior to the start of the study to establish the most effective way to capture data with the least patient burden. These interviews were designed to ensure patient comprehension of the questions asked. Additional information to describe terms included in the survey were included based on patient advice.

### Recruitment, patients and data collection

Potential participants from a UK patient panel database (Opinion Health) were contacted about taking part in the study. This is an extensive database of patients with a variety of medical conditions, who gave prior consent to be contacted for research purposes. Patients are recruited into the Opinion Health panel from various channels, including direct mailing, bespoke telephone recruitment, peer/healthcare provider referral, magazine/newspaper advertising, and from relevant charities/associations/communities. The wide range of recruitment methods employed has led to a strong and nationally representative sample of the general population of which 18 % are aged over 65 years (30 % who are 55+ years), over 35 % are from lower household income bands with 17 % from Social Grade D or E.

These potential participants were provided with the survey address and unique identifier, which they could use to access the online survey. Participants who followed the link were presented with a study screening form to assess their eligibility. Patients (≥18 years of age), currently residing in the UK, with a self-reported clinical diagnosis by a medical professional of SAR and currently experiencing rhinitis symptoms, were recruited after informed consent. Currently symptomatic patients were selected to minimize recall error, enabling patients to draw on current symptomatic experience. Patients who experienced AR symptoms all year round (i.e. perennial allergic rhinitis) with no seasonal flare-ups were excluded.

The survey was sent to 1300 potential participants. The aim was to recruit 1000 SAR participants, 200 mild and 800 moderate/severe. For the purpose of screening, disease severity was graded using the ARIA-defined criteria of sleep disturbance, impairment of daily activities including leisure/sports, impairment of work/study and presence of troublesome symptoms [1].

## Surveys

All eligible participants were granted online access to the main survey to be completed at their own pace. Patients next completed symptom severity and socio-demographic/healthcare utilisation questionnaires (see Additional file 1). Symptom severity was assessed by EMA and FDA endorsed efficacy endpoints 12 h reflective total nasal symptom score (rTNSS; consisting of nasal congestion, itching, rhinorrhea and sneezing) and 12 h reflective total ocular symptom score (rTOSS; comprising ocular itch, redness and watering). These reflective scores assess symptom severity for the previous 12 h. Patients rated all symptoms as 'none = 0', 'mild = 1', 'moderate = 2' or 'severe = 3', both for symptoms 'today' and for symptoms 'at their worst'. Socio-demographic Information collected included patients' age, gender, ethnicity and educational level. The healthcare resource utilisation survey included questions on duration and number of SAR symptom episodes, SAR medication usage, GP visits, impact on co-morbid asthma, absenteeism and presenteeism. These latter two items were based on the Work Productivity and Activity Impairment (WPAI) questionnaire. The full WPAI questionnaire was not used in order to minimise participant burden. Symptom episode was defined for patients as 'an episode is a period of time when you experience symptoms (or need to take medication to treat symptoms) continuously'.

Participants received £10 upon completion of the survey. All subjects were free to withdraw from participation in this study at any time, and for any reason.

## Statistics

Statistical analyses were conducted in STATA 12 to compare baseline characteristics and exposures for mild disease to moderate/severe disease. For the purpose of analysis, participants with moderate/severe AR were defined as those who scored a rTNSS $\geq$8 out of 12, including a congestion score $\geq$2/3, when describing their 'worst symptoms'. These rTNSS and nasal congestion score cut-offs were chosen in order to align with moderate/severe definitions from a recently conducted clinical trial [38]. Participants with mild disease were the remaining patients. The number of patients with mild and moderate/severe AR in both groups was very similar whether severity was classified according to rTNSS and congestion scores or according to the ARIA definition.

Student t tests and Wilcoxon rank-sum tests were used to compare continuous outcomes for the two SAR severities, for parametric and non-parametric data, respectively. Results are presented with means and standard deviations, unless significant skew was observed in the outcome, in which case medians are presented. Chi-squared tests and Fisher's exact tests (where cell frequency was less than 5) were used to compare categorical outcomes to investigate differences between the two SAR severities and results presented as frequencies and percentages. Odds ratios were calculated for moderate/severe versus mild SAR for a given exposure with reference to no exposure. For all analyses p values <0.05 were judged to be statistically significant.

## Results

### Survey response

The survey was sent to 1300 potential participants. Data collection was stopped once 1000 patients completed the survey.

### Demographic and socioeconomic characteristics

One thousand SAR patients were recruited (mild: n = 254; moderate/severe: n = 746). The average age was 42.6 [standard deviation (SD) 12.1] years, with female gender and white ethnicity predominating (Table 1). Most participants were in full or part-time employment or self-employed (69.1 %), with over three quarters (76.9 %) educated to A-level standard (i.e. international baccalaureate level or above).

### Sensitization pattern

Grass and tree pollen were the most commonly reported sensitizing allergens, but indoor allergen (e.g. to animal dander, mites) and mould sensitization was also common. A high level of polysensitization was apparent particularly in the moderate/severe group (Table 1). Significantly (p < 0.001) more patients with moderate/severe disease were aware of their sensitizing allergen (Table 1).

### Episode pattern and duration

Patients with moderate/severe AR experienced significantly more symptomatic episodes/year than those with mild disease (median 8.0 vs 6.0; p = 0.025) with each of these episodes lasting significantly longer (12.5 vs 9.8 days; p = 0.0041; Table 1).

### Medication usage

Almost all patients reported taking medication to treat their rhinitis symptoms (90.6 and 96.2 % of patients with mild and moderate/severe AR, respectively). Oral H1-antihistamines were the medications most commonly reported, followed by INS (Table 2). Patients with moderate/severe AR were more likely to report nasal spray use (66.7 %) than those with mild disease [58.3 %;

**Table 1 Participant demographic and baseline data**

| | Allergic rhinitis severity | | p value |
|---|---|---|---|
| | Mild (n = 254) | Moderate/severe (n = 746) | |
| Age, mean (sd) | 44.1 (13.0) | 42.1 (11.8) | 0.0274 |
| Gender, n (%) female | 175 (68.9) | 503 (67.4) | 0.665 |
| *Ethnicity, n (%)* | | | |
| White | 226 (89.0) | 666 (89.3) | 0.894 |
| Asian | 16 (6.3) | 41 (5.5) | 0.633 |
| Black | 3 (1.2) | 25 (3.4) | 0.070 |
| Mixed | 5 (2.0) | 5 (0.7) | 0.072 |
| No response | 4 (1.6) | 9 (1.2) | 0.654 |
| *Allergen sensitivity (self-reported)* | | | |
| Grass pollen | 165 (65.0) | 579 (77.6) | <0.001 |
| Tree pollen | 119 (46.9) | 462 (61.9) | <0.001 |
| Weed pollen | 56 (22.0) | 259 (34.7) | <0.001 |
| Animals | 57 (22.4) | 231 (31.0) | <0.001 |
| Mites | 29 (11.4) | 163 (21.8) | <0.001 |
| Moulds | 25 (9.8) | 152 (20.4) | <0.001 |
| Not sure | 57 (22.4) | 96 (12.9) | <0.001 |
| Other | 25 (9.8) | 83 (11.1) | 0.569 |
| No. symptom episodes/year, median | 6.0 | 8.0 | 0.025 |
| *No. days/episode* | | | |
| Mean (SD) | 9.8 (18.1) | 12.5 (20.2) | 0.0041 |
| Median | 4.0 | 5.0 | 0.013 |
| Asthma diagnosis, n (%) | 70 (30.4) | 257 (35.8) | 0.1368 |

SAR severity: participants with moderate/severe AR were defined as those who scored a rTNSS $\geq 8$ out of 12, including a congestion score $\geq 2/3$, when describing their 'worst symptoms'. Participants with mild AR included all remaining patients

*SD* standard deviation

odds ratio (OR) 1.44; 95 % confidence interval (CI) 1.05–1.97; p = 0.0196]. One-third of patients in both groups used ocular medication (Table 2). Only 0.9 and 1.7 % of patients with mild or moderate/severe disease, respectively, reported use of injections (either immunotherapy or systemic corticosteroids) to treat their AR.

Most patients reported the use 2 or more AR medications (56.1 % of patients with mild AR and 70.5 % of patients with moderate/severe AR), but were nearly twice as likely to do so if they had moderate/severe disease (OR: 1.87; 95 % CI 1.36–2.56; p = 0.0001) (Table 2). The search for better nasal symptom relief, was the most common reason reported by patients for taking 2 or more AR medications. This was particularly evident in the moderate/severe group, where 58.3 % of patients cited the need for more effective nasal treatment as the reason for co-medicating compared to 42.6 % of those with mild AR (OR 1.88; 95 % CI 1.25–2.84; p = 0.0014) (Table 2). More effective ocular symptom relief was another important determinant governing co-prescribing behaviour, reported by over 40 % of patients in both

groups (Table 2). This was in line with the proportion of patients who reported ocular medication use (mild: 31.3 %; moderate/severe: 38.3 %). The search for faster response also drove AR treatment choice, with almost 35 % of patients with moderate/severe AR citing this as their reason for co-medicating (Table 2).

**Symptom burden**

The symptom burden reported by these patients was high, even though over 90 % of them were taking an AR medication. On the day of assessment, participants in both severity groups reported significant nasal and ocular symptoms. However, this burden (both nasal and ocular) was significantly higher in those with moderate/severe disease (Fig. 1). Patients with moderate/severe disease also reported a significantly (p < 0.0001) higher overall nasal symptom burden when symptoms were at their worst (10.0 [SD 1.5] vs 5.9 [SD 1.9]).

On the day of assessment (June–July 2011), many patients were experiencing 'moderate' or 'severe' nasal itch,

**Table 2** Medication usage in mild and moderate/severe seasonal allergic rhinitis patients

| | SAR severity | | | |
| --- | --- | --- | --- | --- |
| | Mild (n = 254) | Moderate/severe (n = 746) | Odds ratio (95 % CI) | P value |
| Taking medication, n (%) | 230 (90.6) | 718 (96.2) | 2.68 (1.45, 4.89) | 0.0004 |
| *Oral medications, n (%)* | *184 (80.0 %)* | *605 (84.3 %)* | *1.34 (0.89, 1.98)* | *0.1322* |
| Cetirizine | 82 (44.6) | 313 (51.7) | 1.33 (0.94, 1.89) | 0.0885 |
| Loratadine | 61 (33.2) | 195 (32.2) | 0.96 (0.67, 1.39) | 0.8153 |
| Chlorphenamine | 61 (33.2) | 178 (29.4) | 0.84 (0.58, 1.22) | 0.3349 |
| Pseudoephedrine | 14 (7.6) | 92 (15.2) | 2.18 (1.19, 4.25) | 0.0081 |
| Phenylephrine | 7 (3.8) | 33 (5.5) | 1.46 (0.62, 3.97) | 0.3716 |
| Acrivastine | 20 (10.9) | 82 (13.6) | 1.29 (0.75, 2.28) | 0.3420 |
| Levocetirizine | 0 (0) | 19 (3.1) | – | 0.011 |
| Fexofenadine | 10 (5.4) | 38 (6.3) | 1.17 (0.56, 2.68) | 0.6741 |
| Desloratadine | 3 (1.6) | 24 (4.0) | 2.49 (0.74, 13.06) | 0.1651 |
| Other | 17 (9.2) | 57 (9.4) | 1.02 (0.57, 1.93) | 0.9408 |
| *Nasal sprays, n (%)* | *134 (58.3 %)* | *479 (66.7 %)* | *1.44 (1.05, 1.97)* | *0.0196* |
| Fluticasone propionate | 96 (71.6) | 338 (70.6) | 0.95 (0.60, 1.47) | 0.8083 |
| Beclomethasone | 33 (24.6) | 110 (23.0) | 0.91 (0.57, 1.48) | 0.6875 |
| Mometasone | 4 (3.0) | 31 (6.5) | 2.25 (0.77, 8.92) | 0.1241 |
| Fluticasone furoate | 4 (3.0) | 12 (2.5) | 0.89 (0.26, 3.84) | 0.8401 |
| Flunisolide | 1 (0.8) | 12 (2.5) | 3.42 (0.50, 147.15) | 0.2116 |
| Budesonide | 2 (1.5) | 10 (2.1) | 1.41 (0.29, 13.36) | 0.6602 |
| Ipratropium bromide | 0 (0) | 5 (1.0) | – | 0.29 |
| Other | 18 (13.4) | 48 (10.0) | 0.72 (0.39, 1.36) | 0.2600 |
| Oxymetazoline | 9 (6.7) | 39 (8.1) | 1.23 (0.57, 2.97) | 0.5871 |
| Azelastine | 25 (18.7) | 106 (22.1) | 1.23 (0.75, 2.10) | 0.3860 |
| *Ocular medications, n (%)* | *72 (31.3 %)* | *275 (38.3 %)* | *1.36 (0.98, 1.90)* | *0.0552* |
| Sodium cromoglicate | 14 (19.4) | 82 (29.8) | 1.76 (0.91, 3.61) | 0.0798 |
| Antazoline | 12 (16.7) | 50 (18.2) | 1.11 (0.54, 2.44) | 0.7651 |
| Xylometazoline | 9 (12.5) | 36 (13.1) | 1.05 (0.47, 2.62) | 0.8943 |
| Azelastine | 3 (4.2) | 13 (4.7) | 1.14 (0.30, 6.41) | 0.8400 |
| Olopatadine | 3 (4.2) | 17 (6.2) | 1.52 (0.42, 8.29) | 0.5137 |
| Lodoxamide trometamol | 1 (1.4) | 9 (3.3) | 2.40 (0.32, 106.74) | 0.3950 |
| Other | 33 (45.8) | 98 (35.6) | 0.65 (0.37, 1.15) | 0.1121 |
| *Co-medicating, n (%)* | *129 (56.1)* | *506 (70.5)* | *1.87 (1.36, 2.56)* | *0.0001* |
| Reported reason for co-medicating, n (%) | | | | |
| More effective nasal treatment | 55 (42.6) | 295 (58.3) | 1.88 (1.25, 2.84) | 0.0014 |
| More effective ocular treatment | 54 (41.9) | 209 (41.3) | 0.98 (0.65, 1.48) | 0.9089 |
| Faster nasal response | 22 (17.1) | 116 (22.9) | 1.45 (0.86, 2.52) | 0.1490 |
| Faster ocular | 13 (10.1) | 57 (11.3) | 1.13 (0.59, 2.33) | 0.7007 |
| Other | 18 (19.0) | 48 (9.5) | 0.65 (0.35, 1.23) | 0.1378 |

SAR severity: paricipants with moderate/severe AR were defined as those who scored a rTNSS ≥8 out of 12, including a congestion score ≥2/3, when describing their 'worst symptoms'. Participants with mild AR included all remaining patient

*SAR* seasonal allergic rhinitis, *CI* confidence interval

congestion, rhinorrhea and sneezing as well as ocular itch, watering and redness, despite treatment, with significantly more patients with moderate/severe AR experiencing greater symptom severity for each nasal and ocular symptom (Table 3; Fig. 2). Congestion appeared to be the most bothersome nasal symptom; with 61.5 % of participants with moderate/severe AR rating its severity as 'moderate' or 'severe' on the day of assessment compared to 33.5 % of those with mild disease (Fig. 2). Ocular itch was the most bothersome ocular symptom; 59.4 % patients with moderate/

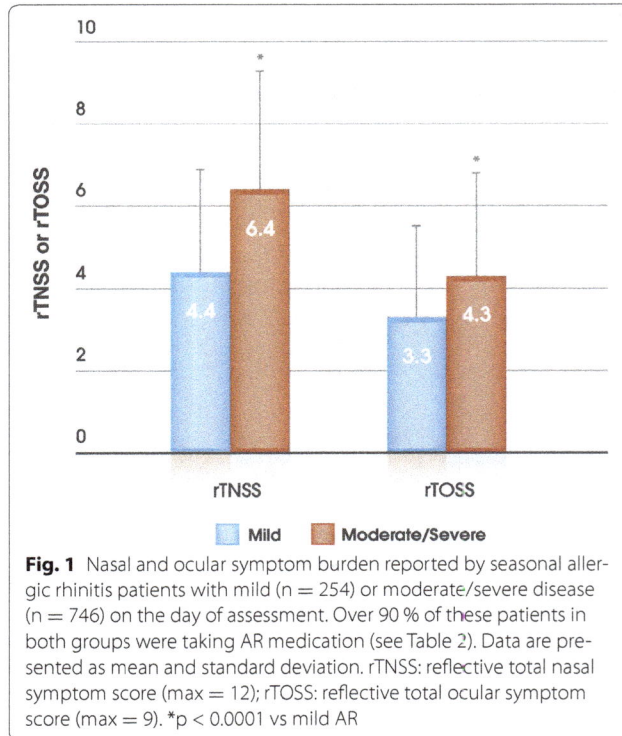

**Fig. 1** Nasal and ocular symptom burden reported by seasonal allergic rhinitis patients with mild (n = 254) or moderate/severe disease (n = 746) on the day of assessment. Over 90 % of these patients in both groups were taking AR medication (see Table 2). Data are presented as mean and standard deviation. rTNSS: reflective total nasal symptom score (max = 12); rTOSS: reflective total ocular symptom score (max = 9). *p < 0.0001 vs mild AR

severe AR rated its severity as 'moderate' or 'severe' on the day of assessment compared to 39.7 % of those with mild AR (Fig. 2).

### Health care visits
Participants with moderate/severe AR reported visiting their GP for their SAR more frequently than those with mild AR (1.61 vs 1.19 times/year; OR 1.49; 95 % CI 1.11–2.01; p = 0.0061). In both groups, dissatisfaction with treatment was a primary reason for the visit; 28 % of visits for patients with mild AR versus 35 % of visits for those with moderate/severe disease, with patients with moderate/severe AR being significantly more likely to report treatment dissatisfaction than those in the mild group (OR 1.49; 95 % CI 1.06–2.13; p = 0.0194).

### Impact on asthma
Many AR participants reported co-morbid asthma; 30.4 and 35.8 % of participants with mild and moderate/severe AR, respectively, and reported modifying their asthma medication (both reliever and controller) if they failed to take their AR medication. Patients with moderate/severe AR were twice as likely to describe this behaviour. For asthma reliever medication, 45.7 % of patients with mild AR with co-morbid asthma (n = 70) reported increased use compared to 53.7 % of patients with moderate/severe AR (n = 257) (OR 1.93;

95 % CI 1.01–3.68; p = 0.0303). Similarly, 15.7 % of patients with mild AR with co-morbid asthma reported the need to increase their controller medication if they failed to take their AR medication, rising to 19.5 % of patients in the moderate severe group (OR 2.04; 95 % CI 0.86–5.03; p = 0.0781).

### Absenteeism and presenteeism
Patients with moderate/severe AR reported absenteeism from work due to their SAR on 4.1 (SD 16.4) days/year compared to 2.5 (SD 7.7) days/year for patients in the mild group (OR: 1.34; 95 % CI: 0.87-2.11; p = 0.1708). This was significantly more likely for patients with moderate/severe AR who reported 37.7 (SD 53.0) days/year when their productivity was affected by their SAR symptoms, almost double that noted by patients with mild disease (21.0 days [SD 29.9]; OR: 1.71; 95 % CI: 1.15-2.54; p = 0.0048).

Participants with mild AR did report some negative impact on their productivity, clustered predominantly at the lower impact end of the productivity scale (i.e. < 50 % impact). The negative impact on participant-reported work productivity due to SAR symptoms was much more apparent for those with moderate/severe disease. These patients were almost 4 times more likely to experience > 50 % negative impact on their work productivity than those with mild disease (32.8 % vs 12.2 %; OR: 3.52; 95 % CI: 2.10-6.13; p < 0.0001) (Fig. 3).

### Discussion
This study provides a comprehensive view of the AR burden and unmet need in the UK. A complete dataset has been collected from a medically- diagnosed, symptomatic, SAR patient population (of similar disease severity to those included in a recent SAR study) [39] including information on SAR episode pattern and duration, medication/co-medication usage, reasons for co-medication, residual symptoms on treatment, number of healthcare visits, absenteeism and productivity loss in patietns with mild and moderate/severe AR. It, therefore, represents a complete assessment of AR burden and unmet need in a single survey.

This was a relatively large survey, including 1000 AR patients with wide representation of age, educational level and employment status. Survey content was broad and informed by several world-renowned experts in the field of AR. As this was an online survey, there was no interviewer bias. Responders were free to answer the questions in a time convenient to them and at their own pace. Patients were initially screened for severity using the Allergic Rhinitis and its Impact on Asthma (ARIA) severity classification system yielding 200 patients with mild AR and 800 patients with moderate/severe AR to ensure adequate representation of patients with moderate/severe AR in the survey (i.e. patients most likely to

**Table 3 Nasal and ocular symptom burden of patients with mild and moderate/severe AR on the day of assessment**

| Symptom | Symptom severity | SAR severity | | P value |
|---------|-----------------|--------------|--------------|---------|
| | | Mild (n = 254) | Moderate/severe (n = 746) | |
| *Nasal symptoms of the rTNSS* | | | | |
| Nasal itch, n (%) | None | 63 (24.8) | 87 (11.7) | <0.001 |
| | Mild | 128 (50.4) | 298 (39.9) | 0.004 |
| | Moderate | 54 (21.3) | 283 (37.9) | <0.001 |
| | Severe | 9 (3.5) | 78 (10.5) | 0.001 |
| Nasal congestion, n (%) | None | 67 (26.4) | 61 (8.2) | <0.001 |
| | Mild | 102 (40.2) | 226 (30.3) | 0.004 |
| | Moderate | 67 (26.4) | 312 (41.8) | <0.001 |
| | Severe | 18 (7.1) | 147 (19.7) | <0.001 |
| Rhinorrhea, n (%) | None | 82 (32.3) | 111 (14.9) | <0.001 |
| | Mild | 102 (40.2) | 241 (32.3) | 0.023 |
| | Moderate | 56 (22.0) | 279 (37.4) | <0.001 |
| | Severe | 14 (5.5) | 115 (15.4) | <0.001 |
| Sneezing, n (%) | None | 55 (21.7) | 68 (9.1) | <0.001 |
| | Mild | 108 (42.5) | 256 (34.3) | 0.019 |
| | Moderate | 75 (29.5) | 281 (37.7) | 0.019 |
| | Severe | 16 (6.3) | 141 (18.9) | <0.001 |
| *Ocular symptoms of the rTOSS* | | | | |
| Ocular itch, n (%) | None | 51 (20.1) | 97 (13.0) | 0.006 |
| | Mild | 102 (40.2) | 206 (27.6) | <0.001 |
| | Moderate | 74 (29.1) | 276 (37.0) | 0.023 |
| | Severe | 27 (10.6) | 167 (22.4) | <0.001 |
| Ocular watering, n (%) | None | 70 (27.6) | 154 (20.6) | 0.022 |
| | Mild | 102 (40.2) | 220 (29.5) | 0.002 |
| | Moderate | 64 (25.2) | 239 (32.0) | 0.040 |
| | Severe | 18 (7.1) | 133 (17.8) | <0.001 |
| Ocular redness, n (%) | None | 91 (35.8) | 183 (24.5) | <0.001 |
| | Mild | 106 (41.7) | 316 (42.4) | 0.861 |
| | Moderate | 51 (20.1) | 209 (28.0) | 0.013 |
| | Severe | 6 (2.4) | 38 (5.1) | 0.067 |

SAR severity: paricipants with moderate/severe AR were defined as those who scored a rTNSS ≥8 out of 12, including a congestion score ≥2/3, when describing their 'worst symptoms'. Participants with mild AR included all remaining patients

Symptom severity: Assessed by individual symptom scores of the rTNSS and rTOSS; 0 = none, 1 = mild, 2 = moderate, 3 = severe

*SAR* seasonal allergic rhinitis, *rTNSS* reflective total nasal symptom score, *rTOSS* reflective total ocular symptom score

visit their healthcare provider). However, to align with moderate/severe definition commonly employed in AR clinical trials, severity was also classified using rTNSS and congestion score cut offs for the purpose of data analysis. Very similar numbers were reported using this method of categorization; 254 and 746 for patients with mild and moderate/severe AR, respectively. This confirms the robustness of the ARIA severity definition as a quick, simple and accurate method of severity categorization, and also that the moderate/severe definition used in the present analysis largely conforms to ARIA.

Although the data relates to the UK in terms of allergen exposure, as well as treatment and referral patterns, the results also have a broader relevance for clinical trial design in general. For example, knowledge of the duration of a typical mild and moderate/severe SAR symptom episode could inform trial duration decisions and also encourage contextualization of efficacy endpoints with a temporal focus. A potential limitation of this survey was that patients were recruited from a patient panel. These panels include a varied and heterogeneous patient population. Panel patients are not subjected to stringent

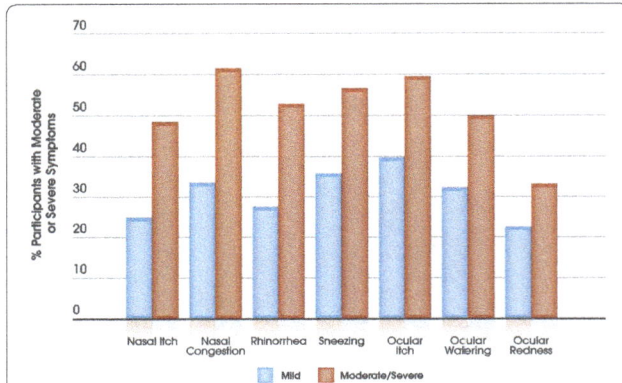

**Fig. 2** Proportion of patients with mild (n = 254) or moderate severe AR (n = 746) scoring a '2' (moderate) or '3' (severe) for individual nasal and ocular symptom scores on the day of assessment. Over 90 % of these patients in both groups were taking AR medication (see Table 2). Significance values for mild vs moderate/severe groups are given for each level of symptom severity in Table 3

intermittent/persistent). These classifications are not interchangeable [1], and whilst the SAR/PAR classification is still widely used in primary care, the newer (and more therapeutically relevant) ARIA classification system should be promoted at both the patient and physician level. By design, most patients included in the survey had moderate/severe disease and so represent the type of patients who present to physicians [2, 4, 17, 23]. Also, patients were included in this survey based on a reported medical diagnosis of SAR, rather than a medically-confirmed diagnosis. No data were collected on irritant exposure or smoking history. It would have been interesting to examine their impact on symptom burden and therapeutic response. As with all surveys of this nature there was a reliance on patient recall. Variability was noted for some responses as evidenced by large standard deviations around the mean. Where this occurred, median values were used.

inclusion/exclusion criteria and have a relaxed ecology of care making the information they provide more indicative of the real world. Conversely, AR patients recruited into randomized controlled trials (RCTs) are poorly representative of those seen in primary care [40]. In the present study AR was classified according to time of year when symptoms appeared (i.e. SAR) rather than the ARIA classification based on symptom longevity (i.e.

The survey found that patients experienced several symptomatic bursts throughout the year, each lasting for some days, with participants with moderate/severe AR reporting significantly greater symptom episode frequency and duration than their milder counterparts. There was a clear symptom burden shift from patients with mild to those with moderate/severe AR, the latter, more likely to report more and longer episodes/year. These facts were previously unrecognised. The symptom burden shift provides evidence of the quality of the survey data and its

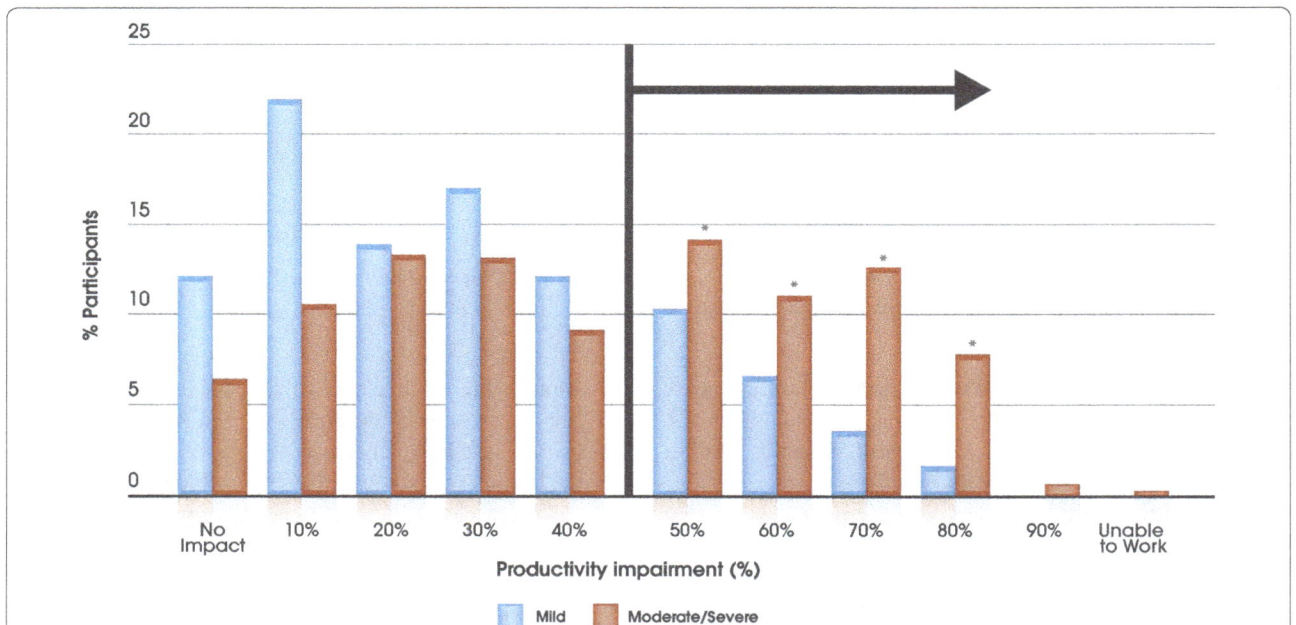

**Fig. 3** Presenteeism due to SAR reported by patients with mild disease (n = 164) and those with moderate/severe disease (n = 521). *p ≤ 0.0093 vs mild AR. Patients with moderate/severe AR significantly (OR 3.52; CI 2.10–6.13; p < 0.0001) more likely than those with mild AR to have a >50 % impairment in their work productivity due to their SAR symptoms

sensitivity to discriminate according to disease symptom severity. Knowledge of duration and frequency of AR symptom episodes is important to know when assessing the symptomatic and economic burden of AR, and when considering treatment choice. It indicates that rapid relief of symptoms is important to control the disease.

The extent to which patients co-medicate is underestimated by physicians and payers alike, since over the counter medications are frequently added to prescription medications. This finding has also been observed in Spain and France [3, 26, 27]. The majority of participants who took part in this survey reported using 2 or more AR medications (most commonly an INS plus an oral H1-antihistamine) in an attempt to achieve better and faster nasal and ocular symptom relief. This was true for both the participants with moderate/severe disease (70.5 %) and those with mild AR (56.1 %), although significantly more likely in those with more severe disease. Therefore, the direct cost of AR may be higher than previously thought, as patients supplement with multiple treatments, driven by their search for better efficacy. This search for a faster and more effective nasal therapy was more in evidence as a driver for those patients with moderate/severe AR emphasizing the higher symptom burden of this group, not only in terms of symptom severity, but also in terms of episode frequency and duration. The fact that over half of patients with mild AR co-medicated was an unexpected finding. This result showed that monotherapy provides insufficient symptom relief for a substantial proportion of patients with mild AR too, suggesting that they may underestimate the true severity of their disease and/or rely on over-the-counter AR medications, being resistant to attending their physician in order to receive a more effective treatment option, or indeed a more accurate severity diagnosis. Others have confirmed that co-mediation prescribing behaviour has been steadily rising in the UK in the last 2 decades; dual therapy has doubled since 1992, whilst use of triple therapy has increased eight-fold [41].

However, co-medication does not appear to provide the symptom relief, which AR patients seek. Logically, one would assume that use of several medications from different classes would provide improved pathologic coverage leading to better symptom control. But, this does not appear to be the case. The present survey results confirm the results obtained in randomized clinical trials [29, 30]. Both patients with mild and moderate/severe AR included in this survey remained symptomatic, with those with more severe disease more likely to be so, even though > 90 % of patients were on AR treatment, and many were co-medicating. In other words, patients' symptoms were still of moderate severity, on average, despite treatment. Nasal congestion and ocular itching remained problematic for 60 % of patients with

moderate/severe disease and were difficult to control with mono or multiple therapies. A similar pattern of mono- and multiple-therapy insufficiency has also been observed in other countries [4]. There is, therefore, a clear need for a faster and more effective AR treatment option with wide symptomatic and pathologic coverage, which provides more complete and rapid symptom control. MP29-02, comprising azelastine hydrochloride, fluticasone propionate and a novel formulation in a single spray, is the newest addition to the AR treatment arsenal and is promising in this regard [39, 42]. Allergen-specific immunotherapy should be strongly considered for patients who fail to respond to symptomatic therapy, particularly for those patients for whom symptoms are predominantly caused by one allergen [43], and may significantly reduce the burden of AR in these patients.

This survey also serves to highlight the large indirect burden of AR in the UK; the hidden costs associated with this disease are substantial. Many patients with AR also have asthma, with failure to control one having a detrimental effect on control of the other [1]. In the present survey, asthma medication usage (both reliever and controller) was likely to be increased by participants if they failed to use their AR medication, and more likely to occur in those with moderate/severe AR. Other indirect costs reported included absenteeism and presenteeism. On average, patients with moderate/severe AR reported 4 days/year absent from work due to their SAR. Assuming an average cost of £71 for each lost day [44], this amounts to £1.14 billon/year in the UK alone. This figure does not take presenteeism into consideration, which was reportedly negatively impacted on 38 days/year and carries a substantial indirect cost [19].

Knowledge of AR symptom patterns is vital when considering relevancy of clinical trial data and appropriateness of clinical trial design. Patients with intermittent AR (as categorized by ARIA) experience symptoms for <4 days/week or for less than 4 consecutive weeks [1]. Based on the results presented here, we now have corresponding information for SAR (i.e. average symptom episode lasts 9.8 days for mild SAR and 12.5 days for moderate/severe SAR). Therefore, SAR trials of 14 days duration are sufficiently long to assess the clinical efficacy of medications in most patients; since this timeframe spans a single episode, and thus reflects the real-world situation. Additionally, any improvements afforded by AR medications in patients with moderate/severe AR should now be contextualized and assessed for clinical relevancy within a 12.5 day time frame. It is also clear that direct head-to-head trials of active comparators are needed, not simply comparisons versus placebo, since the vast majority of patients with moderate/severe AR are treated, and most are co-medicating. Therefore, studies versus placebo only, in those patients with moderate/severe disease are not clinically-relevant, may provide a distorted view of the effectiveness of active comparators, and are likely to increase the number of insufficiently effective drugs registered, failing to meet patient expectations of treatment. The results of our study support the request of ARIA to conduct clinical trials against gold standard therapy in order to show clinically relevant improvements that will lower the burden of AR and improve its management. A recently published state of the art analysis of a new AR therapy, is an important first step in this direction [39]; (1) patients included in the trial had moderate/severe disease, representing the type of patient commonly seen in practice, (2) first-line AR medications were used as active comparators (in addition to placebo), (3) results were contextualised within a typical symptom episode window and (4) data were analysed to show not only superior efficacy to established first line therapies but also a faster response, which is what patients want [33, 45].

The impact of patients' attitudes on their AR health outcomes and their decision processes when considering which AR medication to take are interesting avenues for additional research. More information on patient knowledge (both about the disease and available treatments) as well as incidence of co-morbidities (e.g. food allergy, asthma, atopic dermatitis) would also provide a more global look at burden of care. Finally, patients should be empowered to take responsibility for their own AR control, encouraged to improve their disease awareness and knowledge of AR therapeutic options and improve concordance with their treatment regimen. In this regard, the importance of a common AR control concept and language (for both patients and physicians) has been recognized [46]. MACVIA ARIA has recently launched an app, called Allergy Diary, which uses a simple visual analogue scale (VAS) to assess control and will use this same VAS in an app for health care providers (called Allergy Diary Companion) and in the updated guideline to guide AR treatment decisions [46].

## Conclusions
This cross-sectional online questionnaire-based study represents a comprehensive assessment of the burden and unmet need of AR in the UK in a large patient population. Knowledge of the results of study should be used to inform clinical trial design and relevancy of clinical findings, and to assess the potential impact of AR treatments on the true burden and unmet need in this highly prevalent condition.

**Abbreviations**
AR: allergic rhinitis; ARIA: allergic rhinitis in asthma; CI: confidence interval; INS: intranasal corticosteroid; OR: odds ratio; RCT: randomized controlled trial; rTNSS: reflective total nasal symptom score; rTOSS: reflective total ocular symptom score; SAR: seasonal allergic rhinitis; SCUAD: severe chronic upper airway disease; SD: standard deviation; WPAI: work productivity and activity impairment.

**Authors' contributions**
All authors have been involved in the analysis and interpretation of data. SA and RP also contributed to the conception and design of the survey. All authors were involved in the drafting of the manuscript, critically revised each draft and gave their final approval for publication. All authors agree to be accountable for all aspects of this work and have participated sufficiently to take public responsibility for the content. All authors read and approved the final manuscript.

**Authors' information**
DP is Professor of Primary Care Respiratory Medicine at the University of Aberdeen, co-founder of the Respiratory Effectiveness Group (http://www.effectivenessevaluation.org) and Director of Observational and Pragmatic Research Institute Singapore. GS is Hon. Consultant Rhinologist and Allergist at the Royal National TNE Hospital, London and Hon. Senior Lecturer at University College, London. DR has had a career-long interest in respiratory allergy and was twice chairman of the UK Primary Care Respiratory Society. He is a member of ARIA and current Chairman of the Primary care Interest Group of EAACI. CB is an ENT specialist and allergologist at the Ghent University Hospital, and runs the Upper Airways Research Laboratory, Ghent University. He is also affiliated with the Karolinska Institute in Stockholm, Sweden. GWC is Professor of Respiratory Medicine and Director of Allergy & Respiratory Disease Clinic, Dept Internal Medicine, University of Genoa, IRCCS AOU San Martino, Genoa Italy. JM is an ENT specialist and Director of the Rhinology Unit and Smell Clinic, ENT Department, Hospital Clínic de Barcelona; and Professor of Research and Head of the Laboratory Clinical and Experimental Respiratory Immunoallergy at IDIBAPS. Barcelona, Catalonia, Spain. LK is Director of the Center for Rhinology and Allergology, Wiesbaden, Germany (http://www.Allergiezentrum.org), Vice-President of the German Academy of Allergology and Clinical Immunology, Vice-President of the German Union of Allergologists and Professor at Heidelberg University, Germany. RP is an employee of Icon plc. SA is the director of a Clinical Outcomes Assessment research consultancy. RM is the director of a Medical and Scientific research consultancy. JB is a Professor Emeritus at the University of Montpellier in France. He is recognized as past chairman of the Global Initiative for Asthma (GINA) and as the founder and Chairman of ARIA (Allergic Rhinitis and its Impact on Asthma), in collaboration with the World Health Organization. Prof Bousquet is also past Chairman of the WHO Global Alliance Against Chronic Respiratory Diseases (GARD), Director of the WHO Collaborating Centre for Asthma and Rhinitis in Montpellier, and coordinator of several projects of the European Union in research, health and ICT. Professor Bousquet's current interests lie with the European Innovation Partnership on Active and Health Aging, and updating how chronic diseases like allergic rhinitis are managed using an integrated care pathway.

**Author details**
[1] University of Aberdeen, Aberdeen, UK. [2] The Royal National Throat, Nose and Ear Hospital, London, UK. [3] Woodbrook Medical Centre, Loughborough, UK. [4] University of Edinburgh, Edinburgh, UK. [5] Upper Airways Research Laboratory, Ghent University Hospital, Ghent, Belgium. [6] Allergy and Respiratory Clinic, IRCCS AOU S. Martino, Genoa, Italy. [7] Hospital Clínic, IDIBAPS, CIBERES, Barcelona, Catalonia, Spain. [8] Center for Rhinology and Allergology, Wiesbaden, Germany. [9] ICON, Oxford, UK. [10] Acaster Consulting, London, UK. [11] Medscript Ltd, Dundalk, Ireland. [12] University Hospital, Montpellier, France. [13] MACVIA-LR, Contre les Maladies Chronique spour un Vieillissement Actif en Languedoc Roussilon, European Innovation Partnership on Active and Healthy Ageing Reference Site, Montpellier, France. [14] INSERM, VIMA : Ageing and Chronic Diseases, Epidemiological and Public Health Approaches, U1168, Paris, France. [15] UVSQ, UMR-S 1168, Université Versailles St-Quentin-en-Yvelines, Versailles, France.

**Acknowledgements**
We thank Icon Plc for statistically analysing the results.

**Funding**
Funding for this survey was provided by Meda Pharma.

**Competing interests**
DB has Board Membership with Aerocrine, Almirall, Amgen, AstraZeneca, Boehringer Ingelheim, Chiesi, Meda, Mundipharma, Napp, Novartis, and Teva. Consultancy: A Almirall, Amgen, AstraZeneca, Boehringer Ingelheim, Chiesi, GlaxoSmithKline, Meda, Mundipharma, Napp, Novartis, Pfizer, and Teva; Grants and unrestricted funding for investigator-initiated studies from UK National Health Service, British Lung Foundation, Aerocrine, AKL Ltd, Almirall, AstraZeneca, Boehringer Ingelheim, Chiesi, Eli Lilly, GlaxoSmith-Kline, Meda, Merck, Mundipharma, Napp, Novartis, Orion, Pfizer, Respiratory Effectiveness Group, Takeda, Teva, and Zentiva; Payments for lectures/speaking: Almirall, AstraZeneca, Boehringer Ingelheim, Chiesi, Cipla, GlaxoSmithKline, Kyorin, Meda, Merck, Mundipharma, Novartis, Pfizer, SkyePharma, Takeda, and Teva; Payment for manuscript preparation: Mundipharma and Teva; Patents (planned, pending or issued): AKL Ltd.; Payment for the development of educational materials: GlaxoSmithKline, Novartis; Stock/Stock options: Shares in AKL Ltd which produces phytopharmaceuticals and owns 80 % of Research in Real Life Ltd and its subsidiary social enterprise Optimum Patient Care; received Payment for travel/accommodations/meeting expenses from Aerocrine, Boehringer Ingelheim, Mundipharma, Napp, Novartis, and Teva; Funding for patient enrolment or completion of research: Almirral, Chiesi, Teva, and Zentiva; and Peer reviewer for grant committees: Medical Research Council (2014), Efficacy and Mechanism Evaluation programme (2012), HTA (2014). GS has received research grants from GSK and ALK as well as honoraria for articles, consulting, lectures/chairing and/or advisory boards from ALK, Bausch & Lomb, Church & Dwight, Circassia, GSK, Groupo Uriach, Meda, Merck, Ono, Shionogi and Stallergenes. DS has been paid consultancy fees by Stallergenes, Uriach and TEVA. He has lectured on behalf of MEDA, GSK, AZ, Chiesi, Thermo-Fisher, Boehringer, Novartis and Almirall. He is Director of Health Strategy at Optimum Patient Care. CB is on the speaker's bureau for Meda. GWC has received honoraria for lectures or scientific advisory boards: ALK, Allergy Therapeutics, AstraZeneca, Boston Scientific, Bruschettini, Chiesi, Circassia, Faes, GSK, Meda, Menarini, Mundifarma, Novartis, Recordati, Roche, Sanofi-Aventis, Uriach, Stallergènes, Thermo Fisher, Teva and Valeas. JM is or has been a member of national and international scientific advisory Boards (consulting), received fees for lectures, or grants for research projects from ALK-Abelló, Boheringer-Ingelheim, FAES, GSK, Hartington Pharmaceuticals, Hyphens, Johnson & Johnson, MEDA Pharma, Menarini, MSD, Novartis, Pierre Fabre, Sanofi, UCB, and Uriach Group. LK has received research grants from ALK-Abelló, Allergopharma, Bionorica, Dr. Pfleger, Stallergenes, HAL, Artu Biologicals, Allergy Therapeutics/Bencard, Hartington, Lofarma, MEDA, MSD, Novartis/Leti, ROXALL, GSK, Essex-Pharma, Cytos, Curalogic, and has served on the speaker's bureau for the above mentioned pharmaceutical companies. RP has no conflict of interest to report. SA was employed by Oxford Outcomes who were commissioned by Meda to conduct this research. SA now works for Acaster Consulting Ltd, which receives fees for research and consultancy from Meda. RM has received consultancy fees from GSK, Meda, MACVIA-ARIA and Research in Real life. JB has received honoraria for: Scientific and advisory boards: Almirall, Meda, Merck, MSD, Novartis, Sanofi-Aventis, Takeda, Teva, Uriach. Lectures during meetings: Almirall, AstraZeneca, Chiesi, GSK, Meda, Menarini, Merck, MSD, Novartis, Sanofi-Aventis, Takeda, Teva, Uriach. Board of Directors: Stallergènes.

**References**
1. Bousquet J, Khaltaev N, Cruz AA, Denburg J, Fokkens WJ, Togias A, et al. Allergic Rhinitis and its impact on asthma (ARIA) 2008 update (in collaboration with the World Health Organization, GA(2)LEN and AllerGen). Allergy. 2008;63(Suppl 86):8–160.
2. Canonica GW, Bousquet J, Mullol J, Scadding GK, Virchow JC. A survey of the burden of allergic rhinitis in Europe. Allergy. 2007;62(Suppl 85):17–25.
3. Mullol J. A survey of the burden of allergic rhinitis in Spain. J Investig Allergol Clin Immunol. 2009;19:27–34.
4. Bousquet PJ, Demoly P, Devillier P, Mesbah K, Bousquet J. Impact of allergic rhinitis symptoms on quality of life in primary care. Int Arch Allergy Immunol. 2013;160:393–400.
5. Canonica GW, Mullol J, Pradalier A, Didier A. Patient perceptions of allergic rhinitis and quality of life: findings from a survey conducted in europe and the United States. World Allergy Organ J. 2008;1:138–44.
6. Meltzer EO, Gross GN, Katial R, Storms WW. Allergic rhinitis substantially impacts patient quality of life: findings from the Nasal Allergy Survey Assessing Limitations. J Fam Pract. 2012;61:S5–10.
7. Nathan RA. The burden of allergic rhinitis. Allergy Asthma Proc. 2007;28:3–9.
8. European Academy of Allergy and Clinical Immunology (EAACI). Beware of Allergy Campaign. http://www.bewareofallergy.com. Accessed Aug 2015.
9. Antonescu E, Childres N, Gardini E, Grossetete F, Juvin P, Parvanova A, et al. Written declaration on recognising the burden of allergic disease. European Parliament. http://www.eaaci.org. Accessed June 2015.
10. Samolinski B, Fronczak A, Kuna P, Akdis CA, Anto JM, Bialoszewski AZ, et al. Prevention and control of childhood asthma and allergy in the EU from the public health point of view: Polish Presidency of the European Union. Allergy. 2012;67:726–31.
11. Bousquet J, Addis A, Adcock I, Agache I, Agusti A, Alonso A, et al. Integrated care pathways for airway diseases (AIRWAYS-ICPs). Eur Respir J. 2014;44:304–23.
12. Bousquet J, Michel J, Standberg T, Crooks G, Iakovidis I, Gomez M. The European Innovation Partnership on Active and Healthy Aging: the European Geriatric Medicine introduces the EIP on AHA Column. Eur Geriatr Med. 2014;5:361–2.
13. Valovirta E, Myrseth SE, Palkonen S. The voice of the patients: allergic rhinitis is not a trivial disease. Curr Opin Allergy Clin Immunol. 2008;8:1–9.
14. Kremer B, den Hartog HM, Jolles J. Relationship between allergic rhinitis, disturbed cognitive functions and psychological well-being. Clin Exp Allergy. 2002;32:1310–5.
15. Braido F, Baiardini I, Scichilone N, Musarra A, Menoni S, Ridolo E, et al. Illness perception, mood and coping strategies in allergic rhinitis: are there differences among ARIA classes of severity? Rhinology. 2014;52:66–71.
16. Green RJ, Davis G, Price D. Concerns of patients with allergic rhinitis: the Allergic Rhinitis Care Programme in South Africa. Prim Care Respir J. 2007;16:299–303.
17. Mullol J, Bartra J, del CA, Izquierdo I, Munoz-Cano R, Valero A. Specialist-based treatment reduces the severity of allergic rhinitis. Clin Exp Allergy. 2013;43:723–9.
18. Lamb CE, Ratner PH, Johnson CE, Ambegaonkar AJ, Joshi AV, Day D, et al. Economic impact of workplace productivity losses due to allergic rhinitis compared with select medical conditions in the United States from an employer perspective. Curr Med Res Opin. 2006;22:1203–10.
19. Hellgren J, Cervin A, Nordling S, Bergman A, Cardell LO. Allergic rhinitis and the common cold–high cost to society. Allergy. 2010;65:776–83.
20. Small M, Piercy J, Demoly P, Marsden H. Burden of illness and quality of life in patients being treated for seasonal allergic rhinitis: a cohort survey. Clin Transl Allergy. 2013;3:33.
21. Walker S, Khan-Wasti S, Fletcher M, Cullinan P, Harris J, Sheikh A. Seasonal allergic rhinitis is associated with a detrimental effect on examination performance in United Kingdom teenagers: case-control study. J Allergy Clin Immunol. 2007;120:381–7.
22. Clatworthy J, Price D, Ryan D, Haughney J, Horne R. The value of self-report assessment of adherence, rhinitis and smoking in relation to asthma control. Prim Care Respir J. 2009;18:300–5.
23. Schatz M. A survey of the burden of allergic rhinitis in the USA. Allergy. 2007;62(Suppl 85):9–16.
24. Bousquet J, Annesi-Maesano I, Carat F, Leger D, Rugina M, Pribil C, et al. Characteristics of intermittent and persistent allergic rhinitis: DREAMS study group. Clin Exp Allergy. 2005;35:728–32.
25. Bachert C, Van CP, Olbrecht J, van SJ. Prevalence, classification and perception of allergic and nonallergic rhinitis in Belgium. Allergy. 2006;61:693–8.

26. Demoly P, Allaert FA, Lecasble M. ERASM, a pharmacoepidemiologic survey on management of intermittent allergic rhinitis in every day general medical practice in France. Allergy. 2002;57:546–54.

27. Navarro A, Valero A, Rosales MJ, Mullol J. Clinical use of oral antihistamines and intranasal corticosteroids in patients with allergic rhinitis. J Investig Allergol Clin Immunol. 2011;21:363–9.

28. Anolik R, Mometasone Furoate Nasal Spray With Loratadine Study Group. Clinical benefits of combination treatment with mometasone furoate nasal spray and loratadine vs monotherapy with mometasone furoate in the treatment of seasonal allergic rhinitis. Ann Allergy Asthma Immunol. 2008;100:264–71.

29. Ratner PH, van Bavel JH, Martin BG, Hampel FC Jr, Howland WC III, Rogenes PR, et al. A comparison of the efficacy of fluticasone propionate aqueous nasal spray and loratadine, alone and in combination, for the treatment of seasonal allergic rhinitis. J Fam Pract. 1998;47:118–25.

30. Esteitie R, deTineo M, Naclerio RM, Baroody FM. Effect of the addition of montelukast to fluticasone propionate for the treatment of perennial allergic rhinitis. Ann Allergy Asthma Immunol. 2010;105:155–61.

31. Hellings PW, Dobbels F, Denhaerynck K, Piessens M, Ceuppens JL, De GS. Explorative study on patient's perceived knowledge evel, expectations, preferences and fear of side effects for treatment for allergic rhinitis. Clin Transl Allergy. 2012;2:9.

32. Ciprandi G, Incorvaia C, Scurati S, Puccinelli P, Soffia S. Frati F, et al. Patient-related factors in rhinitis and asthma: the satisfaction with allergy treatment survey. Curr Med Res Opin. 2011;27:1005–11.

33. Valovirta E, Ryan D. Patient adherence to allergic rhinitis treatment: results from patient surveys. Medscape J Med. 2008;10:247.

34. Mosges R, Klimek L. Today's allergic rhinitis patients are different: new factors that may play a role. Allergy. 2007;62:969–75.

35. Settipane RA, Lieberman P. Update on nonallergic rhinitis. Ann Allergy Asthma Immunol. 2001;86:494–507.

36. Bousquet PJ, Bachert C, Canonica GW, Casale TB, Mullol J, Klossek JM, et al. Uncontrolled allergic rhinitis during treatment and its impact on quality of life: a cluster randomized trial. J Allergy Clin Immunol. 2010;126:666–8.

37. Meltzer EO, Blaiss MS, Derebery MJ, Mahr TA, Gordon BR, Sheth KK, et al. Burden of allergic rhinitis: results from the Pediatric Allergies in America survey. J Allergy Clin Immunol. 2009;124:S43–70.

38. Carr W, Bernstein J, Lieberman P, Meltzer E, Bachert C, Price D, et al. A novel intranasal therapy of azelastine with fluticasone for the treatment of allergic rhinitis. J Allergy Clin Immunol. 2012;129:1282–9.

39. Meltzer E, Ratner P, Bachert C, Carr W, Berger W, Canonica GW, et al. Clinically relevant effect of a new intranasal therapy (MP29-02) in allergic rhinitis assessed by responder analysis. Int Arch Allergy Immunol. 2013;161:369–77.

40. Costa DJ, Amouyal M, Lambert P, Ryan D, Schunemann HJ, Daures JP, et al. How representative are clinical study patients with allergic rhinitis in primary care? J Allergy Clin Immunol. 2011;127:920–6.

41. Price D, Scadding G, Bachert C, Saleh H, Nasser S, Bichel K, et al. Dynamics of treatment within a year in patients diagnosed with either allergic, non-allergic rhinitis or hay fever over the period 1992–2012. Allergy. 2014;69:A284.

42. Klimek L, Bachert C, Mosges R, Munzel U, Price D, Virchow JC, et al. Effectiveness of MP29-02 for the treatment of allergic rhinitis in real-life: results from a noninterventional study. Allergy Asthma Proc. 2015;36:40–7.

43. Scadding GK, Durham SR, Mirakian R, Jones NS, Leech SC, Farooque S, et al. BSACI guidelines for the management of allergic and non-allergic rhinitis. Clin Exp Allergy. 2008;38:19–42.

44. UK Healthcare: The case for health benefits. http://www.ukhealthcare.org.uk/the-case-for-health-benefits. Accessed June 2015.

45. Acaster S, Ali S, Breheny K, Bachert C, Bousquet J, Price D. Treatment preferences in patients with moderate/severe seasonal allergic rhinitis: findings of a discrete choice experiment. Allergy. 2012;67:A891.

46. Bousquet J, Schunemann HJ, Fonseca J, Samolinski B, Bachert C, Canonica GW et al. MACVIA-ARIA Sentinel NetworK for allergic rhinitis (MASK-rhinitis): The new generation guideline implementation. Allergy. 2015 **[Epub ahead of print]**.

# 7

# Consideration of methods for identifying mite allergens

Yubao Cui* 🄌, Qiong Wang and Haoyuan Jia

**Abstract**

House dust mites are small arthropods that produce proteins—found in their feces, body parts, and eggs—that are major triggers of human allergies worldwide. The goal of this review is to describe the current methods used to identify these allergens. A literature search for allergen identification methods employed between 1995 and 2016 revealed multiple techniques that can be broadly grouped into discovery and confirmation phases. The discovery phase employs screening for mite proteins that can bind IgEs in sera from animals or patients allergic to dust mites. The confirmation phase employs biochemical methods to isolate either native or recombinant mite proteins, confirms the IgE binding of the purified allergens, and uses either in vitro or in vivo assays to demonstrate that the purified antigen can stimulate an immune response. The methods used in the two phases are defined and their strengths and weaknesses are discussed. The majority of HDM-allergic patients may respond to just a small subset of proteins, but new protein discovery methods are still warranted in order to develop a complete panel of HDM allergens for component resolved diagnosis and patient-tailored therapies.

**Keywords:** Allergen identification, Allergen classification, Dust mite allergen, Mite allergen, Mite allergy

## Background

Sensitization and ongoing exposure to house dust mite (HDM) allergens causes acute reactions including asthma, rhinitis, atopic dermatitis, or other allergic responses [1]. The most common sources of these allergens are the two major HDM species, *Dermatophagoides pteronyssinus* and *Dermatophagoides farinae*, but other dust and storage mite species also contribute [2]. Mite species have differing geographic distributions with *D. pteronyssinus* and *D. farinae* typically overlapping in temperate regions, and with the storage mite *Blomia tropicalis* in the tropics [3].

Almost all body parts of the mites, including the gut, feces, cuticles, and eggs [4–6], contain allergens, triggering allergy in 85% of individuals with asthma. Mite gastrointestinal tract proteins often cause chronic allergy [7, 8] particularly airway allergy, as these proteins are deposited in fecal pellets, which can become airborne and are inhaled. Proteins from the mite cuticle and dermis appear more likely to stimulate atopic dermatitis, as these allergens probably act through skin contact [4]. Importantly, in addition to mite-derived proteins, research is beginning to show potential allergenicity to mite-borne bacteria and fungi, although not to the same level [9].

Over 20 HDM allergens have been characterized to date [10]. The International Union of Immunological Societies (IUIS)—which catalogs allergens by using the first 3 letters of the source of the allergen (e.g., Der for *Dermatophagoides*), the first or second letter of the species (e.g., p for *pteronyssinus*), and finally an Arabic number corresponding to the order in which the allergen was discovered, its clinical significance, or both—has catalogued allergens from four species of dust mites (*D. pteronyssinus, D. farinae, Euroglyphus maynei,* and *Dermatophagoides microceras*) and six species of storage mites (*Acarus siro, B. tropicalis, Chortoglyphus arcuatus, Glycyphagus domesticus, Lepidoglyphus destructor,* and *Tyrophagus putrescentiae*). Proteins from these groups have all been reported to bind (to differing extents) IgEs from serum of patients allergic to dust mites, but the

*Correspondence: ybcui1975@hotmail.com
Department of Clinical Laboratory, Wuxi People's Hospital Affiliated to Nanjing Medical University, No. 299, Qingyang Road, Wuxi 214023, Jiangsu Province, People's Republic of China

role of most of these proteins in stimulating an allergic response has yet to be defined.

For dust mites, the best characterized allergens are the group 1 and 2 proteins. These represent the so-called major allergens, meaning that the majority of HDM-allergic patients have high levels of high- affinity IgEs directed against these proteins. In a Chinese study of 200 patients, 89% had IgE-reactivity against Der p 1 and 84% had IgE-reactivity against Der p 2 [11]. In an additional study of *D. farinae* extracts, 95% of the patients had specific IgE reactivity against Der f 1 and 95% of patients had IgE reactivity against Der f 2 [12]. The *D. farinae* and *D. pteronyssinus* group 1 and 2 proteins can bind over 50% of the IgEs in HDM-reactive sera (reviewed in [10]). Seven dust mite homologues of the group 1 and 2 proteins are now listed by the IUIS and there are species-specific as well as cross-reactive epitopes [13, 14]. However, for storage mite species, the group 1 proteins are not major allergens; instead the major IgE-binding component in *B. tropicalis* extracts appears to be Blo t 5 [14, 15].

The major dust mite allergens have been well studied [10], hence this review will focus on the techniques used to identify, isolate, and characterize newer allergens. Well-designed discovery and isolation procedures are necessary to establish a complete panel of dust mite allergens for patient-specific diagnostic and therapeutic applications and to provide tools for assessing indoor, outdoor, and occupational environments for mite allergy burden. Ideally, these discovery techniques should be applied to as many mite species as possible. Morgan et al. [16], in

assessing human sera for reactivity to *E. maynei*, concluded that this species produces many potent allergens with unique allergenic epitopes, making it "essential that individuals allergic to mites be tested with and treated for all mite species present in the local environment".

In order to stimulate efforts to find new allergens, particularly from lesser- studied mite species as proposed by Morgan et al. [16], this review summarizes the techniques used to discover and confirm the allergenicity of various mite proteins. The structure of the review is shown in Fig. 1. It progresses from the consideration of techniques used to identify candidate allergens to techniques used to isolate and confirm that candidate proteins induce an allergic response.

## Discovery phase
### Identification of potential allergens by IgE binding
Using blood serum samples, researchers are able to identify antibodies, in particular IgEs, resulting from reaction to allergen exposure. It is the most common way to identify an allergic response in humans or animals. Early studies used human sera and crossed radioimmunoelectrophoresis to estimate the number of IgE-reactive species in crude mite extracts. CRIE first separates native proteins based on charge, followed by orthogonal electrophoresis into a gel containing sera where antibody protein precipitates form. Subsequent blotting with radiolabeled anti-IgE reveals reactive peaks. When Chinese HDM allergic patients were screened using this

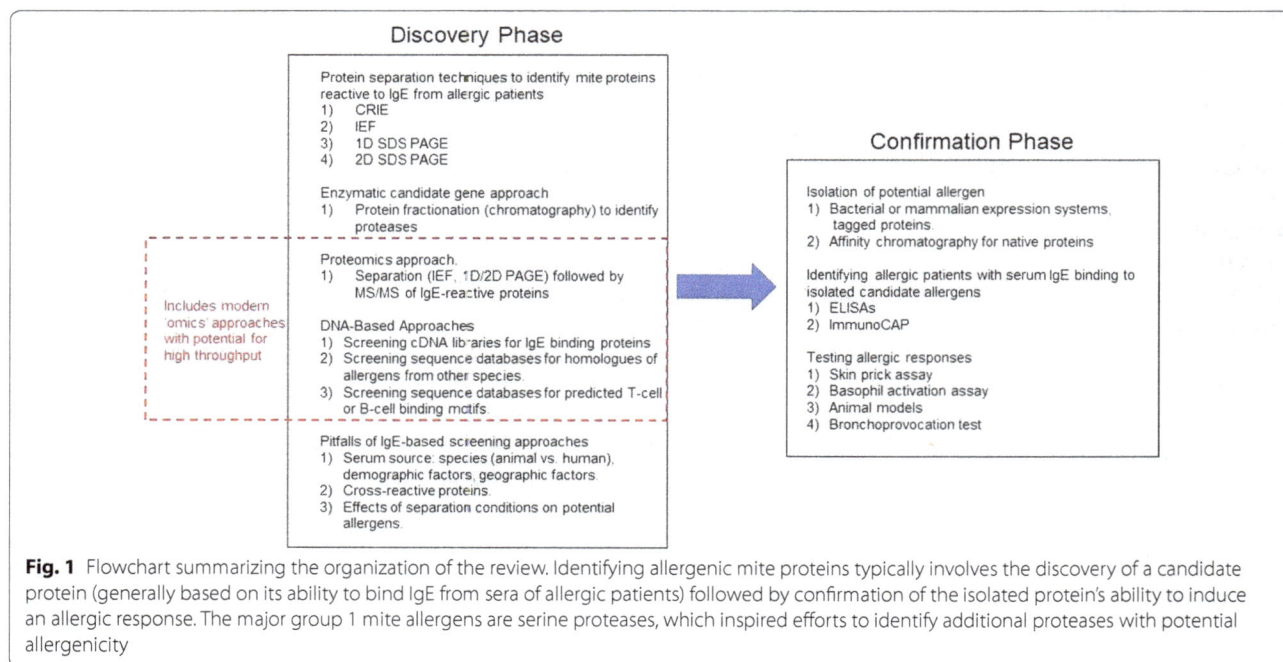

**Fig. 1** Flowchart summarizing the organization of the review. Identifying allergenic mite proteins typically involves the discovery of a candidate protein (generally based on its ability to bind IgE from sera of allergic patients) followed by confirmation of the isolated protein's ability to induce an allergic response. The major group 1 mite allergens are serine proteases, which inspired efforts to identify additional proteases with potential allergenicity

technique, 23 allergen-IgE precipitates were detected in *D. pteronyssinus* and 17 in *D. farinae* extracts [17].

More recent discovery attempts used additional forms of protein separation (isoelectric focusing (IEF), one dimensional sodium dodecyl sulfate polyacrylamide gel electrophoresis (1D SDS-PAGE), two dimensional SDS-PAGE (2D SDS-PAGE), or chromatography) or DNA-based tools (cDNA libraries or genomic approaches) coupled with IgE-binding to identify potential allergens. These studies along with the allergens of interest are found in Table 1 and are displayed chronologically to reveal how the discovery techniques have evolved.

Ferrandiz et al. [18] used 1D SDS-PAGE and western blotting to detect 13 IgE-reactive components from extracts of the poorly studied mite *D. siboney*, a species present in Cuba and recently identified in China [19]. This study went on to purify group 1 and 2 homologues from *D. siboney* by using affinity chromatography with cross-reactive antibodies raised against group one and two proteins from other mite species. Morgan et al. [16] used preparative IEF followed by non-reducing 1D SDS-PAGE and blotting using sera from 16 individual patients to identify 47 potential allergens in the mite *E. maynei*. The percentage of patients with IgEs reactive to a given allergen varied from 6 to 88%, thus helping to prioritize major and minor reactive species. Morgan et al. went on

to identify a group 2 homologue by using cross-reactive monoclonal antibodies raised against other group 2 proteins. These studies serve as examples of how candidate gene approaches can be used to identify species-specific homologues of known mite allergens.

Candidate gene approaches based on expected biochemical activity can also be used to identify potential novel allergens. The major group 1 allergens are serine proteases whose enzymatic activities are proposed to enhance the immune response by affecting the barrier function of the mucosa [20]. Based on previous studies suggesting that there were at least three distinct serine proteases in *D. pteronyssinus* fecal extracts, King et al. [6] used chromatography to separate and identify the collagenolytic protease Der p 9 based on its enzymatic activity and weak IgE binding. Additionally, Harris et al. [21] used fluorogenic substrates to perform a large-scale screen for active cysteine and serine *D. pteronyssinus* proteases, but this approach merely resulted in the identification of the known Der p 1 protein indicating that predictions based on proteolytic activity may not be particularly powerful. Alternatively, native and recombinant active proteases may have autolysis activity that interferes with detecting IgE binding [22].

Separation techniques coupled with protein sequencing (a.k.a. proteomics) [23] are capable of identifying a

**Table 1  Methods for identifying mite allergens in the discovery phase**

| Authors | Methods | PubMed ID | Allergen[a] | Year |
|---|---|---|---|---|
| Aki et al. [28] | cDNA library screen | 7622766 | Der f 10 | 1995 |
| Ferrandiz et al. [18] | 1D SDS-PAGE/western blotting | 8556562 | Der s 1 and 2 | 1995 |
| Fujikawa et al. [25] | cDNA library screen | 8649452 | Der f 14 | 1996 |
| King et al. [6] | Chromatography (protease activity) | 8876548 | Der p 9 | 1996 |
| Morgan et al. [16] | IEF, 1D SDS-PAGE/western blotting | 9275144 | Eur m 2 | 1997 |
| Wey et al. [53] | Chromatography (mAB) | 10592827 | 94kd IgE binding protein | 1997 |
| Le Mao et al. [24] | 2D SDS-PAGE/western blotting | 9802372 | Der f 14, Der f 15 | 1998 |
| Tsai et al. [61] | Chromatography (mAB) | 9723675 | Der f 11 | 1998 |
| Yi et al. [15] | 1D SDS-PAGE/western blotting | 10697258 | Blo t IgE binding proteins | 1999 |
| Binder et al. [44] | cDNA library screen | 11673567 | Plo i 1 | 2001 |
| McCall et al. [62] | 1D SDS-PAGE/western blotting | 11292526 | Der f 15 | 2001 |
| Weber et al. [37] | 1D SDS-PAGE/western blotting | 12847483 | Der f 18 | 2003 |
| Huntley et al. [45] | 2D SDS-PAGE/western blotting | 15679630 | Pso o 10, 11 and 14 | 2004 |
| Angus et al. [31] and Gao et al. [63] | EST screen | 15651897 | Blo t 21 | 2004 |
| Harris et al. [21] | Protease activity screen | 15489163 | Der p 1 | 2004 |
| Weghofer et al. [29] | cDNA library screen | 18445190 | Der p 21 | 2008 |
| Weghofer et al. [30] | cDNA library screen | 23460742 | Der p 23 | 2013 |
| An et al. [27] | Chromatography, 1 and 2D SDS-PAGE/western blotting | 23481662 | Der f 25, 28, 29, 30 | 2013 |
| Chan et al. [32] | Sequence mining, 2D SDS-PAGE/western blotting | 25445830 | Der f 24 | 2015 |
| Martins et al. [26] | IEF, 1 and 2D SDS-PAGE/western blotting | 26015775 | Der p IgE binding proteins | 2015 |
| Choopong et al. [43] | 1 and 2D SDS-PAGE/western blotting | 26754146 | Aconitate hydrase | 2016 |

[a] If a known allergen was identified in an unbiased screen, this was still considered a discovery attempt

larger range of potential allergens than candidate gene approaches. Le Mao et al. [24] separated *D. farinae* extracts by IEF, 1D, or 2D SDS-PAGE followed by blotting with individual patient sera to estimate the number of IgE-reactive species to be 15–16, 7, or 12, respectively. Known allergens were identified in this screen, including multiple isoforms of Der f 2 and Der f 3 detected using monoclonal antibodies against these proteins. Homologues of Der p 4 and Der p 5 were tentatively identified based on amylase activity (Der f 4) and pI (Der f 5). For antigen discovery, the authors excised two high molecular weight species and microsequenced them with Edman degradation to identify a protein resembling Der f 14 [25] and a protein resembling the chitinase allergen from prawns. A similar study used IEF, ID, and 2D electrophoresis to catalogue multiple IgE-binding *D. pteronyssinus* proteins using sera from allergic dogs [26].

An et al. [27] extended and refined the proteomic approach by first separating *D. farinae* extracts into IgE-reactive fractions using a gel filtration step followed by a clean-up step to remove contaminants that might interfere with 2D SDS-PAGE. 2D-separated proteins were transferred to membranes and probed for IgE-binding activity using pooled sera from HDM-sensitive asthmatic patients. Seventeen reactive protein spots were recovered and identified using electrospray ionization (ESI) quadrupole time-of-flight (Q-TOF) mass spectrometry and found to represent twelve different protein species, of which four were known *D. farinae* allergens. Four (Der f 25, Der f 28, Der f 29 and Der f 30) of the eight novel allergens were purified by gel filtration and ion exchange chromatography. Homogeneity of the purified protein samples was inferred by observing a single IgE-band in blots following 1D SDS-PAGE. Using individual patient sera for western blotting and ELISA, An et al. determined that a high proportion of patients (63–76%) had IgEs reactive to the novel potential allergens. A high proportion of patients (60–70%) also had positive skin prick reactions, and the proteins stimulated a response in a basophil activation assay. This study represents a good example of a how modern biochemical methods have improved antigen discovery and the proteins warrant further analysis as part of the confirmation process, particularly in regards to quantitative measurement of specific IgE titers and environmental levels.

Screening of cDNA libraries has also been used to identify both minor and major allergenic components. *D. farinae* cDNA libraries were screened with HDM-immunized rabbit serum to identify Der f 10 [28] and a high molecular weight reactive protein named Mag3 (Der f 14) [25]. Having a cDNA clone enabled Aki et al. to quickly generate sequence information and produce a recombinant GST-tagged protein for purification and

confirmation purposes. Also, once the clone was identified as a tropomyosin homologue, the group was able to use a previously published biochemical purification procedure to isolate the native protein, presumably to a reasonable level of purity. They used dot blots to confirm that approximately 80% of patients had IgEs that recognized native Der f 10 and the major antigens Der f 1 and Der f 2. They used serum from pollen or yeast-sensitive patients as negative controls and followed up the IgE-binding studies with skin prick tests finding that approximately 40% of patients had an immune response to native Der f 10.

More recently, Weghofer et al. screened a *D. pteronyssinus* cDNA library with pooled serum from asthmatic patients to identify new minor (Der p 21) [29] and major (Der p 23) allergens [30]. Again, the cDNA screening approach allowed for rapid production and purification of a recombinant protein, which the authors used in dot blots to examine serum from three different European populations diagnosed with rhinitis, conjunctivitis, and/or asthma. Approximately 70–87% of all patients exhibited Der p 23-specific binding. Using a chip-based Ig-E binding assay demonstrated that only 58% of patients diagnosed with rhinoconjunctivitis had Der p 23-binding IgEs; whereas, 72% of patients with asthma exhibited Der p 23-binding. Quantitation of IgE levels revealed that Der p 23-specific antibodies were present at similar titers to Der p 1 and Der p 2 antibodies, but some patients only reacted to one of the three proteins. They demonstrated the allergenic activity of Der p 23 using a basophil activation assay, confirmed its presence in mite feces, and were able to detect it at low levels in house dust samples. This study is a strong example of a combined discovery and confirmation approach that yielded exciting results.

Other DNA-based approaches, such as whole genome sequencing or cataloguing expressed sequence tags (ESTs), have been used to identify mite allergens but have lagged behind other methods. This is hardly surprising since until recently less than 1% of the potential genomic information from dust mites was publicly available [31]. A draft sequence now allows up to 95% of genes to be identified and provides a scaffold for DNA fragment assembly [32]. The availability of comprehensive sequence data from mites and mite-associated microorganisms have been exploited by using a candidate gene approach to identify species specific homologues of allergens identified from other sources [31, 32]. Chan et al. also coupled their genomic sequencing efforts to 2D SDS-PAGE followed by immunoblotting to identify twelve new *D. farinae* proteins with IgE-binding activity. They used their sequence information to rapidly clone and express six of these twelve candidates and found that only one of the recombinant proteins (Der f 24) bound

IgE from the majority of HDM-allergic patients without binding in serum from non-allergic or pollen-allergic controls. Der f 24 was found to induce a positive skin prick reaction in 50% of the tested patients.

A bioinformatic approach was used to mine the human genome to identify substrates for the scabies mite protein Sar s 3 in an effort to identify skin proteins that might be affected by scabies infestation [33]. B and T cell epitopes are less well understood than protease sites, however mite sequences may eventually be mined to identify novel mite allergens based on algorithms used to identify these epitopes. Initial models for linear B cell binding motifs had predictive power only slightly better than random, but newer approaches, particularly ones incorporating multiple models, will likely prove more powerful [34]. Lin et al. [35] used such models to define the molecular characteristics of the allergen Der f 29 for the prediction of four peptides comprising B cell epitopes and five peptides comprising T cell epitopes. This led to the identification of a novel subtype of dust mite allergen, Der f 29b.

In the future, the most powerful discovery techniques will likely combine the genomic and proteomic approaches discussed above, i.e., using protein separation techniques such as 2D gel electrophoresis to identify IgE-reactive components followed by protein sequencing (Edmann Degradation) and now, more commonly, tandem mass spectrometry (MS/MS) (with various peptide fragmentation (e.g., trypsinization), ionization (e.g., ESI, matrix assisted laser desorption), and mass detection techniques (e.g., time of flight (TOF)) in combination with deep RNA or DNA sequencing. Briefly, the differing MS/MS applications generate ionized protein fragments that are categorized by mass and charge and then subjected to a further round of fragmentation and categorization. The resulting mass information of the given fragments is used to identify proteins predicted via the RNA and/or DNA sequencing strategies. These approaches allow for the comprehensive and high throughput identification of multiple IgE-binding proteins from mite body or feces extracts. Recently, this technique was used successfully to identify new IgE binding proteins in both *D. pteronyssinus* and *D. farinae* [36] and could be considered a model approach for use in additional mite species.

### Pitfalls of discovery techniques

As discussed above, there are a wide range of techniques available to discover new potential allergens, and these discovery methods have both general and specific pitfalls. For all screening strategies, it is important to consider the source of serum. Animal models are useful because they can provide a non-limiting supply of reagents and can provide antibodies for later purification purposes. For

this reason, early screening methods often used serum from rabbits immunized with whole mite extracts [25, 28] or monoclonal antibodies derived from HDM-sensitized mice to identify potential allergens, which were then confirmed using patient sera. However, this approach can be limiting since animals and humans respond to different mite proteins. For example, the major group 1 and group 2 allergens in humans are not major allergens in dogs [37].

When considering pooling patient sera for screening purposes, it should be noted that patients with different allergic presentations and/or age may exhibit different patterns of IgE reactivity. Of note, allergic symptoms may represent a time course with AD appearing and subsiding in childhood, with appearance of allergic rhinitis and possibly asthma later in life [38]. IgE-binding may also follow a time course.

Geographic differences should also be considered when comparing results of previous studies and when considering new screening efforts. Patients from different geographic areas are exposed to allergens from different mite species and from other invertebrates, and this influences their IgE-binding profiles. Additionally, dust mites, even from the same species, may have regional geographic polymorphisms. Yi et al. [15] reported differences in the IgE-binding patterns from *B. tropicalis* extracts derived from Columbia and Singapore, suggesting possible differences in mite subpopulations. Additionally, naturally occurring variations in IgE binding sites have been identified in Blo t 5 [39].

A particular confounding factor for identifying dust mite causal allergens is the presence of IgEs generated by allergic responses to other invertebrate (i.e., helminth, cockroach, or prawn). This can impact the screening process as allergic patients with low titers of HDM-specific IgEs but high titers of non-HDM-related IgEs can yield false positive binding. This is particularly true for allergens with shared epitopes (i.e., glycosylation) [40]. This issue has raised concerns over whether the group 10 proteins are *bona fide* HDM allergens, as it is known that tropomyosin has IgE-reactive glycosylation sites [41]. Aki et al. [28], who discovered Der f 10, noted that the IgE-binding of recombinant Der f 10 was 25× less than the IgE-binding of the native protein, which could indicate differences in glycosylation as proteins synthesized in *E. coli* lack such modifications. A later study in the same geographic area detected very low titers of recombinant Der f 10-reactive IgEs in asthmatic patients and little activity in a bronchoprovocation test, which indicates that Der f 10 may play little role in respiratory HDM allergies [42]. In contrast, a recent study using 2D SDS-PAGE followed by immunoblotting with sera from patients with allergic rhinitis detected native Der f 10 as a major Ig-E binding species [43]. In this study, 75% of patients had IgEs reactive to Der f 10 while only 50% reacted to Der f 2. The varying results obtained for Der f 10 could be due to differences in the native and recombinant forms of the protein or differing patient populations. For example, Banerjee et al. [4] found that only 10% of asthmatic patients but 67% of patients with atopic dermatitis had recombinant Der p 10-reactive IgEs. Alternatively, patients with high reactivity to group 10 proteins may have been sensitized to tropomyosin homologues from other species [11].

In some cases, cross-reactivity has been used as a tool to identify new dust mite allergens. Binder et al. [44] screened a cDNA library to identify allergens from the Indian meal moth isolating a clone encoding for an arginine kinase (termed Plo i 1). They generated recombinant Plo i 1 in *E. coli* and confirmed its allergenicity using basophil activation and skin prick assays. Intriguingly, they found that their recombinant protein could compete away IgE-binding to related proteins in multiple species, including dust mites. This suggests that arginine kinases are pan-allergens, which in dust mites represent the minor group 20 proteins. This cross-species candidate gene approach is not uncommon in the allergen discovery phase [31] and is often in screens from little analyzed species used as the first step to identify proteins resembling known allergens [45].

For protein-based screens, the source of extracts should be carefully considered as well as any confounding effects based on the chosen separation conditions. Of note, there are differences in the number of allergic components identified in whole mite extracts versus feces-specific extracts [46]. This can limit sensitivity for detecting even known allergens. Choopong et al. [43] separated *D. farina* proteins from whole mite body extracts and detected little Der f 1 because, as the authors claim, this protein is enriched in feces. If the goal of a study is to identify allergens specific for a given condition, appropriate patients and extracts should be used. For example, for asthmatics, it may be more appropriate to consider allergens specifically present in feces since this is believed to be the inhaled component. Additionally, techniques such as IEF, which separates proteins based on charge, and SDS-PAGE, which denatures and separates proteins based on size, have resolutions within specific windows of pI and molecular weight that depend on the chosen conditions. Also, conditions which denature proteins may reduce antibody binding. For example, multiple monoclonal antibodies raised against Der f 1 detected proteins from IEF but not from 1D or 2D SDS-PAGE-separated samples, leading Le Mao et al. [24] to conclude that the antibodies recognize the native protein but not heat denatured forms present in the 1D

and 2D PAGE applications. For comprehensive detection of protein species (a.k.a. proteomics) multiple separation techniques should be attempted (see [47]), with the understanding that the number of reactive species can be overestimated due to the presence of multiple isoforms, aggregates, or break-down products of a single expressed protein or underestimated due to separation conditions that affect protein structure and antibody binding.

## Confirmation phase

Screening efforts identify IgE-reactive proteins, but IgE-reactivity is not sufficient to prove that a new allergen has been identified. The confirmation process typically requires purification of native or recombinant candidates, assays (dot blots, western blots, ELISAs or protein microarrays) to determine the percentage of allergic patients that have IgEs reactive to the potential allergen, and use of in vivo or in vitro assays to determine if the purified component can induce an allergic response. Some of these steps are often reported along with the discovery of a new IgE-binding protein (as discussed above), but in many cases the confirmation steps are published in follow-up papers (Table 2).

### Isolation of potential allergens

The majority of papers in Table 2 describe the use of histidine-tagged recombinant proteins synthesized in *E coli* and purified using Ni++ affinity chromatography. GST-tagged Der f 6 [5] and Blo t 3 [48] were purified with glutathione affinity chromatography. The rarity of this approach likely stems from the fact that the GST-tag is bulkier and more likely to interfere with the activity of the purified protein, although the tag can be removed with a standard enzymatic technique [5].

There are few reports of the use of eukaryotic expression systems, e.g. *Pichia pastoris* or *Spodoptera frugiperda* (the baculoviral system), to synthesize dust mite proteins. The touted benefits of these systems include the production of proteins with proper post-translational modifications and proper folding. Misfolding in *E. coli* can lead to the production of insoluble proteins requiring a biochemical refolding step to restore full IgE-biding and/or enzymatic activity. Olsson et al. [49] reported that recombinant Lep d 2 expressed in *E. coli* or in *S. frugiperda* had IgE- binding and basophil activation activities similar to the native protein. Bordas-Le Floch et al. [50] found that recombinant Der p 2 expressed in *E. coli* did have structural differences detected by circular dichroism but had Ig-E binding and basophil stimulation activities comparable to those of the native or recombinant Der p 2 expressed in *P. pastoris*. In contrast, Der p 1 or Der f 1 expressed in *E coli* had significantly less IgE-binding activity when compared to the native form [51].

**Table 2 Methods for identifying mite allergens in the confirmation phase**

| Authors | Protein type | Expression system | Method of isolation | % Patients with IgE binding | Test for allerginicity (% Positive) | PubMed ID | Allergen | Year |
|---|---|---|---|---|---|---|---|---|
| Ferrandiz et al. [18] | N | | Affinity chromatography (mAB) | 80–91 | NA | 8556562 | Der s1 Der s2 | 1995 |
| King et al. [6] | N | | Chromatography (protease activity) | 92 | NA | 8876548 | Der p 9 | 1996 |
| Fujikawa et al. [25] | N | | Affinity chromatography (AB) | | | | Der f 14 | 1996 |
| Wey et al. [53] | N | | Affinity chromatography (mAB) | 37.50 | Skin prick (45%) | 10592827 | Der p 94 kD | 1997 |
| Tsai et al. [61, 64] | N | | Affinity chromatography (mAB) | > 80 | NA | 9723675 | Der f 11 Der p 11 | 1998 |
| Olsson et al. [49] | N and R | E. coli and Baculovirus | Affinity chromatography (His-tagged) | | Basophil activation | 9756203 | Lep d 2 | 1998 |
| Kawamoto et al. [5] | R | E. coli | Affinity chromatography (GST-tagged) | 39 | Basophil activation | 10381565 | Der f 6 | 1999 |
| Binder et al. [44] | R | E. coli | Affinity chromatography (His-tagged) | 25 | Basophil activation skin prick | 11673567 | Plo i 1 (group 20 homologue) | 2001 |
| Cheong et al. [48] | R | E. coli | Affinity chromatography (GST-tagged) | 50 | Skin prick | 12708986 | Blo t 3 | 2003 |
| Ramos et al. [52] | N | | Affinity chromatography (mAB) | 63 | NA | 15080814 | Blo t 1 | 2004 |
| Cai et al. [65] | R | E. coli | Affinity chromatography (His-tagged) | | NA | 17639694 | Der f 3 | 2007 |
| Gao et al. [63] | R | E. coli | Affinity chromatography (His-tagged) | 58.00 | Skin prick | | Blo t 21 | 2007 |
| Weghofer et al. [29] | R | E. coli | Ion exchange chromatography (no tag) | 26 | Basophil activation | 18445190 | Der p 21 | 2008 |
| Weghofer et al. [66] | R | E. coli | Ion exchange chromatography (no tag) | 31 | Basophil activation | 18520154 | Der p 5 | 2008 |
| Beckham et al. [33] | R | E. coli and P. pastoris | Affinity chromatography (His-tagged) ion exchange chromatography | NA | NA | 19812030 | Sar s 3 | 2009 |
| Cui et al. [67] | R | E. coli | Affinity chromatography (His-tagged) | NA | NA | 19951588 | Der f 3 | 2009 |
| Cui et al. [68] | R | E. coli | Affinity chromatography (His-tagged) | NA | NA | 20939383 | Der f 7 | 2010 |
| Bordas-Le Floch et al. [50] | N and R | E. coli. and P. pastoris | Ion exchange chromatography (no tag) | NA | Basophil activation and mouse model | 22286395 | Der p 2 | 2012 |
| Weghofer et al. [30] | R | E. coli | Hydrophobic interaction and ion exchange chromatography (no tag) | 74 | Basophil activation | 23460742 | Der p 23 | 2013 |
| An et al. [27] | N | | Chromatography (gel filtration and ion exchange) | 63–86 | Skin prick (60–70%) and basophil activation | 23481662 | Der f 25 Der f 28–30 | 2013 |
| Banerjee et al. [4] | N and R | E. coli | Affinity chromatography (His-tagged or AB) | 5–67 | NA | | Der p 11 | 2015 |
| Lin et al. [69] | R | E. coli | Affinity chromatography (His-tagged) | NA | Skin prick (42.1%) and mouse model | 26623108 | Der f 27 | 2015 |
| Chan et al. [32] | R | E. coli | Affinity chromatography (His-tagged) | 100 | Skin prick (50%) | 25445830 | Der f 24 | 2015 |

**Table 2  continued**

| Authors | Protein type | Expression system | Method of isolation | % Patients with IgE binding | Test for allerginicity (% Positive) | PubMed ID | Allergen | Year |
|---|---|---|---|---|---|---|---|---|
| Cui et al. [70] | R | *E. coli* | Affinity chromatography (His-tagged) | 41 | NA | 26842967 | Der f 4 | 2016 |
| Lin et al. [35] | R | *E. coli* | Affinity chromatography (His-tagged) | NA | Skin prick (24.3%) | 27158348 | Der f 29b | 2016 |

R: recombinant. N: native. NA: not attempted or too few patients to draw conclusions about prevalence

Hence it is important to consider the structural and post-translational requirements of individual proteins when considering expression systems. For newly discovered allergens, the activity of native and recombinant proteins should be compared.

For isolating native proteins, the most commonly used technique is affinity chromatography using antibodies. Recombinant proteins can be used as antigens to generate specific antibodies which can then be used to isolate the native form [25]. Antibodies can also be generated by immunization with cDNA encoding for the desired target protein [52]. Alternatively, monoclonal antibodies derived by immunizing mice with crude or fractionated mite extracts can serve as tools for purification of potential new native allergens [53]. Additionally, for purification of allergen homologues, cross-reactive antibodies identified in one species can be applied to a new species [18]. In the absence of specific antibodies, alternative chromatography techniques, including ion exchange, gel filtration and hydrophobic exchange, have been used to fractionate whole mite or feces extracts [6, 27, 30, 50]. Fractions were then tested for IgE-binding activity and/or desired enzymatic activity [6] and assayed for homogeneity.

**Testing allergenicity**

Once a potential allergen has been isolated, the majority of studies go on to test for IgE-reactivity in individual patient sera drawn from a specific study population. The percentage of patients who exhibit IgE-binding provides a crude measure of whether a protein is a major, mid-tier, or minor allergen. Unfortunately, this aspect of allergen testing has a great deal of variability in terms of techniques used and outcomes reported. Dot blots, western blots, and ELISA have all been used to measure the prevalence of IgE response to a given allergen, but most data in the literature is qualitative and difficult to compare between groups. Allergic patients often exhibit a wide range of total IgE levels which represents antibodies derived from multiple sensitizing proteins found in the environment, and this is worth considering when performing assays with binary outcomes (a.k.a. binding versus non-binding). Quantitative solid phase assays such as ImmunoCAP [54] are easier to compare between groups and can provide a more comprehensive picture of how relevant a given allergen will be for an individual patient. Naturally, the accuracy of these tests (both qualitative and quantitative) are highly dependent on the quality of the purified proteins. Standardization of techniques used for isolation, verification of purity, and quantification of IgE binding should help reduce some of the variation in the field.

Additionally, it should be noted that simply binding IgEs does not indicate that a protein is an allergen. The ultimate test of allergenicity is when a protein can elicit an immune response. Skin prick tests are considered the gold standard for demonstrating sensitivity to a given allergen [54]. Both positive (histamine) and negative (diluent) controls are necessary and a wheal size > 3 mm larger than the negative control is considered a positive result. In general, there is a good concordance between IgE-binding and skin prick responses [55]. However, An et al. [27] reported that 100% of patients had IgE-reactivity to Der f 24, but only 50% were positive in the skin prick test. The other most common used test for allergenicity, is the basophil activation assay where peripheral blood basophils isolated from allergic patients are tested for upregulation of CD203c when challenged with a purified potential allergen.

Skin prick and basophil activation assays are currently the most frequently used tools to verify an allergic response. However, there are additional models relevant for airway allergies. Animal models have been developed which recapitulate aspects of respiratory allergies in humans. Bordas-Le Floch et al. [50] examined T cells isolated by bronchial lavage from Der p 2-sensitized mice demonstrating that recombinant Der p 2 could stimulate cytokine release. They also used an in vivo mouse model of asthma to test the effectiveness of Der p 2 protein immunotherapy. Sublingual treatment of Derp-2 sensitized mice with recombinant Der p 2 significantly reduced airway hyperreactivity as measured by whole body plethysmography. Airway challenge models have also been used in clinical testing. Minami et al. [42] used a bronchoprovocation test to demonstrate that there was a strong correlation between Der p 1 and Der p 2-specific IgE levels and airway response to an HDM-challenge. There are additional clinical assays for allergen testing relevant to rhinitis, conjunctivitis, or other allergic responses [56].

## Assessing allergens in the environment

Confirming an allergic response under laboratory conditions is an important step towards defining an allergen. However, ultimately, the protein should be able to elicit a response under natural conditions, including the concentrations found in the home or work environments. Also, understanding these local concentrations can help lead to the identification of high risk areas and the development of strategies to mitigate exposure.

The growing availability of isolated allergens offers an opportunity for developing assays (particularly ELISA-based assays) that could be used to quantify allergen levels in dust. Yasueda et al. [57] developed a fluorometric ELISA for detecting the major allergen Der p1/Der f1 and used this technique to assay the levels of this allergen on skin and bedding finding values ranging from 1.1 to 354 ng/m$^2$. A highly sensitive assay was necessary to detect such low levels, and similar or even greater sensitivity may be required for the detection of other putative allergenic mite proteins. Additionally, airborne concentrations of these allergens, which are likely the most relevant form when considering the development of respiratory symptoms, are even more difficult to detect. It should also be noted that studies using environmental sampling typically report considerable variation even when testing different sites in the same room [58], making it difficult to calculate the precise dose experienced by a given patient. This limits our understanding of how environmental exposure contributes to sensitization and development of symptoms and is a major limitation when attempting to definitively demonstrate the allergenicity of a given protein.

## Conclusion

House dust mites are a major source of indoor allergens [59]. More than 80% of humans with allergies to dust mites have high serum levels of IgE antibodies to the group 1 or group 2 proteins (reviewed in [10]). Additional potential allergens have been identified by screens relying on IgE-binding. Also, advances in proteomic and genomic techniques, in particular the availability of the draft sequence of the *D. farinae* genome, should allow multiple potential HDM allergens to be identified [32].

In fact, a recent review proposed that genome sequencing and metabolomics are the future of allergen discovery and treatment [60]. With these techniques, the bottleneck is likely to be the confirmation step which requires production of high quality purified proteins, well-controlled IgE binding studies, and relevant assays to ensure allergenicity. A complete panel of mite allergens should improve the diagnosis and individualized treatment of patients allergic to these species, and specific and well-designed discovery and confirmation techniques (as discussed in this review) are needed to achieve this goal.

**Authors' contributions**
This paper was draft by YC. It was revised following critical review by QW, HJ. All authors read and approved the final manuscript.

**Acknowledgements**
We acknowledge the freelance editor Kathleen Molyneaux for editing in structural and English language.

**Competing interests**
The authors declare that they have no competing interests.

**Funding**
This work was supported by the National Natural Sciences Foundation of China (NSFC31572319).

**References**
1.  Luczynska CM. Identification and quantification of mite allergens. Allergy. 1998;53:54–7.
2.  Zhang C, Li J, Lai X, Zheng Y, Gjesing B, Spangfort MD, Zhong N. House dust mite and storage mite IgE reactivity in allergic patients from Guangzhou, China. Asian Pac J Allergy Immunol. 2012;30:294–300.
3.  Arlian LG, Vyszenski-Moher DL, Fernandez-Caldas E. Allergenicity of the mite, *Blomia tropicalis*. J Allergy Clin Immunol. 1993;91:1042–50.
4.  Banerjee S, Resch Y, Chen KW, Swoboda I, Focke-Tejkl M, Blatt K, Novak N, Wickman M, van Hage M, Ferrara R, et al. Der p 11 is a major allergen for house dust mite-allergic patients suffering from atopic dermatitis. J Invest Dermatol. 2015;135:102–9.
5.  Kawamoto S, Mizuguchi Y, Morimoto K, Aki T, Shigeta S, Yasueda H, Wada T, Suzuki O, Jyo T, Ono K. Cloning and expression of Der f 6, a serine protease allergen from the house dust mite, *Dermatophagoides farinae*. Biochim Biophys Acta. 1999;1454:201–7.
6.  King C, Simpson RJ, Moritz RL, Reed GE, Thompson PJ, Stewart GA. The isolation and characterization of a novel collagenolytic serine protease allergen (Der p 9) from the dust mite *Dermatophagoides pteronyssinus*. J Allergy Clin Immunol. 1996;98:739–47.
7.  Baxi SN, Phipatanakul W. The role of allergen exposure and avoidance in asthma. Adolesc Med State Art Rev. 2010; 21:57–71, viii–ix.

8.   Carrard A, Pichler C. House dust mite allergy. Ther Umsch. 2012;69:249–52.

9.   Gregory LG, Lloyd CM. Orchestrating house dust mite-associated allergy in the lung. Trends Immunol. 2011;32:402–11.

10.  Thomas WR. Hierarchy and molecular properties of house dust mite allergens. Allergol Int. 2015;64:304–11.

11.  Zeng G, Luo W, Zheng P, Wei N, Huang H, Sun B, Zhao X. Component-resolved diagnostic study of Dermatophagoides pteronyssinus major allergen molecules in a Southern Chinese Cohort. J Investig Allergol Clin Immunol. 2015;25:343–51.

12.  Zheng YW, Li J, Lai XX, Zhao DY, Liu XF, Lin XP, Gjesing B, Palazzo P, Mari A, Zhong NS, Spangfort MD. Allergen micro-array detection of specific IgE-reactivity in Chinese allergy patients. Chin Med J (Engl). 2011;124:4350–4.

13.  Gafvelin G, Johansson E, Lundin A, Smith AM, Chapman MD, Benjamin DC, Derewenda U, van Hage-Hamsten M. Cross-reactivity studies of a new group 2 allergen from the dust mite Glycyphagus domesticus, Gly d 2, and group 2 allergens from Dermatophagoides pteronyssinus, Lepidoglyphus destructor, and Tyrophagus putrescentiae with recombinant allergens. J Allergy Clin Immunol. 2001;107:511–8.

14.  Tsai JJ, Yi FC, Chua KY, Liu YH, Lee BW, Cheong N. Identification of the major allergenic components in Blomia tropicalis and the relevance of the specific IgE in asthmatic patients. Ann Allergy Asthma Immunol. 2003;91:485–9.

15.  Yi FC, Chew FT, Jimenez S, Chua KY, Lee BW. Culture of Blomia tropicalis and IgE immunoblot characterization of its allergenicity. Asian Pac J Allergy Immunol. 1999;17:189–94.

16.  Morgan MS, Arlian LG, Barnes KC, Fernandez-Caldas E. Characterization of the allergens of the house dust mite Euroglyphus maynei. J Allergy Clin Immunol. 1997;100:222–8.

17.  Cui YB, Cai HX, Li L, Zhou Y, Gao CX, Shi WH, Yu M. Cloning, sequence analysis and expression in E. coli of the group 3 allergen of Dermatophagoides farinae. Chin Med J (Engl). 2009;122:2657–61.

18.  Ferrandiz R, Casas R, Dreborg S, Einarsson R, Bonachea I, Chapman M. Characterization of allergenic components from house dust mite Dermatophagoides siboney. Purification of Der s 1 and Der s 2 allergens. Clin Exp Allergy. 1995;25:922–8.

19.  Sun JL, Shen L, Chen J, Yu JM, Yin J. Species diversity of house dust mites in Beijing, China. J Med Entomol. 2013;50:31–6.

20.  Wan H, Winton HL, Soeller C, Tovey ER, Gruenert DC, Thompson PJ, Stewart GA, Taylor GW, Garrod DR, Cannell MB, Robinson C. Der p 1 facilitates transepithelial allergen delivery by disruption of tight junctions. J Clin Invest. 1999;104:123–33.

21.  Harris J, Mason DE, Li J, Burdick KW, Backes BJ, Chen T, Shipway A, Van Heeke G, Gough L, Ghaemmaghami A, et al. Activity profile of dust mite allergen extract using substrate libraries and functional proteomic micro-arrays. Chem Biol. 2004;11:1361–72.

22.  Bouaziz A, Walgraffe D, Bouillot C, Herman J, Foguenne J, Gothot A, Louis R, Hentges F, Jacquet A, Mailleux AC, et al. Development of recombinant stable house dust mite allergen Der p 3 molecules for component-resolved diagnosis and specific immunotherapy. Clin Exp Allergy. 2015;45:823–34.

23.  Gonzalez-Buitrago JM, Ferreira L, Isidoro-Garcia M, Sanz C, Lorente F, Davila I. Proteomic approaches for identifying new allergens and diagnosing allergic diseases. Clin Chim Acta. 2007;385:21–7.

24.  Le Mao J, Mayer CE, Peltre G, Desvaux FX, David B, Weyer A, Senechal H. Mapping of Dermatophagoides farinae mite allergens by two-dimensional immunoblotting. J Allergy Clin Immunol. 1998;102:631–6.

25.  Fujikawa A, Ishimaru N, Seto A, Yamada H, Aki T, Shigeta S, Wada T, Jyo T, Murooka Y, Oka S, Ono K. Cloning and characterization of a new allergen, Mag 3, from the house dust mite, Dermatophagoides farinae: cross-reactivity with high-molecular-weight allergen. Mol Immunol. 1996;33:311–9.

26.  Martins LM, Marques AG, Pereira LM, Goicoa A, Semiao-Santos SJ, Bento OP. House-dust mite allergy: mapping of Dermatophagoides pteronyssinus allergens for dogs by two-dimensional immunoblotting. Postepy Dermatol Alergol. 2015;32:73–81.

27.  An S, Chen L, Long C, Liu X, Xu X, Lu X, Rong M, Liu Z, Lai R. Dermatophagoides farinae allergens diversity identification by proteomics. Mol Cell Proteomics. 2013;12:1818–28.

28.  Aki T, Kodama T, Fujikawa A, Miura K, Shigeta S, Wada T, Jyo T, Murooka Y, Oka S, Ono K. Immunochemical characterization of recombinant

and native tropomyosins as a new allergen from the house dust mite, Dermatophagoides farinae. J Allergy Clin Immunol. 1995;96:74–83.

29.  Weghofer M, Dall'Antonia Y, Grote M, Stocklinger A, Kneidinger M, Balic N, Krauth MT, Fernandez-Caldas E, Thomas WR, van Hage M, et al. Characterization of Der p 21, a new important allergen derived from the gut of house dust mites. Allergy. 2008;63:758–67.

30.  Weghofer M, Grote M, Resch Y, Casset A, Kneidinger M, Kopec J, Thomas WR, Fernandez-Caldas E, Kabesch M, Ferrara R, et al. Identification of Der p 23, a peritrophin-like protein, as a new major Dermatophagoides pteronyssinus allergen associated with the peritrophic matrix of mite fecal pellets. J Immunol. 2013;190:3059–67.

31.  Angus AC, Ong ST, Chew FT. Sequence tag catalogs of dust mite-expressed genomes: utility in allergen and acarologic studies. Am J Pharmacogenomics. 2004;4:357–69.

32.  Chan TF, Ji KM, Yim AK, Liu XY, Zhou JW, Li RQ, Yang KY, Li J, Li M, Law PT, et al. The draft genome, transcriptome, and microbiome of Dermatophagoides farinae reveal a broad spectrum of dust mite allergens. J Allergy Clin Immunol. 2015;135:539–48.

33.  Beckham SA, Boyd SE, Reynolds S, Willis C, Johnstone M, Mika A, Simerska P, Wijeyewickrema LC, Smith AI, Kemp DJ, et al. Characterization of a serine protease homologous to house dust mite group 3 allergens from the scabies mite Sarcoptes scabiei. J Biol Chem. 2009;284:34413–22.

34.  Dall'antonia F, Pavkov-Keller T, Zangger K, Keller W. Structure of allergens and structure based epitope predictions. Methods. 2014;66:3–21.

35.  Lin J, Wang H, Li M, Liang Z, Jiang C, Wu Y, Liu Z, Yang P, Liu X. Characterization and analysis of a cDNA coding for the group 29b (Der f 29b) allergen of Dermatophagoides farinae. Am J Transl Res. 2016;8:568–77.

36.  Bordas-Le Floch V, Le Mignon M, Bussieres L, Jain K, Martelet A, Baron-Bodo V, Nony E, Mascarell L, Moingeon P. A combined transcriptome and proteome analysis extends the allergome of house dust mite Dermatophagoides species. PLoS ONE. 2017;12:e0185830.

37.  Weber E, Hunter S, Stedman K, Dreitz S, Olivry T, Hillier A, McCall C. Identification, characterization, and cloning of a complementary DNA encoding a 60-kd house dust mite allergen (Der f 18) for human beings and dogs. J Allergy Clin Immunol. 2003;112:79–86.

38.  Nissen SP, Kjaer HF, Host A, Nielsen J, Halken S. The natural course of sensitization and allergic diseases from childhood to adulthood. Pediatr Allergy Immunol. 2013;24:549–55.

39.  Medina LR, Malainual N, Ramos JD. Genetic polymorphisms and allergenicity of Blo t 5 in a house dust mite allergic Filipino population. Asian Pac J Allergy Immunol. 2016;35:203–11.

40.  Malandain H, Giroux F, Cano Y. The influence of carbohydrate structures present in common allergen sources on specific IgE results. Eur Ann Allergy Clin Immunol. 2007;39:216–20.

41.  Ruan WW, Cao MJ, Chen F, Cai QF, Su WJ, Wang YZ, Liu GM. Tropomyosin contains IgE-binding epitopes sensitive to periodate but not to enzymatic deglycosylation. J Food Sci. 2013;78:C1116–21.

42.  Minami T, Fukutomi Y, Lidholm J, Yasueda H, Saito A, Sekiya K, Tsuburai T, Maeda Y, Mori A, Taniguchi M, et al. IgE Abs to Der p 1 and Der p 2 as diagnostic markers of house dust mite allergy as defined by a bronchoprovocation test. Allergol Int. 2015;64:90–5.

43.  Choopong J, Reamtong O, Sookrung N, Seesuay W, Indrawattana N, Sakolvaree Y, Chaicumpa W, Tungtrongchitr A. Proteome, allergenome, and novel allergens of house dust mite, Dermatophagoides farinae. J Proteome Res. 2016;15:422–30.

44.  Binder M, Mahler V, Hayek B, Sperr WR, Scholler M, Prozell S, Wiedermann G, Valent P, Valenta R, Duchene M. Molecular and immunological characterization of arginine kinase from the Indianmeal moth, Plodia interpunctella, a novel cross-reactive invertebrate pan-allergen. J Immunol. 2001;167:5470–7.

45.  Huntley JF, Machell J, Nisbet AJ, Van den Broek A, Chua KY, Cheong N, Hales BJ, Thomas WR. Identification of tropomyosin, paramyosin and apolipophorin/vitellogenin as three major allergens of the sheep scab mite, Psoroptes ovis. Parasite Immunol. 2004;26:335–42.

46.  Arlian LG, Bernstein IL, Geis DP, Vyszenski-Moher DL, Gallagher JS, Martin B. Investigations of culture medium-free house dust mites. III. Antigens and allergens of body and fecal extract of Dermatophagoides farinae. J Allergy Clin Immunol. 1987;79:457–66.

47.  Sickmann A, Reinders J, Wagner Y, Joppich C, Zahedi R, Meyer HE, Schonfisch B, Perschil I, Chacinska A, Guiard B, et al. The proteome

of *Saccharomyces cerevisiae* mitochondria. Proc Natl Acad Sci USA. 2003;100:13207–12.

48. Cheong N, Yang L, Lee BW, Chua KY. Cloning of a group 3 allergen from *Blomia tropicalis* mites. Allergy. 2003;58:352–6.

49. Olsson S, van Hage-Hamsten M, Whitley P, Johansson E, Hoffman DR, Gafvelin G, Schmidt M. Expression of two isoforms of Lep d 2, the major allergen of *Lepidoglyphus destructor*, in both prokaryotic and eukaryotic systems. Clin Exp Allergy. 1998;28:984–91.

50. Bordas-Le Floch V, Bussieres L, Airouche S, Lautrette A, Bouley J, Berjont N, Horiot S, Huet A, Jain K, Lemoine P, et al. Expression and characterization of natural-like recombinant Der p 2 for sublingual immunotherapy. Int Arch Allergy Immunol. 2012;158:157–67.

51. Sookrung N, Choopong J, Seesuay W, Indrawattana N, Chaicumpa W, Tungtrongchitr A. Allergenicity of native and recombinant major allergen groups 1 and 2 of Dermatophagoides mites in mite sensitive Thai patients. Asian Pac J Allergy Immunol. 2016;34:51–8.

52. Ramos JD, Cheong N, Teo AS, Kuo IC, Lee BW, Chua KY. Production of monoclonal antibodies for immunoaffinity purification and quantitation of Blo t 1 allergen in mite and dust extracts. Clin Exp Allergy. 2004;34:604–10.

53. Wey JJ, Lee HF, Chang TH, Chou CC, Hsieh KH, Huang JH. Purification and characterization of a 94 KD high molecular weight allergen from house dust mite, *Dermatophagoides pteronyssinus*. Zhonghua Min Guo Wei Sheng Wu Ji Mian Yi Xue Za Zhi. 1997;30:228–41.

54. Calabria CW, Dietrich J, Hagan L. Comparison of serum-specific IgE (ImmunoCAP) and skin-prick test results for 53 inhalant allergens in patients with chronic rhinitis. Allergy Asthma Proc. 2009;30:386–96.

55. Sánchez-Borges M, Ivancevich JC, Perez RP, Ansotegui I. Section 4.1. Diagnosis and identification of causative allergens. In: Pawankar R, Caninica GW, Holgate ST, Lockey RF, editors. World Allergy Organization (WAO) white book on allergy. Milwaukee: World Allergy Organization; 2011. p. 101–5.

56. Agache I, Bilo M, Braunstahl GJ, Delgado L, Demoly P, Eigenmann P, Gevaert P, Gomes E, Hellings P, Horak F, et al. In vivo diagnosis of allergic diseases—allergen provocation tests. Allergy. 2015;70:355–65.

57. Yasueda H, Saito A, Nishioka K, Kutsuwada K, Akiyama K. Measurement of Dermatophagoides mite allergens on bedding and human skin surfaces. Clin Exp Allergy. 2003;33:1654–8.

58. Custovic A. To what extent is allergen exposure a risk factor for the development of allergic disease? Clin Exp Allergy. 2015;45:54–62.

59. Platts-Mills TA, Lee BW, Arruda L, Chew FT. Section 3.2. Allergens as risk factors for allergic disease. In: Pawankar R, Caninica GW, Holgate ST, Lockey RF, editors. World Allergy Organization (WAO) white book on allergy. Milwaukee: World Allergy Organization; 2011. p. 79–83.

60. Patel S, Meher BR. A review on emerging frontiers of house dust mite and cockroach allergy research. Allergol Immunopathol (Madr). 2016;44:580–93.

61. Tsai LC, Chao PL, Shen HD, Tang RB, Chang TC, Chang ZN, Hung MW, Lee BL, Chua KY. Isolation and characterization of a novel 98-kd *Dermatophagoides farinae* mite allergen. J Allergy Clin Immunol. 1998;102:295–303.

62. McCall C, Hunter S, Stedman K, Weber E, Hillier A, Bozic C, Rivoire B, Olivry T. Characterization and cloning of a major high molecular weight house dust mite allergen (Der f 15) for dogs. Vet Immunol Immunopathol. 2001;78:231–47.

63. Gao YF, de Wang Y, Ong TC, Tay SL, Yap KH, Chew FT. Identification and characterization of a novel allergen from *Blomia tropicalis*: Blo t 21. J Allergy Clin Immunol. 2007;120:105–12.

64. Tsai LC, Peng HJ, Lee CS, Chao PL, Tang RB, Tsai JJ, Shen HD, Hung MW, Han SH. Molecular cloning and characterization of full-length cDNAs encoding a novel high-molecular-weight *Dermatophagoides pteronyssinus* mite allergen, Der p 11. Allergy. 2005;60:927–37.

65. Cai CY, Bai Y, Liu ZG. Ji KM [Cloning, expression and purification of dust mite allergen Der f 3 and identification of its allergic activity]. Zhongguo Ji Sheng Chong Xue Yu Ji Sheng Chong Bing Za Zhi. 2007;25:22–6.

66. Weghofer M, Grote M, Dall'Antonia Y, Fernandez-Caldas E, Krauth MT, van Hage M, Horak F, Thomas WR, Valent P, Keller W, et al. Characterization of folded recombinant Der p 5, a potential diagnostic marker allergen for house dust mite allergy. Int Arch Allergy Immunol. 2008;147:101–9.

67. Cui YB, Cai HX, Li L, Zhou Y, Gao CX, Shi WH, Yu M. Cloning, sequence analysis and expression in *E. coli* of the group 3 allergen of *Dermatophagoides farinae*. Chin Med J (Engl). 2009;122:2657–61.

68. Cui YB, Cai HX, Zhou Y, Gao CX, Shi WH, Yu M, Li L. Cloning, expression, and characterization of Der f 7, an allergen of *Dermatophagoides farinae* from China. J Med Entomol. 2010;47:868–76.

69. Lin J, Li M, Liu Y, Jiang C, Wu Y, Wang Y, Gao A, Liu Z, Yang P, Liu X. Expression, purification and characterization of Der f 27, a new allergen from *Dermatophagoides farinae*. Am J Transl Res. 2015;7:1260–70.

70. Cui YB, Yu LL, Teng FX, Wang N, Zhou Y, Yang L, Zhang CB. Dust mite allergen Der f 4: expression, characterization, and IgE binding in pediatric asthma. Pediatr Allergy Immunol. 2016;27:391–7.

# 8

# How to manage anaphylaxis in primary care

Alberto Alvarez-Perea[1,2]*(iD), Luciana Kase Tanno[3,4,5] and María L. Baeza[1,2,6]

**Abstract**

Anaphylaxis is defined as a severe life-threatening generalized or systemic hypersensitivity reaction characterized by rapidly developing airway and/or circulaton problems. It presents with very different combinations of symptoms and apparently mild signs and can progress to fatal anaphylactic shock unpredictably. The difficulty in recognizing anaphylaxis is due, in part, to the variability of diagnostic criteria, which in turn leads to a delay in administration of appropriate treatment, thus increasing the risk of death. The use of validated clinical criteria can facilitate the diagnosis of anaphylaxis. Intramuscular epinephrine (adrenaline) is the medication of choice for the emergency treatment of anaphylaxis. Administration of corticosteroids and H1-antihistamines should not delay the administration of epinephrine, and the management of a patient with anaphylaxis should not end with the acute episode. Long-term management of anaphylaxis should include avoidance of triggers, following confirmation by an allergology study. Etiologic factors suspected in the emergency department often differ from the real causes of anaphylaxis. Evaluation of patients with a history of anaphylaxis should also include an assessment of personal data, such as age and comorbidities, which may increase the risk of severe reactions. Special attention should also be paid to co-factors, as these may easily confound the cause of the anaphylaxis. Patients experiencing anaphylaxis should administer epinephrine as soon as possible. Education (including the use of Internet and social media), written personalized emergency action plans, and self-injectable epinephrine have proven useful for the treatment of further anaphylaxis episodes.

**Keywords:** Anaphylaxis, Epinephrine, Management, Primary care

## Background

Anaphylaxis is defined as a severe life-threatening generalized or systemic hypersensitivity reaction [1, 2]. All anaphylaxis guidelines [1–5] highlight the severity of the anaphylactic episode and the risk of death. Since anaphylaxis is characterized by rapidly developing life-threatening airway and/or circulation problems, it must be managed quickly. However, anaphylaxis is often difficult to recognize owing, in part, to the variability of diagnostic criteria, which in turn leads to a delay in administration of appropriate treatment, thus increasing the risk of death. In addition, it hampers reliable epidemiological data since medical records are the basis of national and international registries.

Primary care physicians have a pivotal role in the prevention and treatment of anaphylaxis. However, few studies have covered the management of anaphylaxis in primary care. A systematic review on the management of anaphylaxis identified a number of gaps at this level, most notably a lack of knowledge regarding recognition of the reaction, treatment with epinephrine (adrenaline), and prescription of epinephrine auto-injectors (EAI) [6]. The most common approach to the evaluation of the management of anaphylaxis in primary care has been through questionnaires and case studies. The results of several recent surveys from different countries are based on data from general practitioners, paramedics, and, most frequently, paediatricians and do not differ much from one study to another. There is still much room for improvement with respect to knowledge about epinephrine as the initial treatment of anaphylaxis, intramuscular administration, doses, and prescription of EAIs [7–12]. Studies that reviewed healthcare databases in Canada [13,

*Correspondence: alberto@alvarezperea.com
[1] Allergy Service, Hospital General Universitario Gregorio Marañón, Doctor Esquerdo, 46, 28007 Madrid, Spain
Full list of author information is available at the end of the article

14] and The Netherlands [15] reported similar findings. Interdisciplinary communication and education on anaphylaxis are the most frequently proposed solutions.

Awareness of anaphylaxis as a life-threatening medical condition has been increasing in various specialties, and recent publications indicate that the condition is not as uncommon as previously perceived. Epidemiological data cite incidence rates ranging from 1.5 to 7.9/100,000 person-years in Europe [16] and 1.6 to 5.1/100,000 person-years in the United States [17]. However, epidemiological data on the morbidity and mortality of anaphylaxis are still not optimal. Most studies are biased, mainly because of their limited external validity. Variability in methodology, selection of specific populations, and the frequent use of cumulative incidence rates hamper the extrapolation of results to other populations.

To date, most population-based studies that document allergic reactions using the International Classification of Diseases (ICD) report inconsistent data [17–20], thus hampering determination of the prevalence and incidence of severe allergic reactions, such as anaphylaxis. However, studies have calculated the prevalence of anaphylaxis using different approaches such as emergency department (ED) records or number of EAIs prescribed. Studies on the incidence of anaphylaxis in the ED report rates ranging from 0.04 to 0.5% of visits [20–28]. This remarkable variability is related to differences between populations, characteristics of the ED, difficulties recognizing at-risk and anaphylactic patients, and methodology applied to record the rates. Data on mortality are sparse, and publications show considerable variability, ranging from 0.04 to 2.7 cases/million/year [29–31]. It has been estimated that 1 in every 3000 inpatients in American hospitals experience an anaphylactic reaction with a risk of death of around 1%, that is, 500–1000 deaths annually in the US [32]. Brazilian data suggest that the mortality rate of anaphylaxis is 1.1/million/year and that reactions are triggered mainly by drugs. In addition, deaths typically occurred in hospitals, including both the ED and patients who were dead on arrival [31].

Anaphylaxis typically occurs through an IgE-dependent immunologic mechanism and is most commonly triggered by foods, stinging insect venom, and medications, although pathophysiological events such as IgE-independent immunologic mechanisms and direct mast cell stimulation are also involved [2]. Several studies have demonstrated the complexity of mast and basophil cell signalling and the sensitivity of this system to regulation by specific pathways. A wide variety of molecules contribute to the activation of mast cells and the release of mediators (IgE, IgG, stem cell factor, complement proteins, cytokines, neuropeptides, and opioids), which may interact with receptors on the surface of mast cells,

as summarized by Gurish and Castells [33]. Nevertheless, most of their mechanisms are not fully understood [34–37].

## Diagnosis of anaphylaxis

As anaphylaxis is a rapidly evolving condition affecting several systems, clinical diagnosis is based on consideration of the signs and symptoms that appear within 2 h of exposure to the allergen or trigger [38]. Rapid diagnosis ensures optimal management. The signs and symptoms include respiratory distress, hypotension, tachycardia, cyanosis, urticaria, angioedema, nausea, vomiting, diarrhoea, and abdominal pain. In general, cutaneous manifestations are observed in most cases, followed in frequency by cardiovascular and respiratory symptoms [39]. Diagnosis is more challenging when cutaneous symptoms are absent. Such is the case of hypotensive shock with no other symptoms in the context of contact with a known or suspected allergen. Respiratory (e.g., inspiratory difficulty, dysphonia, and sialorrhoea) and cardiovascular manifestations (e.g., sudden reduced blood pressure and tachycardia) are potentially life-threatening features of anaphylaxis and should be considered warning signs [1–5].

One of the key challenges in recognizing anaphylaxis is that the combination of signs and symptoms is not always the same and reactions with mild and moderate severity may not be easily recognized as anaphylaxis by physicians who are unfamiliar with the condition. Therefore, the use of validated clinical criteria can be helpful when diagnosing anaphylaxis. Previously published criteria (Table 1) have proven to be sufficiently sensitive and accurate for the diagnosis of anaphylaxis in the ED [40].

Over the last few decades, in vitro and in vivo methods have been developed and applied to support the clinical diagnosis of anaphylaxis and to reach the etiological diagnosis of the reaction [41].

Accurate clinical data in the ED, together with available in vitro tools, can ensure a correct diagnosis of anaphylaxis. The in vitro diagnosis of anaphylaxis includes serial measurement of the mediators released during an anaphylactic reaction, namely, tryptase, histamine, chymase, carboxypeptidase A3, platelet-activating factor, and other products from mastocytes. Measurement of serum (or plasma) tryptase levels is recommended in the diagnostic workup of systemic anaphylaxis, although the results should be interpreted on an individual basis and considering the complete allergy workup [41]. During anaphylaxis, serum tryptase peaks 60–90 min after the onset of the reaction and, in general, starts to decrease after 120 min. Therefore, for the diagnosis of anaphylaxis, blood samples should be collected within 1–2 h of the reaction and after 24 h in order to detect this decrease

**Table 1  Diagnostic criteria for anaphylaxis, adapted [1]**

*Diagnostic criteria for anaphylaxis*

Anaphylaxis is highly likely when any *one* of the following three criteria is fulfilled

1. Acute onset of an illness (minutes to several hours) with involvement of the skin, mucosal tissue, or both (e.g., generalized hives, pruritus or flushing, swollen lips–tongue–uvula and at least one of the following

   a. Respiratory compromise (e.g., dyspnea, wheeze–bronchospasm, stridor, reduced PEF, hypoxemia)

   b. Reduced BP or associated symptoms of end-organ dysfunction (e.g., hypotonia [collapse], syncope, incontinence)

2. Two or more of the following that occur rapidly after exposure to a *likely* allergen for that patient (minutes to several hours)

   a. Involvement of the skin–mucosal tissue (e.g., generalized hives, pruritus, flushing, swollen lips–tongue–uvula

   b. Respiratory compromise (e.g., dyspnea, wheeze–bronchospasm, stridor, reduced PEF, hypoxemia)

   c. Reduced BP or associated symptoms (e.g., hypotonia [collapse], syncope, incontinence)

   d. Persistent gastrointestinal symptoms (e.g., crampy abdominal pain, vomiting)

3. Reduced BP after exposure to *known* allergen for that patient (minutes to several hours)

   a. Infants and children: low systolic BP (age specific) or > 30% decrease in systolic BP[a]

   b. Adults: systolic BP of < 90 mmHg or > 30% decrease from that person's baseline

*PEF* peak expiratory flow, *BP* blood pressure

[a] Low systolic blood pressure for children is defined as < 70 mmHg from 1 month to 1 year, less than (70 mmHg + [2 × age]) from 1 to 10 years, and < 90 mmHg from 11 to 17 years

[42]. However, normal levels of serum tryptase in the first sample do not exclude anaphylaxis. Other biomarkers, such as histamine and its metabolites, chymase, carboxypeptidase, cysteinyl leukotrienes, prostaglandins, or platelet-activating factor, have lower and variable positive predictive values for a diagnosis of anaphylaxis than serum tryptase [42].

The identification of agents which trigger the anaphylactic reaction is essential for prevention of new exposure and recurrence. In general, diagnostic testing should be performed 3–4 weeks after the acute episode to allow time for the recovery of mast cell activity [43, 44]. The etiological diagnosis can be supported by serologic methods, e.g., allergen-specific serum IgE, with cellular tests, which measure the release of basophil mediators (leukotrienes, histamine), or with the basophil activation test, in which the expression of basophil markers is analyzed [41]. These techniques offer interesting alternatives in the diagnosis of potential triggers of anaphylaxis. The basophil activation test provides important advantages in patients with anaphylaxis to β-lactams, non-steroidal anti-inflammatory drugs, neuromuscular blocking agents, and drugs for which there is no technique to measure specific IgE [45]. Although in vitro tests are safer, their sensitivity and specificity remain to be determined.

The main in vivo tests currently used to investigate allergy and hypersensitivity reactions are skin tests and provocation tests [41], which follow standard methods and practice parameters and should be requested, performed, and interpreted by experienced professionals.

Co-factors, or augmenting factors, such as concomitant asthma, exercise, or specific drugs (e.g., non-steroidal anti-inflammatory drugs, ACE inhibitors) (Table 2), must always be considered. Co-factors may lead to more severe reactions or to anaphylaxis with lower doses of allergen. Physical exercise is one of the best-known augmenting factors in anaphylaxis. In fact, food-dependent exercise-induced anaphylaxis is considered a distinct clinical syndrome [46]. Sensitization to ω-5 gliadin most commonly presents as wheat-dependent exercise-induced anaphylaxis [47]. In general, the mechanisms underlying the role of co-factors in anaphylaxis remain poorly understood [48].

## Acute management of anaphylaxis

Anaphylaxis is a life-threatening medical emergency, and prompt evaluation and intervention are critical for its management. All health professionals should be prepared

**Table 2  Most common co-factors of anaphylaxis**

| |
| --- |
| Drugs |
|   NSAIDs |
|   ACE inhibitors |
|   β-blockers |
| Alcohol |
| Physical exercise |
| Psychogenic stress |
| Hormonal cycle |
| Concomitant diseases |
|   Asthma |
|   Infections |
|   Cardiovascular disease |
|   Mastocytosis |

*NSAID* non-steroidal anti-inflammatory drug, *ACE* angiotensin-converting enzyme

to identify and treat patients with anaphylaxis. An apparently mild presentation may unpredictably progress to fatal anaphylactic shock in minutes [49]. The severity of an anaphylactic episode can differ from one patient to another, and even in the same patient from one episode to another [50].

The management of a patient with anaphylaxis should start with the removal of exposure to the known or suspected trigger, if still possible [51], followed by the assessment of patient's circulation, airway patency, breathing, mental status, skin, and, if possible, weight [44] (Fig. 1).

After administration of epinephrine, patients with anaphylaxis should be placed supine with their lower limbs elevated. They should not be placed seated, standing, or in the upright position. In cases of vomiting or dyspnoea, the patient should be placed in a comfortable position with the lower limbs elevated. This should prevent distributive shock and empty vena cava/empty ventricle syndrome [52].

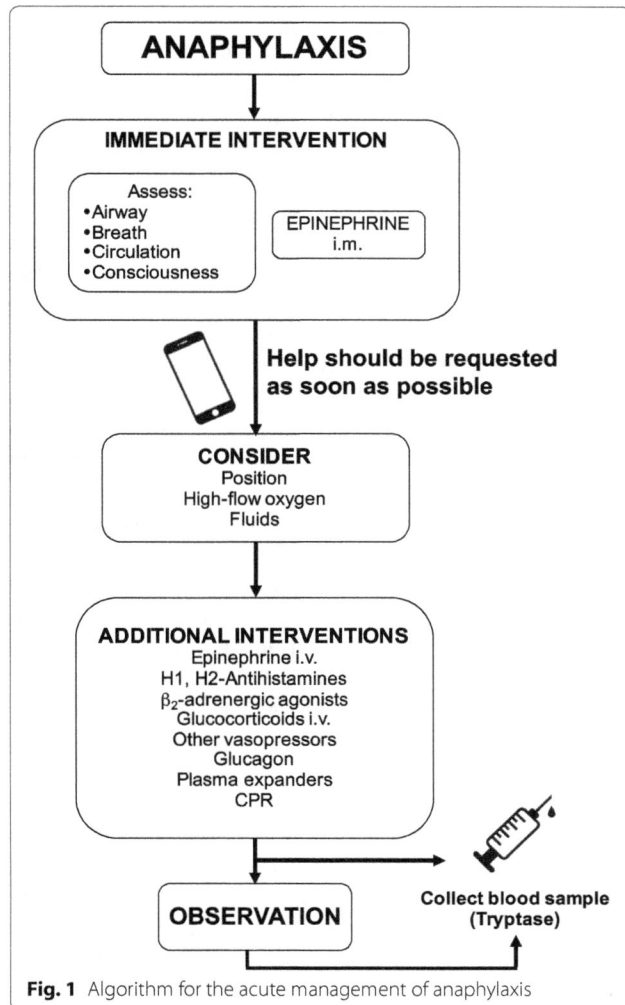

Fig. 1 Algorithm for the acute management of anaphylaxis

Help should be requested as soon as possible. Patients' vital signs (blood pressure, heart frequency, and oxygenation) should be monitored continuously or as often as possible. When indicated, supplemental oxygen and intravenous fluid should be administered and, if necessary, cardiopulmonary resuscitation should be performed [53].

Biphasic anaphylaxis is defined as recurrence of anaphylaxis hours after recovery of the initial symptoms, with no further exposure to the trigger [1]. Given that biphasic anaphylaxis is not uncommon [21, 54], patients overcoming symptoms should undergo monitoring and medical supervision in a centre with trained staff, an ED, and hospital beds available. The duration of monitoring must be tailored to the severity of symptoms [55].

## Pharmacologic treatment of anaphylaxis: epinephrine as the drug of choice

Evidence supporting the use of different medications for the treatment of anaphylaxis is based on observational, epidemiologic, pharmacologic, and animal models, as well as on post-mortem studies [56]. The severity of anaphylaxis makes epinephrine difficult to assess in prospective, randomized, double-masked, placebo-controlled trials [57].

Epinephrine is the medication of choice for the immediate treatment of anaphylaxis [58] and is the only drug that exerts a vasoconstrictor effect, thus reverting airway mucosal edema and hypotension [59]. Additionally, it has inotropic and chronotropic cardiac effects, bronchodilator activity and a stabilization effect on mast cells and basophils [60, 61].

Evidence has shown that delayed injection of epinephrine is associated with higher hospitalization and mortality rates [62, 63]. In contrast, prompt pre-hospital administration of epinephrine is associated with better outcomes [64, 65].

Epinephrine should be injected by the intramuscular route in the *vastus lateralis* muscle (outer thigh) due to its vasodilator effect in skeletal muscle, which facilitates rapid absorption and pharmacologic effects. In contrast, it acts as a vasoconstrictor in the subcutaneous tissue, potentially delaying its absorption [66–68].

The dose of epinephrine for the treatment of anaphylaxis in a health centre is 0.01 mg/kg when administered intramuscularly at a 1:1000 dilution. The maximum dose is 0.3 mg for children and 0.5 for teenagers and adults. With an EAI, patients weighing between 7.5 and 25 kg should receive 0.15 mg, while patients weighing over 25 kg should receive 0.3 mg [3].

The epinephrine injection can be repeated once or twice at 5–15 min intervals in patients who do not respond to the first dose, in patients whose reaction is progressing rapidly, or in biphasic anaphylaxis [69].

A third dose of epinephrine is needed less frequently [70, 71]. Lack of response to epinephrine is an indicator of the need for admission to the intensive care unit, where the patient can receive further care, such as intravenous infusion of epinephrine [72].

Administration of therapeutic doses of epinephrine, as used in anaphylaxis, may induce adverse effects, including transient anxiety, headache, dizziness, tremor, pallor, and palpitations. These symptoms are similar to those caused physiologically by increased endogenous epinephrine levels. However, the adverse effects cannot be dissociated from the beneficial effects of epinephrine [57, 60, 61, 73]. Less frequently, usually due to overdosing or the administration of an intravenous bolus, epinephrine may cause ventricular arrhythmias, pulmonary oedema, malignant hypertension, and intracranial haemorrhage, although these effects are very rare in children and healthy adults [59, 61, 74, 75].

There is no absolute contraindication to epinephrine in the treatment of anaphylaxis [50]. However, the risk–benefit ratio should be assessed in patients with cardiovascular disease [76]. The heart is a potential target organ in anaphylaxis, and acute coronary syndrome can occur during anaphylaxis in the absence of epinephrine [77].

## Second-line drugs for the treatment of anaphylaxis

Antihistamines (both anti-H1 and anti-H2) and corticosteroids are second-line medications for the treatment of anaphylaxis, since they are not life-saving and, therefore, should not be used as initial or only treatment [58, 78, 79].

There is no evidence that supports the use of H1-antihistamines in anaphylaxis. H1-antihistamines relieve itching, flushing, and urticaria, but they do not act on airway obstruction or hypotension. Their onset of action is slower than that of epinephrine. Moreover, recommendations for anaphylaxis, including the doses administered, are extrapolated from those in urticaria. A limited number of first-generation H1-antihistamines is available in parenteral form for use in anaphylaxis. These drugs frequently cause mild side effects (e.g., somnolence, confusion). Severe adverse effects (e.g., seizures, hypotension, cardiac toxic events) are uncommon. Second-generation H1-antihistamines are more secure; however, they are not available for parenteral use. Nevertheless, antihistamines are still the most frequently wrongly used drugs for the treatment of anaphylactic reactions in the ED [58, 80, 81].

There is evidence that the effect of H2-antihistamines, when administered concurrently with H1-antihistamines, could be enhanced in skin symptoms, although their role in anaphylaxis remains unclear [79, 82].

Corticosteroids are traditionally administered to prevent biphasic or protracted anaphylaxis, although these effects have never been proven. Their use in asthma indicates that the onset of pharmacological action may take several hours after administration. Therefore, corticosteroids have little or no effect on initial symptoms or signs [78].

Inhaled beta-2 adrenergic agonists, such as salbutamol or terbutaline, may play a role in anaphylaxis by relieving bronchospasm, in addition to the effect of epinephrine. However, the administration of these drugs should never delay the administration of epinephrine [2].

## Long-term management of anaphylaxis

Management of anaphylaxis continues after resolution of the acute episode. The key to preventing future anaphylactic reactions is a confirmed etiological diagnosis and the avoidance of triggers. In some cases, long-term etiologic treatments may provide protection in case of accidental exposures, such as allergen-specific immunotherapy in cases of *Hymenoptera* venom-induced anaphylaxis. Finally, the patient should know how to treat new symptoms in case they re-appear [2–5, 83].

All patients who experience an episode of anaphylaxis should be advised that their specific triggers must be identified. Important differences between the etiological diagnosis suspected in the ED and the definitive cause of anaphylaxis have been reported in recent studies in adults and children [28, 84, 85]. The triggers of anaphylaxis can be identified by allergy specialists, who will also provide information on possible cross-reacting agents and safe alternatives, especially in the case of drug hypersensitivity. Such an approach has proven useful for reducing the risk of severe anaphylaxis [86]. The tools most commonly used by allergists to this end are a detailed history/documentation of the acute episode, skin tests, detection of allergen-specific IgE, and challenge tests. It is usually accepted that the optimal time for testing is around 4 weeks after the acute episode [5].

Avoidance of some triggers may impact negatively on patients' quality of life [50]. In these cases, immunomodulatory and/or etiological treatments may be available, including drug desensitization [87], insect venom immunotherapy [88], food oral immunotherapy [89], and anti-IgE therapy [90].

Given the unpredictable nature of anaphylaxis, patients should be prepared to act whenever necessary, especially when health care professionals are not present. International guidelines consider written action plans to be a useful tool for optimizing outcome [2–5].

An anaphylaxis action plan is a written document that can guide the patient and caregivers in the event that he or she experiences an allergic reaction in the community (Table 3). The several available action plan models have improved outcomes for other allergic diseases, such as

**Table 3 Summary of data that should be included in a personalized anaphylaxis emergency action plan**

Patient identification (name, address, date of birth, weight)
Photograph
Specific allergens
Specific co-factors and risk factors
Instructions on when to use epinephrine, including dosage
Additional medications, including instructions and dosage
Details of contact person
Telephone number of the local emergency service
Physician (allergist, family doctor)

asthma, and thus have the potential to reduce the frequency and severity of reactions, as well as the anxiety felt by patients and their caregivers [91].

EAIs are the preferred method for administration of epinephrine in the community setting. Given that handling of ampoules, needles, and syringes by patients or their relatives is often subject to error, the EAI could be preferable when commercially available [2–5]. Currently, EAIs administer three doses, namely, 0.15, 0.3 mg, and, in a minority of countries, 0.5 mg. Self-injectable epinephrine may also be used in health care settings [92].

Self-injectable epinephrine should be prescribed to patients with a history of anaphylaxis and a high probability of recurrence, especially when triggered by foods or insects and in patients with idiopathic anaphylaxis. Patients living in isolated areas without access to medical services, and patients with mastocytosis, should also receive EAIs (Table 4) [2–5].

Specific patients with no history of anaphylaxis should also keep an EAI at home. These cases include patients with previous generalized skin reactions after exposure to trace amounts of food and those who are allergic to triggers that are difficult to avoid owing to their ubiquity (e.g., peanut, egg, milk) (Table 4) [2–5].

The number of devices prescribed should be considered. General indications for prescribing 2 or more EAIs include high body weight, fear of possible misuse, a history of biphasic or protracted reactions in the past, and concomitant severe asthma (Table 4) [93].

Nevertheless, prescription of an EAI must be based on objective data from the medical history after the risk–benefit ratio has been properly assessed. Carrying an EAI has been associated with impaired quality of life [94].

There is growing evidence on the benefits of education with the aim of reducing the morbidity and mortality of anaphylaxis, although long-term benefits have yet to be clarified [95, 96]. Education should begin after the resolution of the acute episode, before discharge, and ED health professionals should be well prepared to provide correct guidance. Patients should be taught how to recognize anaphylaxis symptoms, when to inject epinephrine and seek medical assistance, and how to recognize and avoid possible co-factors, which may multiply the risk for severe anaphylaxis [50].

In the last few years, Internet and social media have become highly accessible information sources for health-related queries [97]. The few studies that have focused on the impact of these technologies in patients with anaphylaxis tend to describe the beneficial effects, as in other allergic diseases. The use of Internet, social media, and mobile applications may play a role in future approaches to education in anaphylaxis [98–100].

## Anaphylaxis in special populations

Various groups of patients present particularities that affect how anaphylaxis should be managed in the ED. These particularities should also be taken into account when assessing the risk of anaphylaxis and establishing preventive measures.

Infants may not be able to describe their anaphylaxis symptoms properly, and some signs may be difficult to interpret (irritability, crying, somnolence, etc.), thus delaying diagnosis and treatment. The clinical criteria for diagnosis of anaphylaxis in the ED have not been specifically validated for use in this age group. The differential diagnosis of anaphylaxis in infants must also include congenital abnormalities, aspiration of a foreign body, or food protein-induced enterocolitis syndrome, which seldom occur later in life [101].

Food allergy is the most common cause of anaphylaxis in childhood and has become a common health issue in

**Table 4 Indications for prescription of epinephrine auto-injectors**

| Cases requiring *at least one* epinephrine autoinjector device | Cases requiring *more than one* autoinjector device |
| --- | --- |
| History of a previous anaphylactic reaction | High body weight |
| Allergy to ubiquitous triggers (peanut, egg, milk) | History of anaphylaxis requiring more than one dose of epinephrine |
| Clinical reactions even to tiny amounts of food, excluding oral allergy syndrome | History of protracted or biphasic anaphylaxis |
| Food allergy and unstable or moderate to severe asthma | Fear of possible misuse |
| Remote from medical help and previous mild to moderate reactions | Food allergy and severe asthma |
| Underlying mastocytosis | |

schools [102]. Around 20% of cases of anaphylaxis may occur in this setting [103, 104]. Nevertheless, many schools are insufficiently prepared to manage anaphylaxis [105], with limited availability of emergency action plans, epinephrine, and trained school staff, thus delaying diagnosis and transfer of patients to the ED, where management can be hampered by the lack of reliable information. In order to improve the management of anaphylaxis in schools, individualized measures should include collaboration between parents, school personnel, and allergists or paediatricians [106].

Teenagers are at greater risk for anaphylaxis owing to the intrinsic characteristics of this age group [98, 107, 108]. Adolescents tend to have higher risk behaviour and thus minimize the consequences of transgressions, thus potentially leading them to disregard triggers of anaphylaxis. They also try to hide their allergy problems from others, avoid EAIs, and seek medical care only at late stages of the reaction. These factors may delay the recognition of an episode of anaphylaxis. Management of anaphylaxis in teenagers presenting at the ED may be hampered by misinformation (e.g., lessening of symptoms, hiding triggers) [109, 110]. The first experiences with alcohol may also act as a co-factor of severity [93].

Old age does not seem to increase the risk of anaphylaxis [111]. However, it has been associated with a higher risk of death, possibly as a consequence of comorbidities, polypharmacy, higher risk of hospitalization, and changes in the immune system, which lead to a pro-inflammatory state [112]. In elderly patients with anaphylaxis managed in the ED, age or even a history of cardiovascular disease is not an absolute contraindication for the administration of epinephrine. Nevertheless, the potential advantages and disadvantages must be carefully considered [76].

The prevalence of anaphylaxis, especially idiopathic anaphylaxis, is higher in patients with mastocytosis than in the general population [113]. NSAIDs and hymenoptera venom hypersensitivity are also frequent among these patients. Evaluation of patients with mastocytosis in the ED must take into consideration that anaphylaxis is particularly severe in these cases, with cardiovascular symptoms being very common. In many cases, no eliciting trigger can be identified [114, 115]. Patients with underlying mastocytosis should always be prescribed at least one EAI [116].

## Conclusions

In summary, anaphylaxis may not be as uncommon as previously thought, and epidemiologic publications are prone to discrepancies owing to the different methodologies, target populations, and settings.

Anaphylaxis is not always well recognized, especially if hypotension is the only sign. This multisystemic disease may present as very different combinations of symptoms, and apparently mild signs may unpredictably progress to fatal anaphylactic shock. A rapid diagnosis leads to optimal management. Fast intervention is critical. Estimation of circulatory, respiratory, and mental status and removal of the possible cause should be followed by administration of intramuscular epinephrine, which is the treatment of choice, with no absolute contraindications. Moreover, the risk–benefit ratio should always be assessed in patients with cardiovascular disease. Antihistamines and corticosteroids are second-choice medications. An EAI should always be prescribed after a suspected episode of anaphylaxis.

Etiologic factors suspected in the ED often differ from the real cause. Nonetheless, since the ED is not the appropriate place to study the cause of the anaphylaxis, a meticulous allergy workup should be offered. Special attention should be given to co-factors, as these may easily confound the cause of anaphylaxis.

Finally, anaphylaxis is a complex disease that should be well recognized and handled by any physician. We stress the need for increased awareness of anaphylaxis among health professionals, who should receive appropriate training to diagnose and manage it.

**Abbreviations**
ACE: angiotensin-converting enzyme; BP: blood pressure; EAI: epinephrine auto-injector; ED: emergency department; ICD: International Classification of Diseases; NSAID: nonsteroidal anti-inflammatory drug; PEF: peak expiratory flow.

**Authors' contributions**
AA-P participated in the design of the review and drafted the manuscript. LKT drafted the manuscript and revised it critically. MLB participated in the design of the review, drafted the manuscript and revised it critically. All authors read and approved the final manuscript.

**Author details**
[1] Allergy Service, Hospital General Universitario Gregorio Marañón, Doctor Esquerdo, 46, 28007 Madrid, Spain. [2] Gregorio Marañón Health Research Institute, Madrid, Spain. [3] Hospital Sírio Libanês, São Paulo, Brazil. [4] Division of Allergy, Department of Pulmonology, University Hospital of Montpellier, Montpellier, France. [5] Pierre and Marie Curie Institute of Epidemiology and Public Health, Sorbonne Universités, Paris, France. [6] Biomedical Research Network on Rare Diseases (CIBERER)-U761, Madrid, Spain.

**Competing interests**
The authors declare that they have no competing interests.

**Funding**
The authors declare that no funding was received for the present manuscript.

**References**

1. Sampson HA, Munoz-Furlong A, Campbell RL, Adkinson NF Jr, Bock SA, Branum A, et al. Second symposium on the definition and management of anaphylaxis: summary report—Second National Institute of Allergy and Infectious Disease/Food Allergy and Anaphylaxis Network symposium. J Allergy Clin Immunol. 2006;117:391–7.
2. Simons FER, Ardusso LR, Bilò M, Cardona V, Ebisawa M, El-Gamal YM, et al. International consensus on (ICON) anaphylaxis. World Allergy Organ J. 2014;7:9.
3. Muraro A, Roberts G, Worm M, Bilò MB, Brockow K, Fernández Rivas M, et al. Anaphylaxis: guidelines from the European Academy of Allergy and Clinical Immunology. Allergy. 2014;69:1026–45.
4. Lieberman P, Nicklas RA, Oppenheimer J, Kemp SF, Lang DM, Bernstein DI, et al. The diagnosis and management of anaphylaxis practice parameter: 2010 update. J Allergy Clin Immunol. 2010;126:442–77.
5. Simons FER, Ardusso LRF, Bilò MB, El-Gamal YM, Ledford DK, Ring J, et al. World Allergy Organization guidelines for the assessment and management of anaphylaxis. World Allergy Organ J. 2011;4:13–37.
6. Kastner M, Harada L, Waserman S. Gaps in anaphylaxis management at the level of physicians, patients, and the community: a systematic review of the literature. Allergy. 2010;65:435–44.
7. Wang J, Sicherer SH, Nowak-Wegrzyn A. Primary care physicians' approach to food-induced anaphylaxis: a survey. J Allergy Clin Immunol. 2004;114:689–91.
8. Krugman SD, Chiaramonte DR, Matsui EC. Diagnosis and management of food-induced anaphylaxis: a national survey of pediatricians. Pediatrics. 2006;118:e554–60.
9. Lowe G, Kirkwood E, Harkness S. Survey of anaphylaxis management by general practitioners in Scotland. Scott Med J. 2010;55:11–4.
10. Erkoçoğlu M, Civelek E, Azkur D, Özcan C, Öztürk K, Kaya A, et al. Knowledge and attitudes of primary care physicians regarding food allergy and anaphylaxis in Turkey. Allergol Immunopathol (Madr). 2013;41:292–7.
11. Baççioğlu A, Yilmazel Uçar E. Level of knowledge about anaphylaxis among health care providers. Tuberk Toraks. 2013;61:140–6.
12. Gómez Galán C, Ferré Ybarz L, Peña Peloche MA, Sansosti Viltes A, de la Borbolla Morán JM, Torredemer Palau A, et al. Intention to prescribe self-injectable epinephrine: are there differences depending on who assesses the patient post-reaction? Allergol Immunopathol (Madr). 2015;43:286–91.
13. Chung T, Gaudet L, Vandenberghe C, Couperthwaite S, Sookram S, Liss K, et al. Pre-hospital management of anaphylaxis in one Canadian Urban Centre. Resuscitation. 2014;85:1077–82.
14. Kimchi N, Clarke A, Moisan J, Lachaine C, La Vieille S, Asai Y, et al. Anaphylaxis cases presenting to primary care paramedics in Quebec. Immun Inflamm Dis. 2015;3:406–10.
15. Saleh-Langenberg J, Dubois AEJ, Groenhof F, Kocks JWH, van der Molen T, Flokstra-de Blok BMJ. Epinephrine auto-injector prescriptions to food-allergic patients in primary care in The Netherlands. Allergy Asthma Clin Immunol. 2015;11:28.
16. Panesar SS, Javad S, De Silva D, Nwaru BI, Hickstein L, Muraro A, et al. The epidemiology of anaphylaxis in Europe: a systematic review. Allergy. 2013;68:1353–61.
17. Wood RA, Camargo CA, Lieberman P, Sampson HA, Schwartz LB, Zitt M, et al. Anaphylaxis in America: the prevalence and characteristics of anaphylaxis in the United States. J Allergy Clin Immunol. 2014;133:461–7.
18. Tanno LK, Ganem F, Demoly P, Toscano CM, Bierrenbach AL. Undernotification of anaphylaxis deaths in Brazil due to difficult coding under the ICD-10. Allergy. 2012;67:783–9.
19. Tanno LK, Calderon MA, Goldberg BJ, Akdis CA, Papadopoulos NG, Demoly P. Categorization of allergic disorders in the new World Health Organization International Classification of Diseases. Clin Transl Allergy. 2014;4:42.
20. Moro Moro M, Tejedor Alonso MA, Esteban Hernandez J, Mugica Garcia MV, Rosado Ingelmo A, Vila Albelda C. Incidence of anaphylaxis and subtypes of anaphylaxis in a general hospital emergency department. J Invest Allergol Clin Immunol. 2011;21:142–9.
21. Smit DV, Cameron PA, Rainer TH. Anaphylaxis presentations to an emergency department in Hong Kong: incidence and predictors of biphasic reactions. J Emerg Med. 2005;28:381–8.
22. Bellou A, Manel J, Samman-Kaakaji H, de Korwin JD, Moneret-Vautrin DA, Bollaert PE, et al. Spectrum of acute allergic diseases in an emergency department: an evaluation of one years' experience. Emerg Med. 2003;15:341–7.
23. Brown AF, McKinnon D, Chu K. Emergency department anaphylaxis: a review of 142 patients in a single year. J Allergy Clin Immunol. 2001;108:861–6.
24. Campbell RL, Luke A, Weaver AL, St Sauver JL, Bergstralh EJ, Li JT, et al. Prescriptions for self-injectable epinephrine and follow-up referral in emergency department patients presenting with anaphylaxis. Ann Allergy Asthma Immunol. 2008;101:631–6.
25. Beyer K, Eckermann O, Hompes S, Grabenhenrich L, Worm M. Anaphylaxis in an emergency setting—elicitors, therapy and incidence of severe allergic reactions. Allergy. 2012;67:1451–6.
26. Cianferoni A, Novembre E, Mugnaini L, Lombardi E, Bernardini R, Pucci N, et al. Clinical features of acute anaphylaxis in patients admitted to a university hospital: an 11-year retrospective review (1985–1996). Ann Allergy Asthma Immunol. 2001;87:27–32.
27. Poachanukoon O, Paopairochanakorn C. Incidence of anaphylaxis in the emergency department: a 1-year study in a university hospital. Asian Pac J Allergy Immunol. 2006;24:111–6.
28. Alvarez-Perea A, Tomás-Pérez M, Martínez-Lezcano P, Marco G, Pérez D, Zubeldia JMM, et al. Anaphylaxis in adolescent/adult patients treated in the emergency department: differences between initial impressions and the definitive diagnosis. J Invest Allergol Clin Immunol. 2015;25:288–94.
29. Turner PJ, Gowland MH, Sharma V, Ierodiakonou D, Harper N, Garcez T, et al. Increase in anaphylaxis-related hospitalizations but no increase in fatalities: an analysis of United Kingdom national anaphylaxis data, 1992–2012. J Allergy Clin Immunol. 2015;135:956–.
30. Liew WK, Williamson E, Tang MLK. Anaphylaxis fatalities and admissions in Australia. J Allergy Clin Immunol. 2009;123:434–42.
31. Tanno LK, Bierrenbach AL, Calderon MA, Sheikh A, Simons FER, Demoly P, et al. Decreasing the undernotification of anaphylaxis deaths in Brazil through the International Classification of Diseases (ICD)-11 revision. Allergy. 2017;72:120–5.
32. Neugut AI, Ghatak AT, Miller RL. Anaphylaxis in the United States. Arch Intern Med. 2001;161:15.
33. Gurish M, Castells M. Mast cells: surface receptors and signal transduction. UpToDate. 2017. http://www.uptodate.com. Accessed 1 Oct 2017.
34. Metcalfe DD, Peavy RD, Gilfillan AM. Mechanisms of mast cell signaling in anaphylaxis. J Allergy Clin Immunol. 2009;124:639–46.
35. Strait RT, Morris SC, Yang M, Qu X-W, Finkelman FD. Pathways of anaphylaxis in the mouse. J Allergy Clin Immunol. 2002;109:658–68.
36. Rivera J, Gilfillan AM. Molecular regulation of mast cell activation. J Allergy Clin Immunol. 2006;117:1214–25.
37. Muñoz-Cano R, Pascal M, Bartra J, Picado C, Valero A, Kim D-K, et al. Distinct transcriptome profiles differentiate nonsteroidal anti-inflammatory drug-dependent from nonsteroidal anti-inflammatory drug-independent food-induced anaphylaxis. J Allergy Clin Immunol. 2016;137:137–46.
38. Muraro A, Werfel T, Hoffmann-Sommergruber K, Roberts G, Beyer K, Bindslev-Jensen C, et al. EAACI food allergy and anaphylaxis guidelines: diagnosis and management of food allergy. Allergy. 2014;69:1008–25.
39. Worm M, Edenharter G, Ruëff F, Scherer K, Pföhler C, Mahler V, et al. Symptom profile and risk factors of anaphylaxis in Central Europe. Allergy Eur J Allergy Clin Immunol. 2012;67:691–8.
40. Harduar-Morano L, Simon MR, Watkins S, Blackmore C. Algorithm for the diagnosis of anaphylaxis and its validation using population-based data on emergency department visits for anaphylaxis in Florida. J Allergy Clin Immunol. 2010;126:98–104.e4.
41. Tanno LK, Calderon MA, Li J, Casale T, Demoly P. Updating allergy and/or hypersensitivity diagnostic procedures in the WHO ICD-11 revision. J Allergy Clin Immunol Pract. 2016;4:650–7.

42.  Sala-Cunill A, Cardona V. Biomarkers of anaphylaxis, beyond tryptase. Curr Opin Allergy Clin Immunol. 2015;15:329–36.

43.  Simons FE, Frew AJ, Ansotegui IJ, Bochner BS, Golden DB, Finkelman FD, et al. Risk assessment in anaphylaxis: current and future approaches. J Allergy Clin Immunol. 2007;120:S2–24.

44.  Simons FE. Anaphylaxis. J Allergy Clin Immunol. 2010;125:S161–81.

45.  Mayorga C, Celik G, Rouzaire P, Whitaker P, Bonadonna P, Rodrigues-Cernadas J, et al. In vitro tests for drug hypersensitivity reactions: an ENDA/EAACI Drug Allergy Interest Group position paper. Allergy. 2016;71:1103–34.

46.  Ansley L, Bonini M, Delgado L, Del Giacco S, Du Toit G, Khaitov M, et al. Pathophysiological mechanisms of exercise-induced anaphylaxis: an EAACI position statement. Allergy Eur J Allergy Clin Immunol. 2015;70:1212–21.

47.  Palosuo K, Varjonen E, Nurkkala J, Kalkkinen N, Harvima R, Reunala T, et al. Transglutaminase-mediated cross-linking of a peptic fraction of ω-5 gliadin enhances IgE reactivity in wheat-dependent, exercise-induced anaphylaxis. J Allergy Clin Immunol. 2003;111:1386–92.

48.  Muñoz-Cano RM, Bartra J, Picado C, Valero A. Mechanisms of anaphylaxis beyond IgE. J Invest Allergol Clin Immunol. 2016;26:73–82.

49.  Dhami S, Panesar SS, Roberts G, Muraro A, Worm M, Bilò MB, et al. Management of anaphylaxis: a systematic review. Allergy. 2014;69:168–75.

50.  Simons FER, Ebisawa M, Sanchez-Borges M, Thong BY, Worm M, Tanno LK, et al. 2015 update of the evidence base: World Allergy Organization anaphylaxis guidelines. World Allergy Organ J. 2015;8:32.

51.  Dhami S, Sheikh A, Muraro A, Roberts G, Halken S, Fernandez Rivas M, et al. Quality indicators for the acute and long-term management of anaphylaxis: a systematic review. Clin Transl Allergy. 2017;7:15.

52.  Pumphrey RSH. Fatal posture in anaphylactic shock. J Allergy Clin Immunol. 2003;112:451–2.

53.  Soar J, Pumphrey R, Cant A, Clarke S, Corbett A, Dawson P, et al. Emergency treatment of anaphylactic reactions—guidelines for healthcare providers. Resuscitation. 2008;77:157–69.

54.  Tole JW, Lieberman P. Biphasic anaphylaxis: review of incidence, clinical predictors, and observation recommendations. Immunol Allergy Clin N Am. 2007;27:309–26.

55.  Lee S, Bellolio MF, Hess EP, Erwin P, Murad MH, Campbell RL. Time of onset and predictors of biphasic anaphylactic reactions: a systematic review and meta-analysis. J Allergy Clin Immunol Pract. 2015;3:408–416e2.

56.  Simons FE, Sheikh A. Evidence-based management of anaphylaxis. Allergy. 2007;62:827–9.

57.  Simons FER. Pharmacologic treatment of anaphylaxis: can the evidence base be strengthened? Curr Opin Allergy Clin Immunol. 2010;10:384–93.

58.  Sheikh A, Ten Broek V, Brown SG, Simons FE. H1-antihistamines for the treatment of anaphylaxis: Cochrane systematic review. Allergy. 2007;62:830–7.

59.  Simons KJ, Simons FE. Epinephrine and its use in anaphylaxis: current issues. Curr Opin Allergy Clin Immunol. 2010;10:354–61.

60.  Kemp SF, Lockey RF, Simons FE. Epinephrine: the drug of choice for anaphylaxis. A statement of the World Allergy Organization. Allergy. 2008;63:1061–70.

61.  McLean-Tooke APC, Bethune CA, Fay AC, Spickett GP. Adrenaline in the treatment of anaphylaxis: what is the evidence? BMJ. 2003;327:1332–5.

62.  Brown SGA. Cardiovascular aspects of anaphylaxis implications for treatment and diagnosis. Curr Opin Allergy Clin Immunol. 2005;5:359–64.

63.  Anchor J, Settipane RA. Appropriate use of epinephrine in anaphylaxis. Am J Emerg Med. 2004;22:488–90.

64.  Fleming JT, Clark S, Camargo CA, Rudders SA. Early treatment of food-induced anaphylaxis with epinephrine is associated with a lower risk of hospitalization. J Allergy Clin Immunol Pract. 2015 3:57–62.

65.  Xu YS, Kastner M, Harada L, Xu A, Salter J, Waserman S. Anaphylaxis-related deaths in Ontario: a retrospective review of cases from 1986 to 2011. Allergy Asthma Clin Immunol. 2014;10:38.

66.  Simons FE, Roberts JR, Gu X, Simons KJ. Epinephrine absorption in children with a history of anaphylaxis. J Allergy Clin Immunol. 1998;101:33–7.

67.  Simons FE, Gu X, Simons KJ. Epinephrine absorption in adults: intramuscular versus subcutaneous injection. J Allergy Clin Immunol. 2001;108:871–3.

68.  Campbell RL, Bellolio MF, Knutson BD, Bellamkonda VR, Fedko MG, Nestler DM, et al. Epinephrine in anaphylaxis: higher risk of cardiovascular complications and overdose after administration of intravenous bolus epinephrine compared with intramuscular epinephrine. J Allergy Clin Immunol Pract. 2015;3:76–80.

69.  Manivannan V, Campbell RL, Bellolio MF, Stead LG, Li JTC, Decker WW. Factors associated with repeated use of epinephrine for the treatment of anaphylaxis. Ann Allergy Asthma Immunol. 2009;103:395–400.

70.  Korenblat P, Lundie MJ, Dankner RE, Day JH. A retrospective study of epinephrine administration for anaphylaxis: how many doses are needed? Allergy Asthma Proc. 1999;20:383–6.

71.  Järvinen KM, Sicherer SH, Sampson HA, Nowak-Wegrzyn A. Use of multiple doses of epinephrine in food-induced anaphylaxis in children. J Allergy Clin Immunol. 2008;122:133–8.

72.  Bautista E, Simons FER, Simons KJ, Becker AB, Duke K, Tillett M, et al. Epinephrine fails to hasten hemodynamic recovery in fully developed canine anaphylactic shock. Int Arch Allergy Immunol. 2002;128:151–64.

73.  Simons FER. First-aid treatment of anaphylaxis to food: focus on epinephrine. J Allergy Clin Immunol. 2004;113:837–44.

74.  Kanwar M, Irvin CB, Frank JJ, Weber K, Rosman H. Confusion about epinephrine dosing leading to iatrogenic overdose: a life-threatening problem with a potential solution. Ann Emerg Med. 2010;55:341–4.

75.  Sicherer SH, Simons FER. First-aid management of anaphylaxis. Pediatrics. 2017;139:e20164006.

76.  Lieberman P, Simons FER. Anaphylaxis and cardiovascular disease: therapeutic dilemmas. Clin Exp Allergy. 2015;45:1288–95.

77.  Triggiani M, Patella V, Staiano RI, Granata F, Marone G. Allergy and the cardiovascular system. Clin Exp Immunol. 2008;153:7–11.

78.  Choo KJ, Simons E, Sheikh A. Glucocorticoids for the treatment of anaphylaxis: Cochrane systematic review. Allergy. 2010;65:1205–11.

79.  Nurmatov UB, Rhatigan E, Simons FER, Sheikh A. H2-antihistamines for the treatment of anaphylaxis with and without shock: a systematic review. Ann Allergy Asthma Immunol. 2014;112:126–31.

80.  Boyce JA, Assa'ad A, Burks AW, Jones SM, Sampson HA, NIAID-Sponsored Expert Panel JA, et al. Guidelines for the diagnosis and management of food allergy in the United States: report of the NIAID-sponsored expert panel. J Allergy Clin Immunol. 2010;126:S1–58.

81.  Park JH, Godbold JH, Chung D, Sampson HA, Wang J. Comparison of cetirizine and diphenhydramine in the treatment of acute food-induced allergic reactions. J Allergy Clin Immunol. 2011;128:1127–8.

82.  Lin RY, Curry A, Pesola GR, Knight RJ, Lee HS, Bakalchuk L, et al. Improved outcomes in patients with acute allergic syndromes who are treated with combined H1 and H2 antagonists. Ann Emerg Med. 2000;36:462–8.

83.  Waserman S, Chad Z, Francoeur MJ, Small P, Stark D, Vander Leek TK, et al. Management of anaphylaxis in primary care: Canadian expert consensus recommendations. Allergy Eur J Allergy Clin Immunol. 2010;65:1082–92.

84.  Campbell RL, Park MA, Kueber MA, Lee S, Hagan JB. Outcomes of allergy/immunology follow-up after an emergency department evaluation for anaphylaxis. J Allergy Clin Immunol Pract. 2015;3:88–93.

85.  Alvarez-Perea A, Ameiro B, Morales C, Zambrano G, Rodriguez A, Guzman M, et al. Anaphylaxis in the Pediatric Emergency Department: analysis of 133 cases after an allergy workup. J Allergy Clin Immunol Pract. 2017;5:1256–63.

86.  Altman AM, Camargo CAJ, Simons FER, Lieberman PPL, Sampson HA, Schwartz LB, et al. Risk factors for severe anaphylaxis in patients receiving anaphylaxis treatment in US emergency departments and hospitals. J Allergy Clin Immunol. 2014;127:461–7.

87.  Castells MC. A new era for drug desensitizations. J Allergy Clin Immunol Pract. 2015;3:639–40.

88.  Alfaya Arias T, Soriano Gómis V, Soto Mera T, Vega Castro A, Vega Gutiérrez J, Alonso Llamazares A, et al. Key issues in hymenoptera venom allergy: an update. J Invest Allergol Clin Immunol. 2017;27:19–31.

89.  Nurmatov U, Dhami S, Arasi S, Pajno GB, Fernandez-Rivas M, Muraro A, et al. Allergen immunotherapy for IgE-mediated food allergy: a systematic review and meta-analysis. Allergy. 2017;72:1133–47.

90. El-Qutob D. Off-label uses of omalizumab. Clin Rev Allergy Immunol. 2016;50:84–96.

91. Wang J, Sicherer SH. Guidance on completing a written allergy and anaphylaxis emergency plan. Pediatrics. 2017;139:e20164005.

92. Campbell R, Bellolio M, Motosue M, Sunga K, Lohse C, Rudis M. Auto-injectors preferred for intramuscular epinephrine in anaphylaxis and allergic reactions. West J Emerg Med. 2016;172:775–82.

93. Niggemann B, Beyer K. Adrenaline autoinjectors in food allergy: in for a cent, in for a euro? Pediatr Allergy Immunol. 2012;23:506–8.

94. Pinczower GD, Bertalli NA, Bussmann N, Hamidon M, Allen KJ, Dunngal-vin A, et al. The effect of provision of an adrenaline autoinjector on quality of life in children with food allergy. J Allergy Clin Immunol. 2013;131:238–41.

95. Brockow K, Schallmayer S, Beyer K, Biedermann T, Fischer J, Gebert N, et al. Effects of a structured educational intervention on knowledge and emergency management in patients at risk for anaphylaxis. Allergy. 2015;70:227–35.

96. Salter SM, Vale S, Sanfilippo FM, Loh R, Clifford RM. Long-term effective-ness of online anaphylaxis education for pharmacists. Am J Pharm Educ. 2014;78:136.

97. Lee K, Hoti K, Hughes JD, Emmerton LM, Platt T. Interventions to assist health consumers to find reliable online health information: a compre-hensive review. PLoS ONE. 2014;9:e94186.

98. Gallagher M, Worth A, Cunningham-Burley S, Sheikh A. Strategies for living with the risk of anaphylaxis in adolescence: qualitative study of young people and their parents. Prim Care Respir J. 2012;21:392–7.

99. D'Amato G, Vitale C, Mormile M, Vatrella A, D'Amato M. The impact of social and digital media on asthmatic adolescents. Pediatr Allergy Immunol. 2016;27:650–1.

100. González-de-Olano D, Botella-Padilla I. Respiratory allergy buzz on the Internet. J Allergy Clin Immunol Pract. 2017;5:187–8.

101. Simons FER, Sampson HA. Anaphylaxis: unique aspects of clinical diag-nosis and management in infants (birth to age 2 years). J Allergy Clin Immunol. 2015;135:1125–31.

102. Muraro A, Roberts G, Clark A, Eigenmann PA, Halken S, Lack G, et al. The management of anaphylaxis in childhood: position paper of the European academy of allergology and clinical immunology. Allergy. 2007;62:857–71.

103. Sicherer SH, Mahr T. American Academy of Pediatrics Section on Allergy and Immunology. Management of food allergy in the school setting. Pediatrics. 2010;126:1232–9.

104. Muraro A, Clark A, Beyer K, Borrego LM, Borres M, Lødrup Carlsen KC, et al. The management of the allergic child at school: EAACI/GA2LEN Task Force on the allergic child at school. Allergy. 2010;65:681–9.

105. Polloni L, Lazzarotto F, Toniolo A, Ducolin G, Muraro A. What do school personnel know, think and feel about food allergies? Clin Transl Allergy. 2013;3:39.

106. Muraro A, Agache I, Clark A, Sheikh A, Roberts G, Akdis CA, et al. EAACI Food Allergy and Anaphylaxis Guidelines: managing patients with food allergy in the community. Allergy. 2014;69:1046–57.

107. Monks H, Gowland MH, MacKenzie H, Erlewyn-Lajeunesse M, King R, Lucas JS, et al. How do teenagers manage their food allergies? Clin Exp Allergy. 2010;40:1533–40.

108. MacKenzie H, Roberts G, Van Laar D, Dean T. Teenagers' experiences of living with food hypersensitivity: a qualitative study. Pediatr Allergy Immunol. 2009;21:595–602.

109. Sampson MA, Muñoz-Furlong A, Sicherer SH. Risk-taking and coping strategies of adolescents and young adults with food allergy. J Allergy Clin Immunol. 2006;117:1440–5.

110. Gallagher M, Worth A, Cunningham-Burley S, Sheikh A. Epinephrine auto-injector use in adolescents at risk of anaphylaxis: a qualitative study in Scotland, UK. Clin Exp Allergy. 2011;41:869–77.

111. Ventura MT, Scichilone N, Gelardi M, Patella V, Ridolo E. Management of allergic disease in the elderly: key considerations, recommendations and emerging therapies. Expert Rev Clin Immunol. 2015;11:1219–28.

112. González-de-Olano D, Lombardo C, González-Mancebo E. The difficult management of anaphylaxis in the elderly. Curr Opin Allergy Clin Immunol. 2016;16:352–60.

113. González De Olano D, De La Hoz Caballer B, Núñez López R, Sánchez Muñoz L, Cuevas Agustín M, Diéguez MC, et al. Prevalence of allergy and anaphylactic symptoms in 210 adult and pediatric patients with mastocytosis in Spain: a study of the Spanish network on mastocytosis (REMA). Clin Exp Allergy. 2007;37:1547–55.

114. Prieto-García A, Álvarez-Perea A, Matito A, Sánchez-Muñoz L, Morgado JM, Escribano L, et al. Systemic mastocytosis presenting as IgE-medi-ated food-induced anaphylaxis: a report of two cases. J Allergy Clin Immunol Pract. 2015;3:456–8.

115. Schuch A, Brockow K. Mastocytosis and anaphylaxis. Immunol Allergy Clin N Am. 2017;37:153–64.

116. Gülen T, Ljung C, Nilsson G, Akin C, Nilsson G, Noel P, et al. Risk factor analysis of anaphylactic reactions in patients with systemic mastocyto-sis. J Allergy Clin Immunol Pract. 2017;44:1179–87.

# 9

# Tonsillar cytokine expression between patients with tonsillar hypertrophy and recurrent tonsillitis

Emilia Mikola[1], Varpu Elenius[2†], Maria Saarinen[2†], Oscar Palomares[3,4,5], Matti Waris[6,7], Riitta Turunen[2], Tuomo Puhakka[1,8], Lotta Ivaska[1], Beate Rückert[3,4], Alar Aab[3,4], Tero Vahlberg[9], Tytti Vuorinen[6,7], Tobias Allander[10], Carlos A. Camargo Jr[1,12], Mübeccel Akdis[3,4], Cezmi A. Akdis[3,4] and Tuomas Jartti[2*] ⓘ

## Abstract

**Background:** Tonsils provide an innovative in vivo model for investigating immune response to infections and allergens. However, data are scarce on the differences in tonsillar virus infections and immune responses between patients with tonsillar hypertrophy or recurrent tonsillitis. We investigated the differences in virus detection and T cell and interferon gene expression in patients undergoing tonsillectomy due to tonsillar hypertrophy or recurrent tonsillitis.

**Methods:** Tonsils of 89 surgical patients with tonsillar hypertrophy (n = 47) or recurrent tonsillitis (n = 42) were analysed. Patients were carefully characterized clinically. Standard questionnaire was used to asses preceding and allergy symptoms. Respiratory viruses were analysed in tonsils and nasopharynx by PCR. Quantitative real-time PCR was used to analyse intratonsillar gene expressions of IFN-α, IFN-β, IFN-γ, IL-10, IL-13, IL-17, IL-28, IL-29, IL-37, TGF-β, FOXP3, GATA3, RORC2 and Tbet.

**Results:** Median age of the subjects was 15 years (range 2–60). Patients with tonsillar hypertrophy were younger, smoked less often, had less pollen allergy and had more adenovirus, bocavirus-1, coronavirus and rhinovirus in nasopharynx (all $P < 0.05$). Only bocavirus-1 was more often detected in hypertrophic tonsils ($P < 0.05$). In age-adjusted analysis, tonsillar hypertrophy was associated with higher mRNA expressions of IL-37 ($P < 0.05$).

**Conclusions:** Intratonsillar T cell and interferon gene expressions appeared to be relatively stable for both tonsillar hypertrophy and recurrent tonsillitis. Of the studied cytokines, only newly discovered anti-inflammatory cytokine IL-37, was independently associated with tonsillar hypertrophy showing slightly stronger anti-inflammatory response in these patients.

**Keywords:** Allergy, Asthma, Child, Cytokine, Interferon, Interleukin, T helper cell, Tonsil, Virus

## Background

Tonsillar disease is one of the most common disorders in the field of otorhinolaryngology. Different types of tonsillar disease include recurrent tonsillitis and tonsillar hypertrophy, with both leading to symptoms of mouth breathing, snoring, dyspnea, apnea or dysphagia. Treatment is usually antibiotics or tonsillectomy.

Tonsils are secondary lymphoid organs, which are centrally located at the beginning of the respiratory and gastrointestinal tracts where the immune system first comes into contact with infections agents and allergens [1]. Surgically removed palatine tonsils provide a conventional accessible source to study the interplay between foreign pathogens, allergens and the host immune system. Our previous studies demonstrated that tonsils are organs where immune regulation takes

---

*Correspondence: tuomas.jartti@utu.fi
†Varpu Elenius and Maria Saarinen contributed equally as second author
[2] Department of Paediatrics and Adolescent Medicine, Turku University Hospital and Turku University, P.O. Box 52, 20520 Turku, Finland
Full list of author information is available at the end of the article

place in which allergen-specific regulatory T cells can be generated by mechanisms depending on plasmacytoid dendritic cells [2, 3]. The expression of T cell- and interferon specific genes in tonsils has been shown to be closely related to existing viral infections, age, and allergic illnesses [4, 5]. However, data are scarce on the differences in tonsillar virus infections and immune responses between patients with tonsillar hypertrophy or recurrent tonsillitis [6–8].

Tonsils appear to provide a good in vivo model for investigating the mechanisms of inflammatory processes and infections in lymphoid organs [2–5]. Therefore, we studied whether virus detection and T cell and interferon gene expressions differed between the two main indications of surgery, tonsillar hypertrophy or recurrent tonsillitis.

## Methods
### Patients
Human tonsil samples used in this study were acquired from 200 consecutive tonsillectomy patients who underwent tonsillectomy in Satakunta Central Hospital, Pori, Finland between April 2008 and March 2009. The inclusion criteria were elective tonsillectomy according to clinical indication and written informed consent from the study patient and/or his/her guardian. The study protocol was approved by the ethics committee of Satakunta Central Hospital, Pori, Finland. Study was initiated only after obtaining written consent from the participant or his/her guardian.

### Study protocol and sample collection
A standard questionnaire was used to obtain information on allergic diseases and respiratory symptoms within 30 days before the operation (Additional file 1: Table 1). Tonsillectomy was performed according to routine clinical procedure. Internal tonsillar tissue was immediately cut in 3–4 mm cubes, stored in RNA*later* RNA stabilization reagent (Qiagen, Hilden, Germany), incubated at + 4 °C until next working day and finally stored at − 80 °C after removal of the non-absorbed reagent. For viral analyses, a part of the tonsils and a nasopharyngeal aspirate were stored in dry tubes at − 80 °C [4]. Nasopharyngeal aspirate samples were obtained during anaesthesia using a standardized procedure [4]. Serum total 25(OH)D measurement was done using an immunoassay (Abbott Architect, Chicago, USA) and bioavailable levels of 25(OH)D were estimated using additional serum measurements (D-binding protein and albumin) and published formulae.

### Definitions
Tonsillar hypertrophy group was defined as patients who underwent tonsillectomy because of obstructive symptoms such as snoring, breathing difficulties or swallowing problems. There were no tonsillar infection problems in this group. Recurrent tonsillitis group was defined as patients who underwent tonsillectomy because of recurrently infected tonsils (viral or bacterial) during the past 6–12 months. Those operated because of acute infection or peritonsillar abscess were excluded.

### Analysis of viruses and cytokines
In-house real-time PCR assays were used to detect human bocavirus-1, rhinovirus, enterovirus, and respiratory syncytial virus as described previously [4]. Seeplex RV12 ACE Detection (Seegene, Seoul, Korea) multiplex PCR assay was used for detection of adenovirus, coronaviruses (229E/NL63 and OC43/HKU1), influenza A and B viruses, metapneumovirus, parainfluenza virus types 1-3, respiratory syncytial virus group A and B, and rhinovirus [4, 5]. Virus diagnostics were carried out in the Department of Virology, University of Turku, Turku, Finland, and in the Department of Clinical Microbiology, Karolinska University Hospital, Stockholm, Sweden.

To isolate total RNA from palatine tonsils, tissues (previously stabilized in RNA*later*) were homogenized in grinding tubes containing CK28 ceramic beads by using a Precellys 24 homogenizer (Bertin Technologies, Montigny le Bretonneux, France) two times at 6000 rpm for 50 s [4]. Total RNA from cell samples was isolated using the RNeasy mini kit (Qiagen, Hilden, Germany). Reverse transcription was performed with the Revert Aid M-MuLV Reverse Transcriptase (Fermentas, St. Leon-Rot, Germany) using random hexamer primers according to the manufacturers protocol. Gene expressions of IFN-$\alpha$, IFN-$\beta$, IFN-$\gamma$, IL-10, IL-13, IL-17, IL-28, IL-29, IL-37, TGF-$\beta$, FOXP3, GATA3, RORC2 and Tbet were analysed by quantitative real-time PCR using iTaq SYBR Green Supermix with ROX (Bio-Rad, Hercules, CA, USA) on a 7900HT Fast Real-Time PCR instrument (Applied Biosystems, Foster City, CA, USA). Housekeeping gene elongation factor 1$\alpha$ (EF1$\alpha$) was used for normalization. Data are shown as relative expressions, which show $2^{-(\Delta CT)}$ values multiplied by $10^4$, where $\Delta CT$ corresponds to the difference between the CT value for the gene of interest and EF1$\alpha$.

### Statistical analysis
Continuous variables are described as medians and interquartile ranges, and were analysed using Mann–Whitney U test due to skewed distribution. Categorical variables

are expressed as frequencies and percentages, and were analysed using Chi square test or Fisher exact test. Clinical, viral and immunological differences between study groups were analysed using unadjusted and multivariable linear regression analysis. The adjustments for immunologic analyses were chosen using backward stepwise multivariable models that initially included clinical factors and virus infections which significantly differed between the groups (age, self-reported pollen allergy, self-smoking, both adenotomy and tonsillectomy performed, respiratory symptoms one month prior to the operation and bioavailable 25(OH)D level). The final model was adjusted only for age. Before regression analyses, cytokine and transcription factor values were log-transformed because of positively skewed distributions. The mean difference was computed for log-transformed values: a recurrently infected group minus hypertrophic group. Statistical analysis was completed using JMP version 12.0.1 software (SAS Institute Inc. Cary, NC, USA). A two-sided $P < 0.05$ was considered statistically significant.

## Results
### Study population
Originally, 200 patients participated in the study. Of them, 46 subjects did not have remaining tonsil and/or nasopharyngeal samples for the current analysis, and 11 had no intratonsillar virology done in their samples. Another 54 subjects were excluded for having mixed indications of operation other than hypertrophy or tonsillitis (Fig. 1). Thus, 89 patients comprised the analytic cohort. Forty-seven (53%) of them had tonsillar hypertrophy and 42 (47%) had recurrent tonsillitis.

### Patient characteristics
All operations were performed during afebrile period of chronic tonsil condition. Respiratory symptoms on the operation day were present equally in the hypertrophy group and the recurrent tonsillitis group (15 vs. 18%, respectively; $P = 0.72$). The median age of the patients was 8 years (range 2–46) and 20 years (range 7–60), respectively ($P < 0.001$) (Table 1). In addition to being younger, patients in the hypertrophy group had more often adenotomy and tonsillectomy done, had

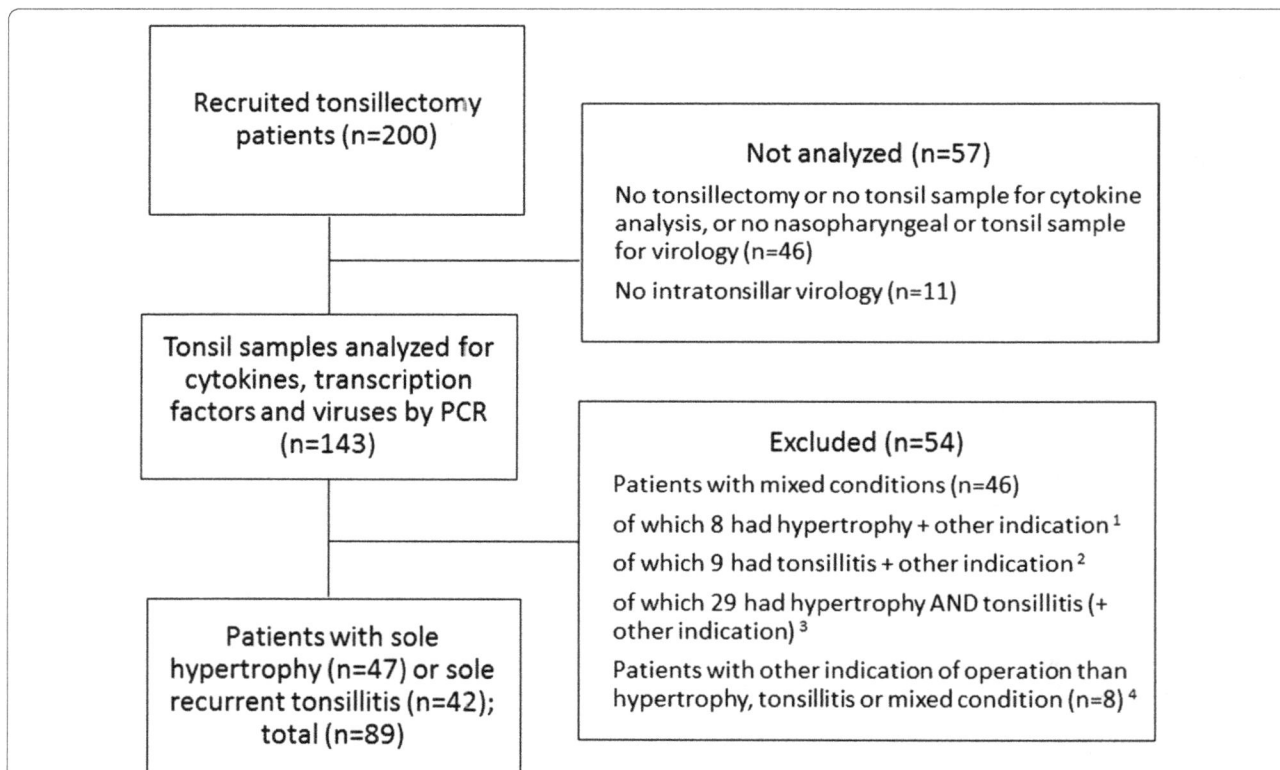

**Fig. 1** Study flow chart. [1]8 had hypertrophy and another indication (recurrent otitis media n = 4; recurrent otitis media and fever n = 3; recurrent fever n = 1). [2]9 had recurrent tonsillitis and another indication (recurrent fever n = 8; recurrent otitis media n = 1). [3]21 had hypertrophy and tonsillitis; 8 had hypertrophy, tonsillitis, and another indication (recurrent fever, n = 5; recurrent otitis media, recurrent fever n = 1; recurrent otitis media n = 2). [4]8 had other indication of operation than hypertrophy or tonsillitis (chronic white patches in tonsils n = 2; accumulation of food remnants, bad smelling breath, and feeling of beat in throat n = 1; recurrent fever n = 1; teeth braces n = 2; throat abscess n = 1; no clear cause n = 1)

**Table 1  Patient characteristics**

| Characteristics | Tonsillar hypertrophy n = 47 | Recurrent tonsillitis n = 42 | P value |
|---|---|---|---|
| Age, years (range) | 8 (2, 46) | 20 (7, 60) | *< 0.0001* |
| Male | 27 (57%) | 23 (55%) | 0.80 |
| Tonsillectomy and adenotomy | 28 (60%) | 5 (12%) | *< 0.0001* |
| Self-reported allergy | 20/43 (47%) | 23/40 (58%) | 0.32 |
| Food | 6/43 (14%) | 3/39 (8%) | 0.38 |
| Drug | 4/43 (9%) | 4/39 (10%) | 0.87 |
| Seasonal, i.e. pollen | 0/43 (0%) | 7/39 (18%) | *0.004* |
| Perennial, i.e. animal or house dust mite | 3/43 (7%) | 2/39 (5%) | 0.74 |
| Other | 2/43 (5%) | 2/39 (5%) | 0.90 |
| Multiple | 5/43 (12%) | 4/39 (10%) | 0.86 |
| Physician-diagnosed atopic dermatitis | 11/44 (25%) | 4/38 (11%) | 0.09 |
| Self-reported allergic rhinitis | 11/44 (25%) | 11/39 (28%) | 0.74 |
| Physician-diagnosed asthma | 6/42 (14%) | 6/39 (15%) | 0.89 |
| Self-smoking | 2/43 (5%) | 14/40 (35%) | *0.0005* |
| Maternal smoking | 15/44 (34%) | 13/41 (32%) | 0.82 |
| Paternal smoking | 16/41 (39%) | 19/36 (53%) | 0.23 |
| Season of the surgery | | | 0.85 |
| Winter (months 12–2) | 7 (15%) | 4 (10%) | |
| Spring (months 3–5) | 14 (30%) | 13 (31%) | |
| Summer (months 6–8) | 8 (17%) | 5 (12%) | |
| Fall (months 9–11) | 18 (38%) | 20 (48%) | |
| Respiratory symptoms | | | |
| The operation day | 6/39 (15%) | 7/38 (18%) | 0.72 |
| Within 2 weeks | 16/42 (38%) | 12/37 (32%) | 0.60 |
| Within 4 weeks | 23/42 (55%) | 18/37 (48%) | 0.59 |
| One month prior the operation | | | |
| Throat pain | 8/39 (21%) | 14/35 (40%) | *0.0005* |
| Rhinitis | 23/39 (59%) | 6/35 (17%) | *0.0002* |
| Cough | 15/39 (38%) | 5/36 (14%) | *0.02* |
| Acute otitis media | 2/39 (5%) | 0/35 (0%) | 0.17 |
| Wheezing | 2/39 (5%) | 0/35 (0%) | 0.17 |
| 25(OH)D level | | | |
| Total (nmol/l) | 56.2 (41.7, 66.9) | 45.7 (34.4, 72.3) | 0.08 |
| Free (pg/ml) | 6.4 (4.9, 8.1) | 5.0 (3.3, 8.8) | 0.14 |
| Bioavailable (ng/ml) | 2.2 (1.7, 2.9) | 1.6 (1.1, 2.7) | *0.01* |

Values are shown as median (interquartile range, except age) or number of subjects (%). Data were analysed by Mann–Whitney U test, Chi square test, or Fisher's Exact test

Significant values are shown in italic

less self-reported pollen allergy, smoked less, and had less throat pain, but had more often rhinitis and cough 1 month prior the operation and higher bioavailable 25(OH)D level than patients in the recurrent tonsillitis group (all $P < 0.01$) (Table 1). Otherwise no significant differences were found between the two groups.

**Viruses detected in nasopharyngeal aspirates and tonsils**

Significantly more patients in the hypertrophy group, compared to the recurrent tonsillitis group, had a virus in their nasopharyngeal aspirates (79 vs. 38%, respectively; $P < 0.001$). In addition, patients in the hypertrophy group had more often adenovirus, bocavirus-1, coronavirus or rhinovirus in nasopharyngeal aspirate (all $P < 0.05$) (Table 2). However, intratonsillar virus detection didn't show statistically significant differences, except for bocavirus-1 which was detected in tonsils in 15% of patients with hypertrophy and only 2% of patients in recurrent tonsillitis group (Table 2). Patients in the hypertrophy group were more often positive for one

**Table 2  Nasopharyngeal and intratonsillar virus detection**

| Virus | Nasopharynx | | P value | Tonsil | | P value |
|---|---|---|---|---|---|---|
| | Tonsillar hypertrophy n = 47 | Recurrent tonsillitis n = 42 | | Tonsillar hypertrophy n = 47 | Recurrent tonsillitis n = 42 | |
| Adenovirus | 9 (19%) | 2 (5%) | *0.03* | 7 (15%) | 2 (5%) | 0.10 |
| Bocavirus-1 | 12 (26%) | 2 (5%) | *0.005* | 7 (15%) | 1 (2%) | *0.03* |
| Coronavirus | 3 (6%) | 0 (0%) | *0.048* | 0 (0%) | 0 (0%) | – |
| Enteroviruses | 4 (9%) | 4 (10%) | 0.87 | 6 (13%) | 4 (10%) | 0.63 |
| Influenza A or B virus | 1 (2%) | 0 (0%) | 0.26 | 0 (0%) | 0 (0%) | – |
| Metapneumovirus | 0 (0%) | 1 (2%) | 0.29 | 1 (2%) | 0 (0%) | 0.26 |
| Parainfluenza virus types 1-4 | 1 (2%) | 1 (2%) | 0.94 | 4 (9%) | 1 (2%) | 0.19 |
| Respiratory syncytial virus | 1 (2%) | 0 (0%) | 0.26 | 2 (4%) | 0 (0%) | 0.11 |
| Rhinovirus species A, B or C | 27 (57%) | 14 (33%) | *0.02* | 2 (4%) | 2 (5%) | 0.91 |
| Number of positive viruses | 37 (79%) | 16 (38%) | *< 0.0001* | 17 (36%) | 8 (19%) | 0.07 |
| Positive for 1 virus | 23 (49%) | 10 (24%) | *0.01* | 9 (19%) | 7 (17%) | 0.76 |
| Positive for 2 viruses | 8 (17%) | 4 (10%) | 0.30 | 5 (11%) | 0 (0%) | *0.01* |
| Positive for 3 viruses | 5 (11%) | 2 (5%) | 0.30 | 2 (4%) | 1 (2%) | 0.62 |
| Positive for 4 viruses | 1 (2%) | 0 (0%) | 0.26 | 1 (2%) | 0 (0%) | 0.26 |
| Positive for ≥ 1 viruses | 37 (79%) | 16 (38%) | | 17 (36%) | 8 (19%) | |
| Positive for ≥ 2 viruses | 14 (30%) | 6 (14%) | | 8 (17%) | 1 (2%) | |
| Positive for ≥ 3 viruses | 6 (13%) | 2 (5%) | | 3 (7%) | 1 (2%) | |
| Positive for ≥ 4 viruses | 1 (2%) | 0 | | 1 (2%) | 0 | |

Values are shown as number of subjects (%). Data were analysed by Chi square test, or Fisher's Exact test

Significant values are shown in italic

virus in their nasopharyngeal aspirates (49 vs. 24%) or two viruses in their tonsils (11 vs. 0%, respectively) (both $P < 0.05$) (Table 2).

### Cytokine and transcription factor expression profiles in tonsils

In unadjusted analysis, patients in the hypertrophy group had stronger tonsillar expression of Tbet ($P = 0.03$) and IL-37 ($P = 0.001$) than patients in the recurrent tonsillitis group (Tables 3, 4). In the multivariable regression analysis, only age remained as a significant co-factor (Table 4). After adjustment for age, the expressions of only IL-37 was independently associated with tonsillar hypertrophy group ($P < 0.05$, Fig. 2). No other differences in cytokine or transcription factor expression were found between the groups.

### Discussion

This study shows differences in virus detections and T cell and interferon gene expressions in patients undergoing tonsillectomy due to tonsillar hypertrophy or recurrent tonsillitis. Patients with tonsillar hypertrophy were typically younger, and had more viral findings, but only bocavirus-1 was more often found in tonsils when compared to patients with recurrent tonsillitis. Respectively, they also had less self-reported pollen allergy, but no differences were found in food allergies between the

**Table 3  Intratonsillar cytokine and transcription factor expression in hypertrophic tonsils and recurrent tonsillitis**

| Cytokine or transcription factor | Tonsillar hypertrophy n = 47 Median (IQR) | Recurrent tonsillitis n = 42 Median (IQR) |
|---|---|---|
| T-helper₁ | | |
| IFN-γ | 58 (37, 90) | 76 (32, 117) |
| Tbet | 54 (31, 83) | 34 (22, 60) |
| T-helper₂ | | |
| IL-13 | 1.2 (0.03, 3.7) | 0.45 (0.02, 2.2) |
| GATA3 | 27 (16, 36) | 18 (12, 39) |
| T-helper₁₇ | | |
| IL-17 | 10 (5.6, 19) | 7.3 (4.1, 13) |
| RORC2 | 15 (7.2, 31) | 20 (10, 28) |
| T-regulatory | | |
| IL-10 | 49 (24, 74) | 35 (21, 64) |
| IL-37 | 0.26 (0.15, 0.37) | 0.14 (0.10, 0.24) |
| FOXP3 | 46 (20, 87) | 48 (24, 80) |
| TGF-β | 163 (105, 232) | 171 (120, 225) |
| Type I/III interferons | | |
| IFN-α | 15 (0.59, 62) | 9.7 (0.27, 56) |
| IFN-β | 24 (2.7, 101) | 22 (2.1, 103) |
| IL-28 | 31 (3.1, 88) | 12 (1.4, 75) |
| IL-29 | 11 (2.3, 34) | 3.7 (1.3, 26) |

Values are arbitrary units × $10^4$ relative to EF1α

IQR, interquartile range; IFN, interferon; Tbet, T-box transcription factor; IL, interleukin; GATA3, GATA-binding factor 3; RORC, RAR-related orphan receptor C; FOXP, forkhead box protein; TGF, tumour growth factor

**Table 4  Differences in cytokine and transcription factor expression between hypertrophic tonsils and recurrent tonsillitis**

| Cytokine or transcription factor | Mean differences recurrently infected minus hypertrophic group | | | | |
| --- | --- | --- | --- | --- | --- |
| | Univariate | | Multivariate | | |
| | n | Difference of means (95% CI) | Adjusted difference of means (95% CI) | Adjustments | |
| T-helper$_1$ | | | | | |
| IFN-γ | 88 | 0.061 (− 0.32, 0.44) P = 0.75 | – | – | |
| Tbet | 89 | *− 0.40 (− 0.76, − 0.034) P = 0.03* | − 0.21 (− 0.61, 0.18) P = 0.29 | Age | |
| T-helper$_2$ | | | | | |
| IL-13 | 89 | − 0.74 (− 1.8, 0.36) P = 0.18 | – | – | |
| GATA3 | 89 | − 0.12 (− 0.42, 0.18) P = 0.43 | – | – | |
| T-helper$_{17}$ | | | | | |
| IL-17 | 89 | − 0.35 (− 0.80, 0.096) P = 0.12 | − 0.087 (− 0.57, 0.40) P = 0.72 | Age | |
| RORC2 | 89 | 0.014 (− 0.35, 0.38) P = 0.94 | – | – | |
| T-regulatory | | | | | |
| IL-10 | 89 | − 0.26 (− 0.61, 0.0871) P = 0.14 | − 0.0070 (− 0.38, 0.36) P = 0.97 | Age | |
| IL-37 | 87 | *− 0.48 (− 0.77, − 0.19) P = 0.001* | *− 0.31 (− 0.63, − 0.0021) P = 0.049* | Age | |
| FOXP3 | 89 | 0.091 (− 0.31, 0.49) P = 0.65 | – | – | |
| TGF-β | 89 | − 0.0077 (− 0.32, 0.30) P = 0.96 | – | – | |
| Type I/III interferons | | | | | |
| IFN-α | 87 | − 0.41 (− 1.5, 0.7) P = 0.47 | – | – | |
| IFN-β | 88 | − 0.21 (− 1.0, 0.61) P = 0.62 | – | – | |
| IL-28 | 89 | − 0.64 (− 1.5, 0.2) P = 0.13 | – | – | |
| IL-29 | 87 | − 0.57 (− 1.5, 0.31) P = 0.15 | – | – | |

Data are expressed as mean differences as a recurrently infected group minus hypertrophic group. The data were analysed using backward stepwise linear regression analysis after logarithmic transformation. Only significant co-factors were used as adjustments in the final model

CI, confidence interval; IFN, interferon; Tbet, T-box transcription factor; IL, interleukin; GATA3, GATA-binding factor 3; RORC, RAR-related orphan receptor C; FOXP, forkhead box protein; TGF, tumour growth factor

Significant values are shown in italic

groups. After age-adjusted analysis, tonsillar hypertrophy was associated with higher tonsillar mRNA expressions of IL-37. Other than age, no other significant co-factors were found.

IL-37 (formerly IL-1 family member 7) is a fundamental inhibitor of innate immunity [9, 10]. It has been shown to be expressed in macrophages, monocytes, plasma and epithelial cells [11]. After ligand activation, IL-37 inhibits inflammatory cytokines (especially IL-1β, but also IL-6, IL-7, IFN-γ, and TNF-α) and augments the level of anti-inflammatory IL-10 and T regulatory cells [11]. We have previously shown that the expression of IL-37 is closely and positively associated with other "immune activation/regulatory" cytokines (IL-10, IL-17, IL-37, TGF-β, FOXP3, GATA3, RORC2, Tbet) in tonsils [2]. The current analysis adds that tonsillar expression of anti-inflammatory cytokine IL-37 is also independently and positively associated with tonsillar hypertrophy.

Interferons (IFN-α, IFN-β, IFN-γ, IL-28, IL-29) are cytokines with antiviral activity and their expression is induced by viral infection. IL-28 and IL-29 are members of IFN-λ family [12, 13]. They are produced by dendritic

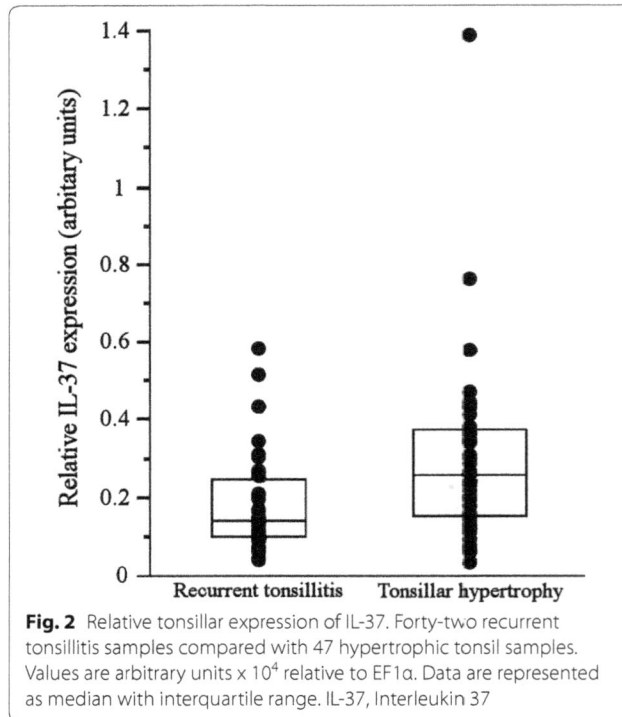

**Fig. 2** Relative tonsillar expression of IL-37. Forty-two recurrent tonsillitis samples compared with 47 hypertrophic tonsil samples. Values are arbitrary units x $10^4$ relative to EF1α. Data are represented as median with interquartile range. IL-37, Interleukin 37

cells and macrophages following viral infection or activation with bacterial components [12–14]. We expected to see differences in IFN expression (lower responses in recurrent tonsillitis than in tonsillar hypertophy group), since they have antiviral properties and they up-regulate the expression of MHC Class II molecules on cells which increases the immune system's ability to recognize viruses [14, 15]. However, we did not observe these differences. We speculate that tonsillar hypertophy may be a consequence of chronic inflammation in tonsils and the same interferon pathways are equally activated in both conditions. We have previously found strong intragroup correlations of tonsillar IFN expression(IFN-α, IFN-β, IFN-γ, IL-28) [2].

Age was the main clinical characteristic differentiating the tonsillectomy indication groups. In agreement with previous findings [16], we found that obstruction due to the hypertrophy is more common with younger children where as adults have more recurrent tonsillitis. The age difference between the groups also explains the differences in smoking and in additional adenotomy performed. Interestingly, Reis and colleagues found no difference between the age distribution of hypertrophy and tonsillitis patients, but the narrow age range of their subjects (ages 2–11 years) may explain the lack of difference [17].

Virus was found in the nasopharynx of 79% of patients with tonsillar hypertrophy group and 38% in recurrent tonsillitis group. Most often detected viruses were

adenovirus, bocavirus-1, coronavirus and rhinovirus. However, intratonsillar virus detection was low and did not show any statistically significant differences except for bocavirus-1. The results of nasopharyngeal and intratonsillar virus detection vs tonsillar cytokine responses are discussed in detail in our previous report [2].

Small differences in cytokine expression may partly be explained by differences concerning tonsillar germinal centers. The mean follicular area has been found to be larger, and the number of germinal centers higher, in the hypertrophy group compared to the recurrent tonsillitis [17–19]. In our study, the samples were taken from inside of the tonsils to minimize the margin of error and the possibility to misinterpreted differences between the groups. Seasonal changes, e.g. pollen and influenza seasons, may affect the expression of peripheral T cells [20], but we found no differences in tonsillar expression of cytokines between the seasons of the surgery. Also, respiratory viruses are continuously detected in children with chronic tonsillitis throughout the year [21–23]. Circulating serum 25(OH)D level has been shown to been positively associated with IL-37 level [3], but here it did not confound the results.

A limitation of the current study is that we did not investigate bacterial colonization of the tonsils in these patients due to fact that the operation was done during an afebrile period of their chronic tonsil condition. The downstream signaling of IL-37 is a complex process and to show functionality of IL-37 by downstream mediators was not in the scope of this study. In addition to forming cell-surface receptor complexes, IL-37 translocates to the nucleus where it binds to nuclear DNA and participate in transcription. [24, 25] IL-37 is regarded as a "dual function" cytokine, similar to IL-1α and IL-33.

## Conclusions
In summary, this study provides new insights about T cell research in lymphoid tissue from the clinical aspect of the surgical indication for tonsillectomy. We found tonsils as a good in vivo model for investigating the mechanisms of inflammatory processes and infections in lymphoid organs. Our data suggest that T-cell and interferon gene expressions appear to relatively stable over the two main indications of tonsillectomy, tonsillar hypertrophy and recurrent tonsillitis. However, anti-inflammatory immune responses, namely IL-37, might be slightly stronger in patients with tonsillar hypertrophy than with patients with recurrent tonsillitis.

## Authors' contributions

The study protocol and manuscript were written by the investigators. Tonsil samples and clinical data were collected by TP, MS and LI. Viral analyses were performed by MW, TVu and TA Cytokine analyses were conducted by OP, RT, BR, AA and supervised by MA and CAA. CAC organized the vitamin D analyses. Data were analyzed by EM, VE, MS and TJ and by statistician TVa. All authors read and approved the final manuscript.

## Author details

[1] Department of Otorhinolaryngology, Turku University Hospital and Turku University, Turku, Finland. [2] Department of Paediatrics and Adolescent Medicine, Turku University Hospital and Turku University, P.O. Box 52, 20520 Turku, Finland. [3] Swiss Institute of Allergy and Asthma Research, University of Zürich, Davos, Switzerland. [4] Christine Kühne-Center for Allergy Research and Education, Davos, Switzerland. [5] Department of Biochemistry and Molecular Biology, School of Chemistry, Complutense University of Madrid, Madrid, Spain. [6] Department of Clinical Virology, Turku University Hospital, Turku, Finland. [7] Department of Virology, University of Turku, Turku, Finland. [8] Department of Otorhinolaryngology, Satakunta Central Hospital, Pori, Finland. [9] Department of Biostatistics, University of Turku and Turku University Hospital, Turku, Finland. [10] Department of Clinical Microbiology, Karolinska University Hospital, Stockholm, Sweden. [11] Department of Emergency Medicine, Massachusetts General Hospital, Harvard Medical School, Boston, USA. [12] Division of Rheumatology, Allergy and Immunology, Department of Medicine, Massachusetts General Hospital, Harvard Medical School, Boston, USA.

## Competing interests

The authors declare that they have no competing interests.

## Funding

TJ and his laboratory are supported by the Academy of Finland (Grants 114034 and 132595), the Finnish Medical Foundation, the Sigrid Juselius Foundation, and the Foundation for Pediatric Research. EM and MS are supported by the Foundation for Pediatric Research. VE is supported by Tampere Tuberculosis Foundation. OP is a Ramon y Cajal Scholar funded by MINECO and the European Social Fund. MA's laboratory is sponsored by EU 7th Framework Program PREDICTA: Post-Infectious Immune Reprogramming and Its Association with Persistence and Chronicity of Respiratory Allergic Diseases (No. 260895). Laboratory of CAA is supported by the Swiss National Science Foundation Grant 32-132899 and Christine Kühne-Center for Allergy Research and Education. The granting agencies covered all costs and played no role in study design, data analysis, or manuscript preparation.

## References

1. Ogra PL. Mucosal immune response in the ear, nose and throat. Pediatr Infect Dis J. 2000;19(5 Suppl):S4–8.
2. Palomares O, Rückert B, Jartti T, Kücüksezer UC, Puhakka T, Gomez E, et al. Induction and maintenance of allergen-specific FOXP3+ Treg cells in human tonsils as potential first-line organs of oral tolerance. J Allergy Clin Immunol. 2012;129(2):510–20.
3. Kücüksezer UC, Palomares O, Rückert B, Jartti T, Puhakka T, Nandy A, et al. Triggering of specific Toll-like receptors and proinflammatory cytokines breaks allergen-specific T-cell tolerance in human tonsils and peripheral blood. J Allergy Clin Immunol. 2013;131(3):875–85.
4. Jartti T, Palomares O, Waris M, Tastan O, Nieminen R, Puhakka T, et al. Distinct regulation of tonsillar immune response in virus infection. Allergy. 2014;69(5):658–67.
5. Elenius V, Palomares O, Waris M, Turunen R, Puhakka T, Rückert B, et al. The relationship of serum vitamins A, D, E and LL-37 levels with allergic status, tonsillar virus detection and immune response. PLoS ONE. 2017;12(2):e0172350.
6. Andersson J, Abrams J, Björk L, Funa K, Litton M, Agren K, et al. Concomitant in vivo production of 19 different cytokines in human tonsils. Immunology. 1994;83(1):16–24.
7. Kim J, Bhattacharjee R, Dayyat E, Snow AB, Kheirandish-Gozal L, Goldman JL, et al. Increased cellular proliferation and inflammatory cytokines in tonsils derived from children with obstructive sleep apnea. Pediatr Res. 2009;66(4):423–8.
8. Woon HG, Braun A, Li J, Smith C, Edwards J, Sierro F, et al. Compartmentalization of total and virus-specific tissue-resident memory CD8+ T cells in human lymphoid organs. PLoS Pathog. 2016;12(8):e1005799.
9. Nold MF, Nold-Petry CA, Zepp JA, Palmer BE, Bufler P, Dinarello CA. IL-37 is a fundamental inhibitor of innate immunity. Nat Immunol. 2010;11(11):1014–22.
10. Banchereau J, Pascual V, O'Garra A. From IL-2 to IL-37: the expanding spectrum of anti-inflammatory cytokines. Nat Immunol. 2012;13(10):925–31.
11. Conti P, Carinci F, Lessiani G, Spinas E, Kritas SK, Ronconi G, et al. Potential therapeutic use of IL-37: a key suppressor of innate immunity and allergic immune responses mediated by mast cells. Immunol Res. 2017;65(5):982–6.
12. Kelm NE, Zhu Z, Ding VA, Xiao H, Wakefield MR, Bai Q, et al. The role of IL-29 in immunity and cancer. Crit Rev Oncol Hematol. 2016;106:91–8.
13. Witte K, Witte E, Sabat R, Wolk K. IL-28A, IL-28B, and IL-29: promising cytokines with type I interferon-like properties. Cytokine Growth Factor Rev. 2010;21(4):237–51.
14. Akdis M, Burgler S, Crameri R, Eiwegger T, Fujita H, Gomez E, et al. Interleukins, from 1 to 37, and interferon-γ: receptors, functions, and roles in diseases. J Allergy Clin Immunol. 2011;127(3):701–21.
15. Commins S, Steinke JW, Borish L. The extended IL-10 superfamily: IL-10, IL-19, IL-20, IL-22, IL-24, IL-26, IL-28, and IL-29. J Allergy Clin Immunol. 2008;121(5):1108–11.
16. Rosenmann E, Rabinowitz R, Schlesinger M. Lymphocyte subsets in human tonsils: the effect of age and infection. Pediatr Allergy Immunol. 1998;9(3):161–7.
17. Reis LG, Almeida EC, da Silva JC, GeA Pereira, VeF Barbosa, Etchebehere RM. Tonsillar hyperplasia and recurrent tonsillitis: clinical-histological correlation. Braz J Otorhinolaryngol. 2013;79(5):603–8.
18. Zhang PC, Pang YT, Loh KS, Wang DY. Comparison of histology between recurrent tonsillitis and tonsillar hypertrophy. Clin Otolaryngol Allied Sci. 2003;28(3):235–9.
19. Agren K, Andersson U, Litton M, Funa K, Nordlander B, Andersson J. The production of immunoregulatory cytokines is localized to the extrafollicular area of human tonsils. Acta Otolaryngol. 1996;116(3):477–85.
20. Jartti T, Burmeister KA, Seroogy CM, Jennens-Clough ML, Tisler CJ, Salazar LP, et al. Association between CD4+CD25(high) T cells and atopy in children. J Allergy Clin Immunol. 2007;120(1):177–83.
21. Proença-Módena JL, Buzatto GP, Paula FE, Saturno TH, Delcaro LS, Prates MC, et al. Respiratory viruses are continuously detected in children with chronic tonsillitis throughout the year. Int J Pediatr Otorhinolaryngol. 2014;78(10):1655–61.
22. Günel C, Kırdar S, Ömürlü İ, Ağdaş F. Detection of the Epstein–Barr virus, human bocavirus and novel KI and KU polyomaviruses in adenotonsillar tissues. Int J Pediatr Otorhinolaryngol. 2015;79(3):423–7.
23. Comar M, Grasso D, dal Molin G, Zocconi E, Campello C. HHV-6 infection of tonsils and adenoids in children with hypertrophy and upper airway recurrent infections. Int J Pediatr Otorhinolaryngol. 2010;74(1):47–9.
24. Sharma S, Kulk N, Nold MF, Gräf R, Kim SH, Reinhardt D, et al. The IL-1 family member 7b translocates to the nucleus and down-regulates proinflammatory cytokines. J Immunol. 2008;180(8):5477–82.
25. Bulau AM, Nold MF, Li S, Nold-Petry CA, Fink M, Mansell A, et al. Role of caspase-1 in nuclear translocation of IL-37, release of the cytokine, and IL-37 inhibition of innate immune responses. Proc Natl Acad Sci USA. 2014;111(7):2650–5.

# 10

# Multi-morbidities of allergic rhinitis in adults: European Academy of Allergy and Clinical Immunology Task Force Report

C. Cingi[1*], P. Gevaert[2], R. Mösges[3], C. Rondon[4], V. Hox[5], M. Rudenko[6], N. B. Muluk[7], G. Scadding[8], F. Manole[9], C. Hupin[10], W. J. Fokkens[11], C. Akdis[12], C. Bachert[2], P. Demoly[13], J. Mullol[14], A. Muraro[15], N. Papadopoulos[16], R. Pawankar[17], P. Rombaux[18], E. Toskala[19], L. Kalogjera[20], E. Prokopakis[21], P. W. Hellings[5] and J. Bousquet[13]

**Abstract**

This report has been prepared by the European Academy of Allergy and Clinical Immunology Task Force on Allergic Rhinitis (AR) comorbidities. The aim of this multidisciplinary European consensus document is to highlight the role of multimorbidities in the definition, classification, mechanisms, recommendations for diagnosis and treatment of AR, and to define the needs in this neglected area by a literature review. AR is a systemic allergic disease and is generally associated with numerous multi-morbid disorders, including asthma, eczema, food allergies, eosinophilic oesophagitis (EoE), conjunctivitis, chronic middle ear effusions, rhinosinusitis, adenoid hypertrophy, olfaction disorders, obstructive sleep apnea, disordered sleep and consequent behavioural and educational effects. This report provides up-to-date usable information to: (1) improve the knowledge and skills of allergists, so as to ultimately improve the overall quality of patient care; (2) to increase interest in this area; and (3) to present a unique contribution to the field of upper inflammatory disease.

**Keywords:** Adenoid hypertrophy, Allergic rhinitis (AR), Asthma, Chronic middle ear effusions, Comorbidities, Disordered sleep, Eczema, Eosinophilic oesophagitis (EoE), Conjunctivitis, Food allergies, Obstructive sleep apnea, Olfaction disorders, Rhinitis, Rhinosinusitis

## Introduction

This report was prepared by the European Academy of Allergy and Clinical Immunology (EAACI) Task Force on "Allergic Rhinitis (AR) comorbidities". This was initiated, based on the rationale that AR is rarely found in isolation and needs to be considered in the context of systemic allergic disease associated with numerous comorbid disorders including asthma, chronic middle ear effusions, sinusitis, lymphoid hypertrophy with obstructive sleep apnea, disordered sleep, and consequent behavioural and educational effects.

AR, which has increased in prevalence over several decades, now affects 10–30% of the population, with the greatest frequency found in children and adolescents [1]. It typically presents after the second year of life but the exact prevalence in early life is unknown. Since children's immune systems develop between the first and fourth years of life, those with an atopic predisposition begin to express allergic disease with a clear $Th_2$ response to allergen exposure, resulting in symptoms, often beginning with atopic dermatitis (AD) and progressing to asthma and rhinitis (the allergic march) [1]. However after early childhood, AR is usually the initial manifestation of allergy [2].

AR is associated with numerous multi-morbid disorders. Those occurring in children have already been discussed in the EAACI Task Force on Paediatric Rhinitis [3]. This paper, by contrast, concerns itself largely with adult AR multimorbidities, but includes relevant paediatric data.

*Correspondence: ccingi@gmail.com
[1] Department of Otorhinolaryngology, Eskisehir Osmangazi University School of Medicine, Eskisehir, Turkey
Full list of author information is available at the end of the article

## Definition

Multimorbidity is the presence of one or more additional disorders (or diseases) *co-occurring* with a primary disease or disorder; or the effect of such additional disorders or diseases [4]. When the primary organ is not known, the term multimorbidity should be used instead of co-morbidity. In allergic diseases, the term should be multimorbidity.

## Multi-morbidities of allergic rhinitis

AR is an organ-specific manifestation of allergic disease. As such, it coexists with other organ-specific disorders that have a common allergic basis. It is therefore rarely found in isolation but frequently has associated multimorbid disorders [5].

These can be subdivided into:

(a) Disorders which are part of the spectrum of allergic diseases, e.g. asthma, AD, food allergy, anaphylaxis;
(b) Disorders anatomically related to the nose: conjunctivitis, sinusitis, middle ear problems, throat and laryngeal effects;
(c) Sleep problems and secondary effects on concentration and behaviour; and
(d) Turbinate hypertrophy.

Although more common in paediatric practice, the occurrence of multi-morbidities in adults is significant and has important implications for quality of life, and work attendance and performance. It is likely that those with severe chronic upper airways disease (SCUAD) suffer more severe co-morbid effects.

## Asthma
### Extent of co-occurrence

A European study of over 20,000 children showed that the co-existence of eczema, asthma and rhinitis in the same child is more frequent than expected if they were independent entities. Those children with one of these diseases at age 4 were 4–7 times more likely to have two or three of them at age 8. Children with two or three allergic diseases at 4 years are 30–60 times more likely to have two or three of these diseases at age 8 [6].

The association between asthma and rhinitis in adults has been recognized for some decades, since the pioneering study of Brydon [7], who showed that the majority of 1000 asthmatics also had rhinitis, which preceded their asthma in 45% of the subjects.

In fact the majority of inflammatory asthma sufferers have some form of upper airway disease (ARIA 2001) [8], either AR, non-allergic rhinitis or rhinosinusitis, usually with nasal polyposis (EPOS 2012) [9]. The extent of

inflammation is usually proportional between upper and lower respiratory tracts with equivalence in eosinophils [10] and clinical severity [11].

Several possible relations exist between AR and asthma: (a) AR may be statistically associated with asthma; (b) AR may exacerbate coexisting asthma; and (c) AR may have a causal role in the pathogenesis of asthma.

Several possible causal mechanisms have been postulated to explain a link between AR and asthma:

- Lack of nasal function, i.e. purifying, warming and humidifying inspired air;
- Nasobronchial reflex (nasal irritants, allergens or cold stimuli);
- Rhinovirus adhesion theory (increased susceptibility to allergic inflammation and intracellular adhesion molecule (ICAM)-1 expression) [12]; and
- "Migration" of T cell responses to other tissues after initial sensitization. Braunstahl [13] has shown that allergen challenge in one part of the airway is followed by a response in all other parts;
- The idea of postnasal drip (carriage of inflammatory cytokines/mediators from nasopharynx to lower airways) has been largely abandoned, since the 'drip' travels to the gut, by virtue of the larynx, not to the lower airway, unless the subject is deeply unconscious.

Certainly the presence of rhinitis, both allergic and non-allergic, is a risk factor for subsequent asthma development [14].

### Effects of co-occurrence

The co-existence of rhinitis is associated with poor asthma control in adults, adolescents and children [15]. Recent studies on AR and asthma are presented in Table 1 [16–19].

## Atopic dermatitis (AD)
### Extent of co-occurrence

In children, there are clear data concerning the co-occurrence of AD and AR, largely from birth cohorts [20].

In one Taiwanese study [21], AR was the most common concomitant atopic disease associated with AD. The group with AD and AR was shown to be more likely to have serum mite-, cockroach- and feather-specific IgE, whereas the positive rates for wheat, peanut and soybean were higher in those with AD without rhinitis.

In a Croatian study [22], the age at onset was younger in the group of AD patients with concomitant AR, suggesting that AD multi-morbidity (although part of the allergic march) may be irrelevant to the later development of isolated respiratory allergy.

**Table 1  Asthma and AR**

| References | Study type | No. patients | Age/Profile | Aim of the study | Results |
|---|---|---|---|---|---|
| Ciprandi et al. [16] | Prospective | 89 (AR), 940 (controls) | Adults | Follow up of patients with AR every 2 years for 8 years to investigate spirometric abnormalities/BHR | 34 of 89 AR patients developed BHR after 8 years<br>Sensitization to mite, birch and parietaria, as well as rhinitis duration are risk factors |
| Navarro et al. [17] | Epidemiologic prospective; multi centre | 942 (with asthma) | Mean age: 35.5; 63% female | Investigate the link between the upper and lower airways | 89.5% had AR<br>Correlation between severity of rhinitis and asthma (p < 0001) and inverse correlation with age (p < 0.0001) and severity of asthma (p < 0.05) |
| Ko et al. [18] | Cross sectional; questionnaire | 600 (with asthma) | 267 male; 333 female | Evaluation of prevalence of AR in asthma | 77% of asthmatics had rhinitis in the past 12 months (of whom 96% were previously diagnosed with AR)<br><br>In patients with asthma and rhinitis, 49% use nasal steroids, resulting in fewer ED visits (13 vs 25%) and fewer hospitalizations for asthma (5 vs 13%) |
| Valero et al. [19] | Cross-sectional international population study; based on questionnaire | 3225; 1 positive skin test | Age range: 10–50; 53% male | Evaluation of the link between AR, asthma and skin test sensitization | Asthma presents in 49% of AR patients<br><br>Asthma severity was associated with length of time from onset and with allergic rhinitis severity<br><br>Patients with asthma have a higher number of allergen sensitizations and higher sensitization intensity than those without asthma (p < 0.01) |

Taken together these observations suggest that sensitization in later onset allergy is not via the skin, but by inhalant allergens acting via the respiratory tract mucosa [2].

### Effects of co-occurrence

While some data suggest that the greater extent of allergic disease promotes more severe reactions [23, 24], other researchers note an inverse relationship between exacerbations in skin and in the respiratory tract [25].

In patients with asthma, AD and AR, the risks of systemic glucocorticoid bioavailability are highest, since treatment is likely to be directed to three sites: skin, bronchi and nose. Absorption occurs (from least to greatest rate) in the nasal mucosa, followed by the bronchi, then the skin. Alternative means of treatment (such as allergen avoidance, saline douching, antihistamines, anti-leukotrienes, immunotherapy and anti-cytokines) may need to be considered.

### Food allergy

#### Extent of co-occurrence

AR can be associated with primary food allergy; however, it is more frequently associated with secondary food allergy, also known as pollen food syndrome (PFS). Some medical professionals refer to pollen food syndrome as oral allergy syndrome (OAS), although strictly

speaking the two are not the same. When the term OAS was first used in 1987 it had no connection with pollen allergy but referred to any allergic symptoms in the mouth that often preceded more serious symptoms. The term pollen food syndrome is preferred when referring to those allergy symptoms to food that are linked to pollen allergy, are limited to the mouth and throat, and are usually mild. [26]. The most typical example is the cross-reactivity in patients with birch pollen AR who develop oral symptoms when eating apples, hazelnut, celery, etc. Typically, when these foods are cooked or processed they can be eaten without causing allergic reactions. Allergic reactions in secondary allergy are usually less severe than in primary food allergy [27]. Common symptoms, which usually come on immediately, include: redness, mild swelling or itching of the lips, tongue, inside of the mouth, soft palate and ears, itching and mild swelling affecting the throat. Occasionally, people might also experience symptoms in the oesophagus (gullet) or stomach, causing abdominal pain, nausea and even vomiting. Sneezing, runny nose, or eye symptoms can also occur.

Those sensitised to both birch and grass pollens are more likely to develop pollen food syndrome [28, 29]. They may also experience symptoms to a wider range of fresh fruits and raw vegetables than those who are sensitised to birch pollen alone.

In one Italian study of pollen sensitive AR subjects aged 4–18 years old, a longer AR duration was significantly associated with moderate-to-severe AR symptoms (p = 0.004), and with co-morbidities such as asthma (p 0.030), PFS was present in 24% (p < 0.001) [30]. In a study of 110 UK adults with spring hay fever, 52 participants (47%) were diagnosed with PFS, which is the commonest form of food allergy in the UK [29].

Interestingly, birth order effects differ for different allergic disorders in a large Japanese study of 14,669 schoolchildren aged 7–15 years [31]. There was no significant difference in the prevalence of BA or AD according to birth order, whereas the prevalence of AR, allergic conjunctivitis and FA decreased significantly as birth order increased. This raises questions about the effects of hygiene on different allergic manifestations.

### Treatment
PFS is usually a mild type of food allergy that occurs upon contact of the mouth and throat with raw fruits or vegetables containing epitopes also present in a pollen to which the subject is sensitized [32].

PFS is a problem in patients sensitized to various pollen allergens. There was clear association between PFS and polyvalent airborne allergy (69%). Cross-reactivity patterns were typical (for example, tree pollen allergy—intolerance of apples, carrots and potatoes; grass pollen allergy—intolerance of kiwi fruit and tomatoes). Subcutaneous SIT significantly alleviated PFS symptoms associated with ingestion of the responsible fruit and vegetables in patients [33].

The treatment is avoidance of the food(s) causing reaction(s). Adrenalin is only indicated if severe reactions are described in the medical history, or if there are reactions to processed food. For primary food allergy an experimental study of SIT using peanuts was suspended because of adverse reactions [34].

SIT for food allergy is reaching the point where it may soon be used routinely in clinical practice. Sublingual immunotherapy is effective for desensitization with a very favorable adverse event profile. Epicutaneous immunotherapy is also effective, most notably in younger children, with a high rate of local reactions. Oral immunotherapy demonstrates high efficacy, but with a higher risk of gastrointestinal and systemic adverse events. The need for long-term application to sustain desensitization is currently unclear. Immunomodulatory adjuvants may be added to enhance or diminish the immunogenicity of proteins, whereas genetic modifications of food allergens are designed to limit the risk of adverse reactions and address the issues of standardization and supply [35].

The most common pollen-fruit cross-reaction is the birch-apple syndrome [36]. Mauro et al. [36] investigated patients with birch-apple syndrome to evaluate the outcome of subcutaneous immunotherapy (SCIT) and sublingual immunotherapy (SLIT). Two of 8 SCIT-treated patients (25%) and 1 of 7 SLIT-treated patients (14.2%) developed complete tolerance to apple. In the remaining patients, an increase in the provocative dose was found in 3 of the SCIT-treated (37.5%) and 2 of the SLIT-treated patients (28.6%). They concluded that different doses of birch extract may be needed in different patients to improve the associated apple allergy and that a finer diagnostic work-up in selecting patients with birch-apple syndrome who are candidates to respond to birch pollen IT also concerning apple allergy is required [36].

## Eosinophilic oesophagitis (EoE)
### Description
EoE is currently defined as a "chronic, immune/antigen-mediated esophageal disease characterized clinically by symptoms related to esophageal dysfunction and histologically by eosinophil-predominant inflammation" [37].

EoE is a clinicopathologic disorder diagnosed by clinicians taking into consideration both clinical and pathologic information:

- Symptoms related to esophageal dysfunction;
- Eosinophil-predominant inflammation on esophageal biopsy, which is required for diagnosis, characteristically consisting of a peak value of $\geq$15 eos per high power field (eos/hpf) [38];
- Response to treatment (dietary elimination; topical corticosteroids) supports, but it is not required, for diagnosis (Strong recommendation, low evidence) [37].

### Extent of co-occurrence
EoE is commonly associated with other atopic diatheses (e.g. food allergy, asthma, eczema, chronic rhinitis, environmental allergies) [39]. In adults, solid food dysphagia is the most common presenting symptom [40, 41], with food impaction necessitating endoscopic bolus removal occurs in 33–54% of adult EoE patients [42]. Other symptoms in adults include chest pain, heartburn and upper abdominal pain [38, 43].

### Treatment
- *Acid suppression* Approximately one-third of patients with suspected eosinophilic esophagitis have a good clinical and histologic response to proton pump inhibitors (PPIs alone, suggesting that GERD, or a PPI-responsive form of esophageal eosinophilia, may be responsible [44, 45].
- *Dietary therapy* is an effective treatment for eosinophilic esophagitis in children and adults. Dietary

therapy is based upon the observation that patients with eosinophilic esophagitis have high rates of food allergies, and that those allergies may contribute to the development of eosinophilic esophagitis [44].

*Topical corticosteroids* have been proven to be an effective therapy for EoE and are a first-line therapy. Whilst available as multi-dose inhalers or aqueous nebulizer solutions for use in asthma, to treat EoE the medication is swallowed rather than inhaled to coat the esophagus and provide topical medication delivery (Recommendation strong, evidence high) [38].

Oral prednisone (a synthetic corticosteroid drug) may be useful to treat EoE if topical steroids are not effective or in patients who require rapid improvement in symptoms (Recommendation conditional, evidence low) [38].

Patients without symptomatic and histologic improvement after topical steroids might benefit from a longer course of topical steroids, higher doses of topical steroids, systemic steroids, an elimination diet or esophageal dilatation (Recommendation conditional, evidence low) [38].

- *Esophageal dilation* Dilation of esophageal strictures is effective for relieving dysphagia, but has no effect on underlying inflammation [46, 47].
- *Other experimental treatments* Prostaglandin D2 receptor antagonist [48], leukotriene inhibitors (Montelukast) [49], Mepolizumab: humanized monoclonal antibody against interleukin (IL)-5 [50], purine analogues (Azathioprine or 6-mercaptopurine) [44, 51].

### Allergic conjunctivitis
#### Extent of co-occurrence
Allergic conjunctivitis is the typical conjunctival reaction in AR. It occurs following exposure to allergens. Ocular symptoms occur in 50–70% of patients with rhinitis, being more common with outdoor than with indoor allergens [52]. Pitt et al. [53] reported that seasonal allergic conjunctivitis (SAC) is associated with significant reductions in both ocular and general quality of life.

#### Effects of co-occurrence
Eye symptoms include itching, watering, redness and difficulty with vision due to these. Ocular symptoms are reduced by nasal air filters [54], suggesting that some eye involvement is secondary to nasal reflexes.

#### Treatment
Some INS reduce eye symptoms as well as nasal ones, the recent molecules appear more consistently effective [55]. The combination of intranasal antihistamine plus INS

shows greater efficacy on rhinoconjunctivitis [56]. The topical ocular antihistamines, antazoline, azelastine, and emedastine, provide rapid relief of the symptoms of allergic conjunctivitis [57].

### Rhinosinusitis
#### Extent of co-occurrence
The extent of co-occurrence of rhinosinusitis is disputed and is likely to be different in acute rhinosinusitis (ARS), chronic rhinosinusitis (CRS) and CRS with nasal polyposis.

#### Effects of co-occurrence
When considering the role of allergy in sinus disease, it can be speculated that nasal inflammation induced by IgE-mediated mechanisms favours the development of acute and/or chronic sinus disease [58, 59].

Several mechanisms could explain the link between allergic inflammation and sinus disease. Allergic inflammation of the nasal mucosa may give rise to mucosal congestion leading to impaired mucus drainage at the ostiomeatal complex in predisposed patients. Ostiomeatal pathology is considered to be essential to the generation of sinus-related symptoms [59].

Certainly, AR sufferers experience common colds (which are a form of acute rhinosinusitis) more severely and for longer than those without underlying minimal persistent inflammation [11]. The contribution of AR to chronic rhinosinusitis is less clear (EPOS 2012) [9]. One study has demonstrated that, in children, the degree of atopy (as reflected by the number of aeroallergen sensitivities or the presence of atopic multi-morbidities) is not associated with progression to CRS in the pediatric age group [60].

Symptoms of IgE-mediated allergic inflammation should be asked for during history taking in patients with CRS and specific allergy evaluation should be performed in case of clinical suspicion. With regard to treatment, it is recommended that anti-allergic therapy is added to the treatment of patients with chronic sinus disease and concomitant allergy [61].

#### Chronic rhinosinusitis with nasal polyps (CRSwNP)
Chronic rhinosinusitis with nasal polyps (CRSwNP) is associated with high concentrations of IgE in nasal polyp (NP) tissue. CRSwNP often coexists with asthma and this group is particularly characterized with tissue eosinophilia and high local IgE levels [62]. Therefore, an allergic aetiology of NPs has been presumed, though never firmly demonstrated. Between 0.5 and 4.5% of subjects with AR have NPs, which compares with the normal population [9]. In a retrospective study by Settipane and Chafee [63], the nasal polyps were present in 4.2% of the total

population of 4986 subjects. Nasal polyp frequency rate was 6.7% in asthmatic patients and 2.2% in the rhinitis alone group. Of the total 211 cases of nasal polyps, 71% had asthma and 29% had rhinitis alone [63]. Pang et al. [64] reported that food allergen intradermal tests were more positive in nasal polyp patients (81%) compared to controls (11%).

In mucosal tissues, mRNA for the ε-chain of IgE was associated with a significant proportion of B cells [65, 66]. Recent evidence has shown local IgE synthesis, local receptor revision, class switch recombination and B-cell differentiation into IgE-secreting plasma cells in NPs [64]. In NPs, the level of IgE is independent of the atopic status of the patient [65, 67, 68] whereas specific IgE in NPs is only partly related to skin prick test positivity [65, 67, 68]. The local IgE in NPs is the result of two types of IgE production: systemic allergic IgE formation and a local polyclonal IgE formation [65, 66]. Local polyclonal IgE correlates with the presence of *Staphylococcus aureus* enterotoxins (SAE) [9, 65–67]. Finally, Gevaert et al. [69] demonstrated that antagonizing IgE by injections of omalizumab is effective for both allergic and nonallergic CRSwNP. The later finding proves the relevance of local mucosal IgE.

CRSwNP is an IgE mediated disease; however, the role of atopy is less clear.

### Otitis media with effusion (OME)
#### Extent of co-occurrence
In one hospital population of children with chronic OME, over 80% had rhinitis [70]. A population survey in Slough schools (in the UK) also demonstrated an association between OME type symptoms and rhinitis [71].

OME is much rarer in adults and is usually found in association with more severe rhinosinusitis (such as aspirin exacerbated respiratory disease, allergic fungal sinusitis and Churg Strauss syndrome) rather than with rhinitis [9].

#### Effects of co-occurrence
The Eustachian tube exerts a major function in middle ear homeostasis via its role in the ventilation and protection of the middle ear and mucociliary clearance. The Eustachian tube contains an allergic inflammatory infiltrate in AR patients [72]. It is therefore not surprising that allergic inflammation with concomitant mucosal swelling may impair the function of the Eustachian tube [73].

Concomitant occurrence of allergic diseases and primary immune deficiencies was reported by Klemola [74]. Klemola [74] reported that 50% of the children with atopic disease had selective IgA deficiency (sIgAD). In allergic diseases such as asthma, atopic dermatitis, allergic rhinitis, and conjunctivitis, there is predisposition to infections resulting from an immunodeficiency [75].

Immune deficiencies and infections may contribute to the development of OME.

#### Treatment
Because of the pathophysiological associations of AR with OME, treatments focusing on allergic inflammation may be helpful in the management of OME [76]. A meta-analysis of 16 randomized controlled trials demonstrated no significant benefit from antihistamines, decongestants, or combined antihistamines and decongestants versus placebo for treatment of OME [77]. Intranasal corticosteroids did reduce the need for surgery in a double blind study in which autoinflation of the middle ear was also effective, but the combination of the two was less efficacious [78].

Atopic status and nasal disease should be evaluated in recurrent or chronic OME patients who have had no response to antibiotic therapy, and INS could be used as an adjunct to treatment of some OME patients. Further studies are needed to elucidate whether atopic status or rhinitis itself may influence the development of OME and the extent of ear involvement in various forms of rhinosinusitis.

### Adenoid hypertrophy (AH)
The adenoid tissue is a peripheral lymphoid organ located in the nasopharynx, forming part of Waldeyer's ring. It contributes to the development of immunity against inhaled micro-organisms in early life. The volume of the adenoid increases with age and is maximal at 5–6 years, followed by a gradual decrease in volume by the age of 8–9 years [79]. Symptoms related to AH are nasal obstruction, open mouth breathing and snoring. 'Adenoid face' can be caused by AH or by severe obstructive rhinitis [61].

#### Extent of co-occurrence
Children with AR appear to have a greater susceptibility to AH than non-allergic children, with IgE-mediated inflammation of the nasal mucosa likely playing a role in both conditions [80].

Adenoid hypertrophy in adults is rare and may indicate underlying malignancy or infection, such as human immune deficiency virus (HIV), rather than allergy.

#### Treatment
Treatment of AR with intranasal corticosteroids has been shown to improve various parameters associated with adenoid hypertrophy [81].

### Olfactory dysfunction
#### Extent of co-occurrence
In a recent study of 51 subjects with AR, half had hyposmia [82]. Half of AR subjects with a normal CT scored

in the 30th percentile in an olfactory test. The degree of olfactory dysfunction does not seem to be related to the degree of nasal obstruction/nasal resistance [82], although with perennial (persistent) AR, the olfactory dysfunction seems to be more stable and more persistent throughout the year [83].

Reduced olfaction is more common in chronic rhinosinusitis, especially when NPs are present [9].

### Effects of co-occurrence

AR may have a negative impact on olfactory function and is considered to be a sinonasal-related origin of chemosensory dysfunction [84]. This is probably secondary to a local inflammation in the nasal fossa and around the olfactory neuroepithelium in the olfactory cleft rather than a nasal obstruction impairing the odours to reach the olfactory cleft [82].

Olfactory function is a global perception of orthonasal and retronasal stimuli and of a stimulation of intranasal trigeminal nerve endings. The trigeminal function is enhanced in patients with AR and a link exists between chemosensory trigeminal function and neuroinflammation [85]. Antidromic activation of the trigeminal nerve after allergen and/or chemosensory stimuli leads to the liberation of neuropeptides and classical trigeminal related symptoms such as sneezing and itching.

### Treatment

Systemic corticosteroid is the first-line-treatment for olfactory dysfunction of sinonasal origin but use must be short term because of side-effects. Topical corticosteroid does not reach the same efficacy but has a good safety profile [86]. Nasal corticosteroids have a positive impact on AR-related olfactory dysfunction [87]. However, most studies have used a visual analogue scale to evaluate olfactory function, which is known to be a poor tool in comparison with other test modalities such as threshold, discrimination or identification tasks in olfactory testing.

Antihistamines also have a positive effect on the olfactory function even if prescribed for a short period of time [88]. Olfactory dysfunction has marked effects on quality of life when severe and needs to be taken into account in the evaluation of comorbidities related to the presence of AR.

### Laryngitis, cough and vocal problems
#### Effects of co-occurrence
The passage of mediators, cytokines and secretions backwards from the nose should not reach the larynx, unless epiglottic function is disturbed. However, many patients with AR do experience throat symptoms, including irritation, the sensation of difficult to shift mucus and cough [89]. In a recent study on AR and laryngeal symptoms,

involving six controls and six adult singers, nasal provocation with pollen extracts caused a rapid induction of laryngeal irritation and globus sensation. However, no objective changes occurred then, nor during the pollen season [90].

### Treatment

Edema of the laryngeal mucosa, laryngeal erythema and candidiasis may all be found in a minority of patients treated with inhaled glucocorticosteroids [91], but are not reported after the prolonged use of a nasal steroid spray.

### Gastro esophageal reflux (GER)

Gastro esophageal reflux (GER) may masquerade as CRS [92]. Associations have been reported between GER and a variety of upper and lower respiratory tract conditions but not with AR [73].

### Obstructive sleep apnea (OSA) and sleep impairment

The effect of AR on sleep can impair quality of life [93]. Patients with AR have more difficulties in falling asleep, take more sleeping drugs, suffer from nocturnal awakenings, and feel that they do not get sufficient sleep when compared to healthy controls [94].

### Treatment

One study [93] has demonstrated an improvement in OSA in a short-term trial of intranasal fluticasone propionate. The mixed/obstructive apnea-hypopnea index decreased by $4.9 \pm 1.0$ events per hour in the fluticasone propionate group and increased by $2.2 \pm 3.3$ events per hour in the placebo group [94]. Craig et al. studied a group of 20 adults with perennial rhinitis and sleep complaints, examining the benefit of twice-daily nasal flunisolide using a double-blind, placebo-controlled, crossover study. They found that nasal congestion and subjective sleep improved significantly in the topical corticosteroid-treated subjects. They concluded that the fatigue in perennial allergies may be a result of nasal congestion and associated sleep fragmentation. Decreasing nasal congestion with nasal steroids may improve sleep, daytime fatigue, and the quality of life of patients with AR [95].

### Fatigue and learning impairment
#### Extent of co-occurrence
Patients with AR frequently complain of disordered sleep, daytime somnolence and inability to concentrate. Recent studies document daytime somnolence in children with AR. Craig et al. [95] reported an association between daytime somnolence and nasal congestion in a group of patients with AR. If nasal symptoms such as

itching, sneezing, rhinorrhea, and congestion are not well controlled during the day, they may contribute to learning problems during school hours. If these symptoms are not well controlled during the night, they may contribute to nocturnal sleep loss, secondary daytime fatigue and learning impairment [96].

### Effects of co-occurrence

Baraniuk et al. [97], in a study of chronic fatigue syndrome, failed to document an increase in AR in these patients. However, patients with AR (unlike the group with rheumatologic disease) had significantly increased symptoms of fatigue intermediate between levels of

**Table 2　Diagnosis of multi-morbidities associated with allergic rhinitis (AR)**

| Multi-morbidities of AR | Definitive medical history, symptoms and signs |
|---|---|
| Asthma | Ask about any history of cough, wheeze, shortness of breath, exercise-induced bronchospasm |
| | Examine the chest for wheeze, hyperexpansion |
| | Assess peak expiratory flows and spirometry in older children preferably with reversibility testing with beta-2 agonists |
| | If in doubt, undertake an exercise, mannitol or methacholine challenge test or measure exhaled nitric oxide (FENO) |
| Conjunctivitis | Ask about a history of red, itchy, watery eyes, eye rubbing |
| | Examine eyes |
| Rhinosinusitis | Ask about a history of nasal obstruction or discharge (purulent) with or without hyposmia, headache, facial pain or cough |
| | Undertake nasendoscopy in older children |
| | CT scan/sinus X-rays not recommended unless there are complications or failed therapy, unilateral symptoms or severe disease unresponsive to medical therapy |
| Otitis media with effusion (OME)/impaired hearing | Ask questions related to immune deficiency and/or recurrent infections |
| | Ask about any speech and language delay, increasing volume of TV, shouting, poor concentration, failing performance at school, frustration, irritability |
| | Examine the ears using a pneumatic otoscope if possible, and Weber and Rinne tests |
| | Use tympanoscopy for evaluation of tympanic membrane and middle ear |
| | Undertake tympanometry |
| | Use a whisper test to screen otitis media with effusion and hearing loss |
| | Use audiometry in older children—pure tones, speech |
| Obstructive sleep apnea and sleep problems | Enquire about any history of disturbed sleep, snoring, apnoea, tiredness, irritability |
| | Assess nasal airway using spatula misting, nasal inspiratory peak flow, visual examination of nostrils and nasendoscopy in older children to view nasal airway and adenoids |
| | Consider sleep study |
| Atopic dermatitis | Ask about skin symptoms of itching, redness, rash |
| Food allergy | Ask about symptoms related to food intake |
| | Ask for oral allergy syndrome (OAS): Allergic reaction that occurs upon contact of the mouth and throat with raw fruits or vegetables which may be tolerated when cooked |
| Eosinophilic oesophagitis | Ask for symptoms related to esophageal dysfunction as solid food dysphagia, chest pain, heartburn and upper abdominal pain |
| | Assess esophageal biopsies |
| Adenoid hypertrophy | Ask about nasal obstruction, open mouth breathing and snoring |
| | Examine the face |
| | Perform posterior rhinoscopy; nasal and nasopharyngeal rigid/flexible endoscopy |
| Olfactory dysfunction | Ask for olfactory dysfunction, hyposmia, anosmia |
| | Evaluate nasal airway and smell function tests |
| Laryngitis, cough and vocal problems | Ask for symptoms including irritation in the throat, the sensation of difficult to shift mucus and cough |
| | Examine throat and larynx, see vocal cords and arytenoids |
| Gastro esophageal reflux | Ask for symptoms of indigestion, regurgitation, cough |
| | Examine throat and larynx |
| Fatigue and learning impairment | Ask about fatigue and learning impairment, school success |
| | Ask about sleep quality, nasal obstruction and nasal discharge |
| Turbinate hypertrophy | Ask about nasal obstruction |
| | Perform anterior rhinoscopy and nasal endoscopy, acoustic rhinometry pre and post decongestant shows whether mucosal lining or bony structure is responsible |

fatigue seen in normal subjects and patients with chronic fatigue syndrome.

AR can reduce driving performance [98]. It can also impair examination performance in adolescents [99].

### Treatment

In a study involving major examinations, sedating antihistamines increased the likelihood of dropping an examination grade [99]. The medications used to treat allergic rhinitis may cause central nervous system adverse effects and contribute to learning impairment. The newer relatively nonsedating medications such as loratadine, cetirizine, and fexofenadine have less potential to impair central nervous system function and learning than their predecessors [96].

### Turbinate hypertrophy
### Extent of co-occurrence

In AR patients, nasal obstruction is a bothersome symptom which is most commonly due to inferior turbinate hypertrophy. The inferior turbinate is the initial deposit point for allergens and undergoes dynamic changes through the allergic cascade, which results in nasal obstruction. Targeting the inferior turbinate to augment the nasal airway is the mainstay of surgical treatment in AR [100].

### Effects of co-occurence

The turbinates are tiny shelf-like bony structures that project into the nasal passageways. They help warm, humidify, and clean the air that passes over them. If turbinate hypertrophy develops, it causes persistent nasal congestion and, sometimes, pressure and headache in the middle of the face and forehead. This condition may require surgery [101].

### Treatment

Turbinate hypertrophy which is multimorbidity of the AR is primarily treated by allergen avoidance and medical treatment, but when these measures fail to control symptoms then surgery to the inferior turbinates of nose can be performed [102]. Outfracture, submucous resection, laser vaporization, radiofrequency ablation, and coblation, cryosurgery, submucous electrocautery, and microdebrider turbinoplasty are treatment options in turbinate hypertrophy related to AR [103].

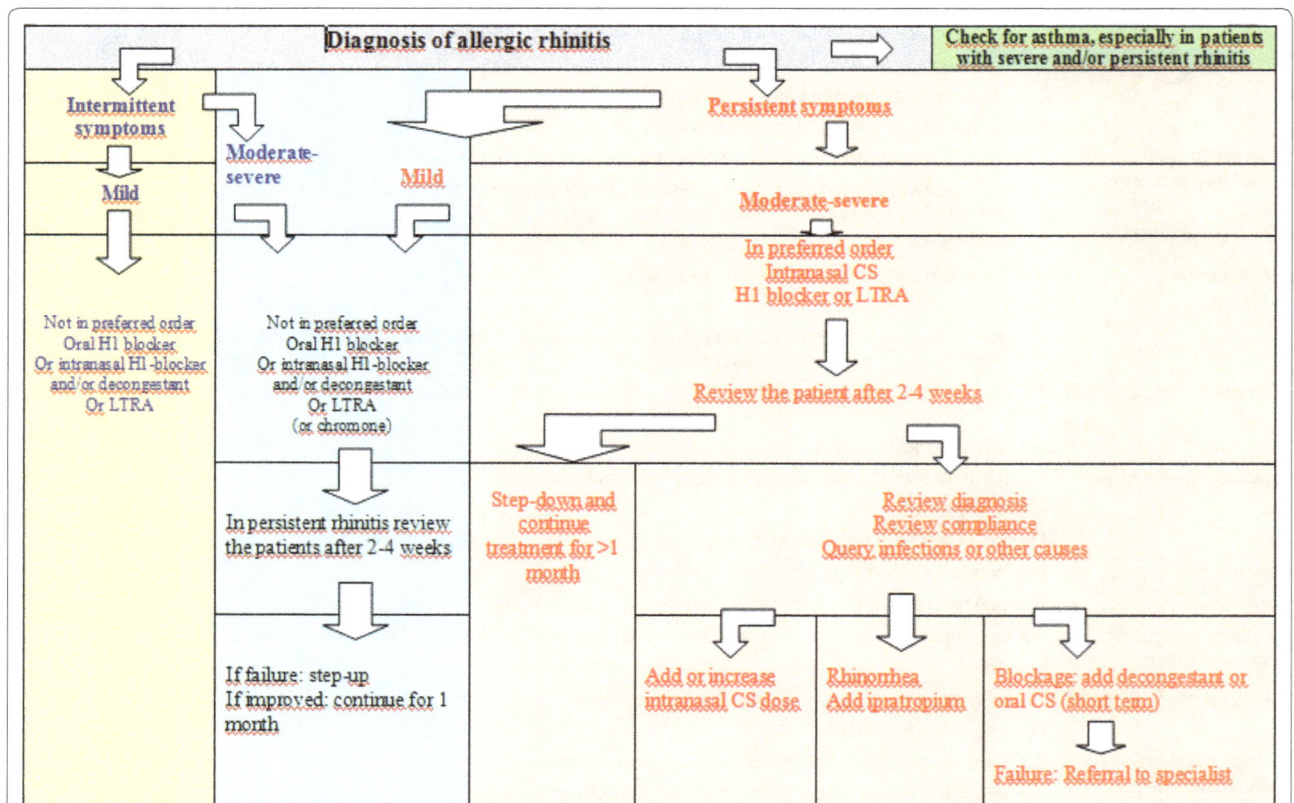

**Fig. 1** Treatment for AR (taken from ARIA 2012) [104]. In addition to the pathways presented in the figure allergen and irritant avoidance may be appropriate; for conjunctivitis, add an oral H1-blocker, intraocular H1-blocker or intraocular cromone (or saline); consider specific immunotherapy when pharmacotherapy fails or is unacceptable to the patient

## Diagnosis

Diagnosis of multi-morbidities of AR are shown in Table 2 [3].

A physical examination of all organ systems potentially affected by allergies, with emphasis on the upper respiratory tract, should be performed in patients with a history of rhinitis.

## Treatment

During the treatment of AR, multi-morbidities (co-morbidities) of AR should be considered. Treatment of AR according to guidelines may cause decreasing the nasal symptoms; and may cause improvement of the co-morbid problems; see Fig. 1 [104].

## Conclusion

This EAACI Task Force Report on AR Multi-morbidities has defined and classified the multi-morbidities associated with AR, together with providing recommendations for diagnosis and treatment. The information provided here should help improve allergists' knowledge and skills, ultimately improving the overall quality of patient care, as well as helping to raise the profile of this important area of work.

### Authors' contributions
All authors contributed to design, planning, literature survey and writing.

### Author details
[1] Department of Otorhinolaryngology, Eskisehir Osmangazi University School of Medicine, Eskisehir, Turkey. [2] Upper Airway Research Laboratory, Ghent University Hospital, Ghent, Belgium. [3] Institute of Medical Statistics, Informatics, and Epidemiology, Medical Faculty, University of Köln, Cologne, Germany. [4] Allergy Unit, IBIMA, Regional University Hospital of Malaga, UMA, Malaga, Spain. [5] Clinical division of Otorhinolaryngology, Head and Neck Surgery, University Hospitals Leuven, Louvain, Belgium. [6] London Allergy and Immunology Centre, London, UK. [7] ENT Department, Faculty of Medicine, Kirikkale University, Kirikkale, Turkey. [8] Royal National Throat, Nose and Ear Hospital, London, UK. [9] Faculty of Medicine, ENT Department, University of Oradea, Oradea, Romania. [10] Institut de Recherche Expérimentale et Clinique (IREC), Pole de Pneumologie, ORL & Dermatologie, Université catholique de Louvain, Louvain-la-Neuve, Belgium. [11] Department of Otorhinolaryngology, Head and Neck Surgery, Academic Medical Centre (AMC), Amsterdam, The Netherlands. [12] Christine Kuhne-Center for Allergy Research and Education, Swiss Institute of Allergy and Asthma Research, University of Zurich, Davos, Switzerland. [13] Hôpital Arnaud de Villeneuve, University Hospital of Montpellier, Montpellier, France. [14] Unitat de Rinologia i Clinica de l'Olfacte, Servei d'Otorinolaringologia, Hospital Clínic, Barcelona, Catalonia, Spain. [15] The Referral Centre for Food Allergy Diagnosis and Treatment Veneto Region, Department of Mother and Child Health, University of Padua, Padua, Italy. [16] Allergy Department, 2nd Pediatric Clinic, University of Athens, Athens, Greece. [17] Nippon Medical School, Tokyo, Japan. [18] Service d'ORL, Cliniques Universitaires St-Luc, Brussels, Belgium. [19] Department of Otorhinolaryngology-Head and Neck Surgery, Temple University, Philadelphia, PA, USA. [20] Department of Otorhinolaryngology and Head and Neck Surgery, University Hospital Sestre milosrdnice, Zagreb, Croatia. [21] Department of Otorhinolaryngology, University Hospital of Crete, Crete, Greece.

### Competing interests
The authors declare that they have no competing interests.

### References
1. Sih T, Mion O. Allergic rhinitis in the child and associated comorbidities. Pediatr Allergy Immunol. 2010;21:e107–13.
2. Scadding GK, Bousquet J. Introduction: allergic rhinitis. Allergy. 2007;62(Suppl 85):3–5.
3. Roberts G, Xatzipsalti M, Borrego LM, Custovic A, Halken S, Hellings PW, et al. Paediatric rhinitis: position paper of the European academy of allergy and clinical immunology. Allergy. 2013;68:1102–16.
4. Comorbidity [Internet]. Wikipedia, the free encyclopedia. http://en.wikipedia.org/wiki/Comorbidity. Accessed 2 Dec 2013.
5. Lack G. Pediatric allergic rhinitis and comorbid disorders. J Allergy Clin Immunol. 2001;108(Suppl 1):S9–15.
6. Pinart M, Benet M, Annesi-Maesano I, von Berg A, Berdel D, Carlsen KC, et al. Comorbidity of eczema, rhinitis and asthma in Ig-E sensitised and non-IgE-sensitised children in MeDALL: a population-based cohort study. Lancet Respir Med. 2014;2:131–40.
7. Brydon MJ. Skin prick testing in general practice. J Adv Nurs. 1998;27:442–4.
8. Bousquet J, Van Cauwenberge P, Khaltaev N, Aria Workshop Group, World Health Organization. Allergic rhinitis and its impact on asthma. J Allergy Clin Immunol. 2001;108(Suppl 5):S147–334.
9. Fokkens WJ, Lund VJ, Mullol J, Bachert C, Alobid I, Baroody F, et al. European Position paper on rhinosinusitis and nasal polyps 2012. Rhinol Suppl. 2012;23:3 p **(preceding table of contents, 1-298)**.
10. Gaga M, Frew AJ, Varney VA, Kay AB. Eosinophil activation and T lymphocyte infiltration in allergen-induced late phase skin reactions and classical delayed-type hypersensitivity. J Immunol. 1991;147:816–22.
11. Katelaris CH, Linneberg A, Magnan A, Thomas WR, Wardlaw AJ, Wark P. Developments in the field of allergy in 2010 through the eyes of clinical and experimental allergy. Clin Exp Allergy. 2011;41:1690–710.
12. Ciprandi G, Pronzato C, Ricca V, Passalacqua G, Bagnasco M, Canonica GW. Allergen-specific challenge induces intercellular adhesion molecule 1 (ICAM-1 or CD54) on nasal epithelial cells in allergic subjects: relationships with early and late inflammatory phenomena. Am J Respir Crit Care Med. 1994;150:1653–9.
13. Braunstahl GJ. United airways concept: what does it teach us about systemic inflammation in airways disease? Proc Am Thorac Soc. 2009;6:652–4.
14. Shaaban R, Zureik M, Soussan D, Neukirch C, Heinrich J, Sunyer J, et al. Rhinitis and onset of asthma: a longitudinal population-based study. Lancet. 2008;372:1049–57.
15. Clatworthy J, Price D, Ryan D, Haughney J, Horne R. The value of self-report assessment of adherence, rhinitis and smoking in relation to asthma control. Prim Care Respir J. 2009;18:300–5.
16. Ciprandi G, Cirillo I, Signori A. Impact of allergic rhinitis on bronchi: an 8-year follow-up study. Am J Rhinol Allergy. 2011;25:e72–6.
17. Navarro A, Valero A, Juliá B, Quirce S. Coexistence of asthma and allergic rhinitis in adult patients attending allergy clinics: ONEAIR study. J Investig Allergol Clin Immunol. 2008;18:233–8.
18. Ko FW, Ip MS, Chu CM, So LK, Lam DC, Hui DS. Prevalence of allergic rhinitis and its associated morbidity in adults with asthma: a multicentre study. Hong Kong Med J. 2010;16:354–61.
19. Valero A, Pereira C, Loureiro C, Martínez-Cócera C, Murio C, Rico P, et al. Interrelationship between skin sensitization, rhinitis, and asthma in patients with allergic rhinitis: a study of Spain and Portugal. J Investig Allergol Clin Immunol. 2009;19:167–72.
20. Mölter A, Simpson A, Berdel D, Brunekreef B, Custovic A, Cyrys J, et al. A multicentre study of air pollution exposure and childhood asthma prevalence: the ESCAPE project. Eur Respir J 2014. [Epub ahead of print].
21. Lee CH, Chuang HY, Shih CC, Jee SH, Wang LF, Chiu HC, et al. Correlation of serum total IgE, eosinophil granule cationic proteins, sensitized allergens and family aggregation in atopic dermatitis patients with or without rhinitis. J Dermatol. 2004;31:784–93.
22. Lugović L, Lipozenćić J. Are respiratory allergic diseases related to atopic dermatitis? Coll Antropol. 2000;24:335–45.
23. Solé D, Camelo-Nunes IC, Wandalsen GF, Melo KC, Naspitz CK. Is rhinitis alone or associated with atopic eczema a risk factor for severe asthma in children? Pediatr Allergy Immunol. 2005;16:121–5.
24. Silverberg JI, Simpson EL. Association between severe eczema in children and multiple comorbid conditions and healthcare utilization. Pediatr Allergy Immunol. 2013;24:476–86.

25. Umeki S. Allergic cycle: relationships between asthma, allergic rhinitis, and atopic dermatitis. J Asthma. 1994;31:19–26.

26. Popescu F-D. Cross-reactivity between aeroallergens and food allergens. World J Methodol. 2015;26(5):31–50. doi:10.5662/wjm.v5.i2.31.

27. Caliskaner Z, Naiboglu B, Kutlu A, Kartal O, Ozturk S, Onem Y, et al. Risk factors for pollen food syndrome in patients with seasonal allergic rhinitis. Med Oral Patol Oral Cir Bucal. 2011;16:e312–6.

28. Asero R, Massironi F, Velati C. Detection of prognostic factors for pollen food syndrome in patients with birch pollen hypersensitivity. J Allergy Clin Immunol. 1996;2:611–6.

29. Skypala IJ, Calderon MA, Leeds AR, Emery P, Till SJ, Durham SR. Development and validation of a structured questionnaire for the diagnosis of pollen food syndrome in subjects with seasonal allergic rhinitis during the UK birch pollen season. Clin Exp Allergy. 2011;41:1001–11.

30. Dondi A, Tripodi S, Panetta V, Asero R, Businco AD, Bianchi A, et al. Pollen-induced allergic rhinitis in 1360 Italian children: comorbidities and determinants of severity. Pediatr Allergy Immunol. 2013;24:742–51.

31. Kusunoki T, Mukaida K, Morimoto T, Sakuma M, Yasumi T, Nishikomori R, et al. Birth order effect on childhood food allergy. Pediatr Allergy Immunol. 2012;23:250–4.

32. Pongdee T. Pollen food syndrome (PFS). The American Academy of Allergy, Asthma & Immunology (AAAAI). https://www.aaaai.org/conditions-and-treatments/library/allergy-library/outdoor-allergies-and-food-allergies-can-be-relate. Accessed 30 Mar 2017.

33. Czarnecka-Operacz M, Jenerowicz D, Silny W. Oral allergy syndrome in patients with airborne pollen allergy treated with specific immunotherapy. Acta Dermatovenerol Croat. 2008;16:19–24.

34. Nelson HS, Lahr J, Rule R, et al. Treatment of anaphylactic sensitivity to peanuts by immunotherapy with injections of aqueous peanuts extract. J Allergy Clin Immunol. 1997;99:744–51.

35. Reisacher WR, Davison W. Immunotherapy for food allergy. Curr Opin Otolaryngol Head Neck Surg. 2017;. doi:10.1097/MOO.0000000000000353 **[Epub ahead of print]**

36. Mauro M, Russello M, Incorvaia C, Gazzola G, Frati F, Moingeon P, Passalacqua G. Birch-apple syndrome treated with birch pollen immunotherapy. Int Arch Allergy Immunol. 2011;156:416–22. doi:10.1159/000323909 **[Epub 2011 Aug 10]**

37. Liacouras CA, Furuta GT, Hirano I, Atkins D, Attwood SE, Bonis PA, et al. Eosinophilic esophagitis: updated consensus recommendations for children and adults. J Allergy Clin Immunol. 2011;128:3–20.

38. Dellon ES, Gonsalves N, Hirano I, Furuta GT, Liacouras CA, Katzka DA, American College of Gastroenterology. ACG clinical guideline: evidenced based approach to the diagnosis and management of esophageal eosinophilia and eosinophilic esophagitis (EoE). Am J Gastroenterol. 2013;108:679–92 **(quiz 693)**.

39. Furuta GT, Liacouras CA, Collins MH, Gupta SK, Justinich C, Putnam PE, et al. Eosinophilic esophagitis in children and adults: a systematic review and consensus recommendations for diagnosis and treatment. Gastroenterology. 2007;133:1342–63.

40. Prasad GA, Talley NJ, Romero Y, Arora AS, Kryzer LA, Smyrk TC, et al. Prevalence and predictive factors of eosinophilic esophagitis in patients presenting with dysphagia: a prospective study. Am J Gastroenterol. 2007;102:2627–32.

41. Mackenzie SH, Go M, Chadwick B, Thomas K, Fang J, Kuwada S, et al. Eosinophilic esophagitis in patients presenting with dysphagia: a prospective analysis. Aliment Pharmacol Ther. 2008;28:1140–6.

42. Desai TK, Stecevic V, Chang CH, Goldstein NS, Badizadegan K, Furuta GT. Association of eosinophilic inflammation with esophageal food impaction in adults. Gastrointest Endosc. 2005;61:795–801.

43. Fass R, Gasiorowska A. Refractory GERD: what is it? Curr Gastroenterol Rep. 2008;10:252–7.

44. Bomis PAL, Furuta GT. Treatment of eosinophilic esophagitis. In: Talley NJ, Grover S, editors. UpToDate. https://www.uptodate.com/contents/treatment-of-eosinophilic-esophagitis#H209980. Accessed 31 Mar 2017.

45. Peterson KA, Thomas KL, Hilden K, et al. Comparison of esomeprazole to aerosolized, swallowed fluticasone for eosinophilic esophagitis. Dig Dis Sci. 2010;55:1313.

46. Schoepfer AM, Gonsalves N, Bussmann C, et al. Esophageal dilation in eosinophilic esophagitis: effectiveness, safety, and impact on the underlying inflammation. Am J Gastroenterol. 2010;105:1062.

47. Robles-Medranda C, Villard F, le Gall C, et al. Severe dysphagia in children with eosinophilic esophagitis and esophageal stricture: an indication for balloon dilation? J Pediatr Gastroenterol Nutr. 2010;50:516.

48. Straumann A, Hoesli S, Bussmann Ch, et al. Anti-eosinophil activity and clinical efficacy of the CRTH2 antagonist OC000459 in eosinophilic esophagitis. Allergy. 2013;68:375.

49. Attwood SE, Lewis CJ, Bronder CS, et al. Eosinophilic oesophagitis: a novel treatment using Montelukast. Gut. 2003;52:181.

50. Straumann A, Conus S, Grzonka P, et al. Anti-interleukin-5 antibody treatment (mepolizumab) in active eosinophilic oesophagitis: a randomised, placebo-controlled, double-blind trial. Gut. 2010;59:21.

51. Netzer P, Gschossmann JM, Straumann A, et al. Corticosteroid-dependent eosinophilic oesophagitis: azathioprine and 6-mercaptopurine can induce and maintain long-term remission. Eur J Gastroenterol Hepatol. 2007;19:865.

52. Bonini S, Coassin M, Aronni S, Lambiase A. Vernal keratoconjunctivitis. Eye (Lond). 2004;18:345–51.

53. Pitt AD, Smith AF, Lindsell L, Voon LW, Rose PW, Bron AJ. Economic and quality-of-life impact of seasonal allergic conjunctivitis in Oxfordshire. Ophthalmic Epidemiol. 2004;11:17–33.

54. O'Meara TJ, Sercombe JK, Morgan G, Reddel HK, Xuan W, Tovey ER. The reduction of rhinitis symptoms by nasal filters during natural exposure to ragweed and grass pollen. Allergy. 2005;60(4):529–32.

55. Keith PK, Scadding GK. Are intranasal corticosteroids all equally consistent in managing ocular symptoms of seasonal allergic rhinitis? Curr Med Res Opin 2009;25:2021–41 **(Review. Erratum in: Curr Med Res Opin 2010; 26:177. Curr Med Res Opin 2010; 26:990)**.

56. Azelastine/fluticasone propionate (Dymista) for seasonal allergic rhinitis. Med Lett Drugs Ther. 2012; 54:85–7.

57. Williams PB, Crandall E, Sheppard JD. Azelastine hydrochloride, a dual-acting anti-inflammatory ophthalmic solution, for treatment of allergic conjunctivitis. Clin Ophthalmol. 2010;7(4):993–1001.

58. Rachelefsky GS, Goldberg M, Katz RM, Boris G, Gyepes MT, Shapiro MJ, et al. Sinus disease in children with respiratory allergy. J Allergy Clin Immunol. 1978;61:310–4.

59. Scadding GK. Recent advances in the treatment of rhinitis and rhinosinusitis. Int J Pediatr Otorhinolaryngol. 2003;67:S201–4.

60. Sedaghat AR, Phipatanakul W, Cunningham MJ. Atopy and the development of chronic rhinosinusitis in children with allergic rhinitis. J Allergy Clin Immunol Pract. 2013;6:689–91.

61. Hellings PW, Fokkens WJ. Allergic rhinitis and its impact on otorhinolaryngology. Allergy. 2006;61:656–64.

62. Bachert C, Zhang N, Holtappels G, De Lobel L, van Cauwenberge P, Liu S, et al. Presence of IL-5 protein and IgE antibodies to staphylococcal enterotoxins in nasal polyps is associated with comorbid asthma. J Allergy Clin Immunol. 2010;126:962–8.

63. Settipane GA, Chafee FH. Nasal polyps in asthma and rhinitis: a review of 6,037 patients. J Allergy Clin Immunol. 1977;59:17–21.

64. Pang YT, Eskici O, Wilson JA. Nasal polyposis: role of subclinical delayed food hypersensitivity. Otolaryngol Head Neck Surg. 2000;122:298–301.

65. Gevaert P, Holtappels G, Johansson SG, Cuvelier C, Cauwenberge P, Bachert C. Organization of secondary lymphoid tissue and local IgE formation to *Staphylococcus aureus* enterotoxins in nasal polyp tissue. Allergy. 2005;60:71–9.

66. Gevaert P, Nouri-Aria KT, Wu H, Harper CE, Takhar P, Fear DJ, et al. Local receptor revision and class switching to IgE in chronic rhinosinusitis with nasal polyps. Allergy. 2013;68:55–63.

67. Van Zele T, Gevaert P, Holtappels G, van Cauwenberge P, Bachert C. Local immunoglobulin production in nasal polyposis is modulated by superantigens. Clin Exp Allergy. 2007;37:1840–7.

68. Bachert C, Gevaert P, Holtappels G, Johansson SGO, Van Cauwenberge P. Total and specific IgE in nasal polyps is related to local eosinophilic inflammation. J Allergy Clin Immunol. 2001;107:607–14.

69. Gevaert P, Calus L, Van Zele T, Blomme K, De Ruyck N, Bauters W, et al. Omalizumab is effective in allergic and nonallergic patients with nasal polyps and asthma. J Allergy Clin Immunol. 2013;131:110–6.

70. Parikh A, Alles R, Hawk L, Pringle M, Darby Y, Scadding GK. Treatment of allergic rhinitis and its impact in children with chronic otitis media with effusion. J Audiol Med. 2000;9:104–17.

71. Umapathy D, Alles R, Scadding GK. A community based questionnaire study on the association between symptoms suggestive of otitis media

with effusion, rhinitis and asthma in primary school children. Int J Pediatr Otorhinolaryngol. 2007;71:705–12.

72. Nguyen LH, Manoukian JJ, Sobol SE, Tewfik TL, Mazer BD, Schloss MD, et al. Similar allergic inflammation in the middle ear and the upper airway: evidence linking otitis media with effusion to the united airways concept. J Allergy Clin Immunol. 2004;114:1110–5.

73. Bousquet J, Khaltaev N, Cruz AA, Denburg J, Fokkens WJ, Togias A, et al. Allergic Rhinitis and its Impact on Asthma (ARIA) 2008 update (in collaboration with the World Health Organization, GA(2)LEN and AllerGen). Allergy. 2008;63(Suppl 86):8–160.

74. Klemola T. Deficiency of immunoglobulin A. Ann Clin Res. 1987;19(4):248–57.

75. Aghamohammadi A, Cheraghi T, Gharagozlou M, et al. IgA deficiency: correlation between clinical and immunological phenotypes. J Clin Immunol. 2009;29:130–6.

76. Caffarelli C, Savini E, Giordano S, Gianlupi G, Cavagni G. Atopy in children with otitis media with effusion. Clin Exp Allergy. 1998;28:591–6.

77. Griffin GH, Flynn C, Bailey RE, Schultz JK. Antihistamines and/or decongestants for otitis media with effusion (OME) in children. Cochrane Database Syst Rev. 2006;4:CD003423.

78. Scadding GK, Darby YC, Jansz AJ, Richards D, Tate H, Hills S, et al. Double-blind, placebo controlled randomised trial of medical therapy in otitis media with effusion. Adv Life Sci Health. 2014;1:58–68.

79. Criscuoli G, D'Amora S, Ripa G, Cinquegrana G, Mansi N, Impagliazzo N, et al. Frequency of surgery among children who have adenotonsillar hypertrophy and improve after treatment with nasal beclomethasone. Pediatrics. 2003;111:e236–8.

80. Huang S-W, Giannoni C. The risk of adenoid hypertrophy in children with allergic rhinitis. Ann Allergy Asthma Immunol. 2001;87:350–5.

81. Scadding G. Non-surgical treatment of adenoidal hypertrophy: the role of treating IgE-mediated inflammation. Pediatr Allergy Immunol. 2010;21:1095–106.

82. Guss J, Doghramji L, Reger C, Chiu AG. Olfactory dysfunction in allergic rhinitis. ORL J Otorhinolaryngol Relat Spec. 2009;71:268–72.

83. Klimek L, Eggers G. Olfactory dysfunction in allergic rhinitis is related to nasal eosinophilic inflammation. J Allergy Clin Immunol. 1997;100:158–64.

84. Fonteyn S, Huart C, Deggouj N, Collet S, Eloy P, Rombaux P. Non-sinonasal-related olfactory dysfunction: a cohort of 496 patients. Eur Ann Otorhinolaryngol Head Neck Dis. 2014;131:87–91.

85. Doerfler H, Hummel T, Klimek L, Kobal G. Intranasal trigeminal sensitivity in subjects with allergic rhinitis. Eur Arch Otorhinolaryngol. 2006;263:86–90.

86. Fleiner F, Goktas O. Topical beclomethasone in the therapy of smelling disorders-a new application technique. Indian J Otolaryngol Head Neck Surg. 2011;63:5–9. doi:10.1007/s12070-010-0063-z.

87. Stuck BA, Blum A, Hagner AE, Hummel T, Klimek L, Hörmann K. Mometasone furoate nasal spray improves olfactory performance in seasonal allergic rhinitis. Allergy. 2003;58:1195.

88. Guilemany JM, García-Piñero A, Alobid I, Centellas S, Mariño FS, Valero A, et al. The loss of smell in persistent allergic rhinitis is improved by levocetirizine due to reduction of nasal inflammation but not nasal congestion (the CIRANO study). Int Arch Allergy Immunol. 2012;158:184–90.

89. Rank MA, Kelkar P, Oppenheimer JJ. Taming chronic cough. Ann Allergy Asthma Immunol. 2007;98:305–13.

90. Verguts MM, Eggermont A, Decoster W, de Jong FI, Hellings PW. Laryngeal effects of nasal allergen provocation in singers with allergic rhinitis. Eur Arch Otorhinolaryngol. 2011;268:419–27. doi:10.1007/s00405-010-1420-y **[Epub 2010 Nov 12]**.

91. DelGaudio JM. Steroid inhaler laryngitis: dysphonia caused by inhaled fluticasone therapy. Arch Otolaryngol Head Neck Surg. 2002;128:677–81.

92. Theodouropoulos DS, Ledford DK, Lockey RF, Pecoraro DL, Rodriguez JA, Johnson MC, et al. Prevalence of upper respiratory symptoms in patients with symptomatic gastroesophageal reflux disease. Am J Respir Crit Care Med. 2001;164:72–6.

93. Canonica GW, Bousquet J, Mullol J, Scadding GK, Virchow JC. A survey of the burden of allergic rhinitis in Europe. Allergy. 2007;62(Suppl 85):17–25.

94. Léger D, Annesi-Maesano I, Carat F, Rugina M, Chanal I, Pribil C, et al. Allergic rhinitis and its consequences on quality of sleep: An unexplored area. Arch Intern Med. 2006;166:1744–8.

95. Craig TJ, Teets S, Lehman EB, Chinchilli VM, Zwillich C. Nasal congestion secondary to allergic rhinitis as a cause of sleep disturbance and daytime fatigue and the response to topical nasal corticosteroids. J Allergy Clin Immunol. 1998;101:633–7.

96. Simons FE. Learning impairment and allergic rhinitis. Allergy Asthma Proc. 1996;17:185–9.

97. Baraniuk JN, Clauw DJ, Gaumond E. Rhinitis symptoms in chronic fatigue syndrome. Ann Allergy Asthma Immunol. 1998;81:359–65.

98. Vuurman EF, Vuurman LL, Lutgens I, Kremer B. Allergic rhinitis is a risk factor for traffic safety. Allergy. 2014;69:906–12.

99. Walker S, Khan-Wasti S, Fletcher M, Cullinan P, Harris J, Sheikh A. Seasonal allergic rhinitis is associated with a detrimental effect on examination performance in United Kingdom teenagers: case–control study. J Allergy Clin Immunol. 2007;120:381–7.

100. Chhabra N, Houser SM. Surgery for allergic rhinitis. Int Forum Allergy Rhinol. 2014;4(Suppl 2):S79–83.

101. Allergic rhinitis University of Maryland Medical Center. http://umm.edu/health/medical/reports/articles/allergic-rhinitis. Accessed 30 July 2015.

102. Jose J, Coatesworth AP. Inferior turbinate surgery for nasal obstruction in allergic rhinitis after failed medical treatment. Cochrane Database Syst Rev. 2010;12:CD005235.

103. Chhabra N, Houser SM. The surgical management of allergic rhinitis. Otolaryngol Clin N Am. 2011;44(3):779–95.

104. Bousquet J, Schünemann HJ, Samolinski B, Demoly P, Baena-Cagnani CE, Bachert C, et al. Allergic rhinitis and its impact on asthma (ARIA): achievements in 10 years and future needs. J Allergy Clin Immunol. 2012;130:1049–62.

# 11

# A common language to assess allergic rhinitis control: results from a survey conducted during EAACI 2013 Congress

Peter W. Hellings[1,2]*, Antonella Muraro[3], Wytske Fokkens[2], Joaquim Mullol[4], Claus Bachert[5], G. Walter Canonica[6], David Price[7], Nikos Papadopoulos[8], Glenis Scadding[9], Gerd Rasp[10], Pascal Demoly[11], Ruth Murray[12] and Jean Bousquet[13,14,15,16]

**Abstract**

**Background:** The concept of control is gaining importance in the field of allergic rhinitis (AR), with a visual analogue scale (VAS) score being a validated, easy and attractive tool to evaluate AR symptom control. The doctors' perception of a VAS score as a good tool for evaluating AR symptom control is unknown, as is the level of AR control perceived by physicians who treat patients.

**Methods:** 307 voluntarily selected physicians attending the annual (2013) European Academy of Allergy and Clinical Immunology (EAACI) meeting completed a digital survey. Delegates were asked to (1) estimate how many AR patients/week they saw during the season, (2) estimate the proportion of patients they considered to have well-, partly- and un-controlled AR, (3) communicate how they gauged this control and (4) assess how useful they would find a VAS as a method of gauging control. 257 questionnaires were filled out completely and analysed.

**Results:** EAACI delegates reported seeing 46.8 [standard deviation (SD) 68.5] AR patients/week during the season. They estimated that 38.7 % (SD 24.0), 34.2 % (SD 20.2) and 20.0 % (SD 16.34) of their AR patients had well-controlled (no AR symptoms), partly-controlled (some AR symptoms), or un-controlled-(moderate/severe AR symptoms) disease despite taking medication [remainder unknown (7.1 %)]. However, AR control was assessed in many ways, including symptom severity (74 %), frequency of day- and night-time symptoms (67 %), activity impairment (57 %), respiratory function monitoring (nasal and/or lung function; 40 %) and incidence of AR exacerbations (50 %). 91 % of delegates felt a simple VAS would be a useful tool to gauge AR symptom control.

**Conclusions:** A substantial portion of patients with AR are perceived as having uncontrolled or partly controlled disease even when treated. A simple VAS score is considered a useful tool to monitor AR control.

**Keywords:** Allergic rhinitis, Control, Digital, Survey, Visual analogue scale, VAS

## Background

Control of disease is considered one of the key outcomes in several medical domains. Although the concept of control is well-defined in asthma, chronic obstructive pulmonary disease and other conditions such as glycaemic control in diabetes, [1] it has only recently gained

significant attention in the field of allergic rhinitis (AR) [2–5]. Indeed, the patients' evaluation of disease control by any type of treatment, leading to a significant reduction of symptom severity, has become one of the novel goals of treatment in different chronic diseases. In AR, there is growing consensus that a visual analogue scale (VAS) score represents a simple, good and valid tool to monitor AR disease control [2, 6]. In 2010, Bousquet and colleagues [7] proposed a simple VAS to evaluate AR control. More sophisticated means of monitoring AR control have been used without showing superiority of one over the

*Correspondence: peter.hellings@med.kuleuven.be
[1] Department of Otorhinolaryngology, University Hospitals Leuven, Leuven, Belgium
Full list of author information is available at the end of the article

other [8]. Therefore, a VAS has been incorporated into the treatment algorithms for AR [2] to guide treatment decisions as part of an integrated care pathway [9]. It has yet to be validated in children. Nowadays, a digital version of the AR control VAS will be rolled out to patients, pharmacists and physicians to encourage better communication (with patients) and referral when appropriate. Physicians of all specialities involved in AR management can use the same VAS, from general practitioners (GPs) and allergists, to ear nose and throat (ENT) specialists, paediatricians, pulmonologists and dermatologists.

A VAS for AR has been shown to assess disease severity according to the Allergic Rhinitis and its Impact on Asthma (ARIA)-guidelines, with a VAS cut off score of 50 mm distinguishing between mild and moderate/severe AR in adults [10]. The VAS score incorporates quality of life (QoL) and reflective total nasal symptom score (rTNSS) [11] and correlates with improvements in AR symptoms and QoL. It can be used to assess AR severity in both intermittent and persistent disease in untreated or treated patients [10]. A change in VAS score of more than 23 mm represents clinically relevant changes in QoL and AR symptoms, possibly reflecting a response to treatment [6].

The major gaps in the current appreciation of VAS as a tool for the evaluation of symptom control are the following: (1) the level of control reached in patients by actual treatment options as perceived by the medical doctors, (2) how disease control is evaluated, and (3) physician perception on the usefulness of a VAS score for the evaluation of symptom control. Physicians often underestimate disease severity and impact on patients' lives, while at the same time over-estimate the effectiveness of treatment [12, 13]. Physician-patient communication is greatly hampered by a lack of a common language to describe AR control and a lack of a universally-accepted definition of what AR control actually means. The aim of this exploratory study was to assess how physicians measure AR symptom control, how they perceive the control status of their patients and how they regard the usefulness of a VAS to gauge disease control.

## Methods

A quantitative, digital survey, designed to collect views of physicians who treat AR routinely in clinical practice, was carried out during the 32nd EAACI Congress (Milan, Italy) from 22nd to 26th June 2013. The survey content was informed by experts in the field of AR (JB, CB and DP) and conducted at the Meda booth by physicians attending the exhibition (see Additional file 1). There was no incentive to take part in the survey.

Those who consented to take part had their EAACI barcode scanned, were allocated a digital ID and were provided with the survey questions on an iPad. Responses to all questions were anonymised and stored on an independent server.

Delegates were asked to:

1. Estimate how many AR patients they saw per week during the season,
2. estimate the proportion of their patients they considered to have well-, partly- and un-controlled disease,
3. communicate how they gauged this control (>1 answer permitted)
4. assess how useful they would find a VAS as a method of gauging control.

A representation of a VAS with marker slider was shown to delegates when considering their response to question 4. Survey questions and representation of the VAS with marker slider are provided in Additional file 1.

Descriptive statistics (mean and standard deviation) were used to summarise survey responses.

## Results

307 EAACI 2013 delegates from 60 different countries and from different specialties (e.g. GPs, allergists, ENT specialists and paediatricians) completed the survey. Valid question responses were obtained for 257 of these. Surveys from 50 delegates were not included as they were incomplete.

On average, respondents reported seeing 46.8 [standard deviation (SD) 68.5] AR patients/week during the season. They estimated that AR was well-controlled, partly-controlled and un-controlled in 38.7 % (SD 24.0), 34.2 % (SD 20.2) and 20.0 % (SD 16.34) of patients, respectively, and unknown for the remainder (7.1 %). Delegates reported assessing disease control in many different ways, including symptom severity (74 %), frequency of day- and night-time symptoms (67 %), activity impairment (57 %), respiratory function monitoring (nasal and/or lung function; 40 %) and incidence of AR exacerbations (50 %) (Fig. 1). 91 % of delegates felt that a VAS was a useful tool to assess disease control.

## Discussion

According to 257 EACCI 2013 delegates, the VAS score is a useful tool to monitor disease control in AR. More than 50 % of AR patients were considered by physicians to have partly-controlled or uncontrolled disease, with many different features of AR, unrelated to nasal symptoms, determining physicians' perception of disease of control. This observation that >50 % of their patients have sub-optimal AR control is in agreement with other surveys [13–15]. The physicians' perception of reaching a good level of control in 38.7 % of patients also

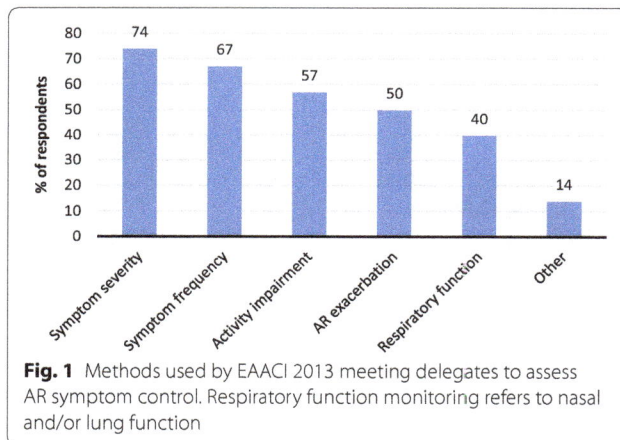

**Fig. 1** Methods used by EAACI 2013 meeting delegates to assess AR symptom control. Respiratory function monitoring refers to nasal and/or lung function

corresponds well with previous reports: A European survey found that, according to physician assessment, good control of nasal and ocular symptoms was achieved in 45.4 and 51.3 % of patients, respectively [13].

It was also apparent that AR control was assessed in multiple ways with no consensus on an optimal method. Of note was the large standard deviation seen around control perception, which shows a wide-ranging response to the question. Interestingly, the determinants of control as perceived by the physicians varied from frequency of day- and night-time symptoms to respiratory function monitoring (nasal and/or lung function). One of the most striking findings was the extra-nasal symptoms, like frequency of day- and night-time symptoms and impaired activity being reported as key determinants of AR control.

91 % of the EAACI delegates who completed this survey agreed upon the validity of a VAS as a useful tool for assessing AR control. In our opinion, it is an intuitive tool for use in clinical studies, and by physicians and patients every day. The VAS is well suited to the task of assessing AR control. It is simple and quick to complete, incorporating assessment of both AR symptoms and quality-of-life [11]. It correlates well with recognized randomized controlled trial endpoints [16], can discriminate according to severity [10] and assess efficacy of treatments [16, 17]. The VAS has also been used to assess effectiveness of treatments in real-life [18] as well as inadequacies of others (including multiple treatments) [19].

Limitations of this survey relate to the fact that the most respondents were specialists (although with experience in treating AR), with relatively few GPs included. Delegates were not provided with an alternative control tool choice and also completed the survey at the Meda

booth, which may have introduced bias. However, no financial or any other incentive was given to complete the survey. Also delegate speciality was not consistently recorded which may have yielded interesting insights into how AR control is assessed across specialities. Finally, information on what proportion of AR patients had concomitant asthma was not captured. This would have provided important information on how disease control was assessed and whether the perception of control was better or worse for those patients with co-morbid disease.

The VAS will form the basis of a new contre les MAladies Chronique pour un VIeillissement Actif (MACVIA)-ARIA AR app directed at patients called 'Allergy Diary' which is now available for free download in many European countries. Users can assess their disease control daily by simply clicking on the VAS in response to the question 'overall how much are your allergic symptoms bothering you today?', from 'not at all bothersome' to 'extremely bothersome'. VAS scores are logged and plotted over time with control assessed as well-, partly- and un-controlled, according to specific VAS score cut-offs. The VAS will also be incorporated into a companion app for healthcare providers as well as into the new AR guideline, and used to guide treatment decisions. Moving to a digital VAS is attractive since in real life, on paper, VAS scores are often wrongly completed by the patient, even after explanation; either by failing to cross the line, putting a cross above or below it or writing a figure. An electronic version would prevent such errors. However, it may not allow for complexity of response such as persistence of a problematical co- morbidity despite good control of AR. The overall aim of 'Allergy Diary', the Allergy Diary companion app and the updated AR guideline (and the VAS contained within them) is to facilitate a top down communication, from guidelines to healthcare providers to patients, allowing doctors to more easily comply with the guidelines, to better tailor AR medications to patients' needs and enable patients to better communicate their needs.

In short, a common language of AR disease control is needed. A simple VAS to measure and assess disease control could meet this need and is welcomed by physicians. It should enable us to move from the illusion to the confirmation of communication.

## Abbreviations
AR: allergic rhinitis; ARIA: allergic rhinitis and its impact on asthma; EAACI: European Academy of Allergy and Clinical Immunology; ENT: ear nose and throat; GP: general practitioner; MACVIA: Contre les MAladie Chronique pour un VIeillissement Actif; QoL: quality of life; rTNSS: reflective total nasal symptom score; SD: standard deviation; VAS: visual analogue scale.

## Authors' contributions
All authors have been involved in the analysis and interpretation of data. JB, CB and DP also designed and approved the content of the questionnaire for the physicians. All authors were involved in the drafting of the manuscript, critically revised each draft and gave their final approval for publication. All authors agree to be accountable for all aspects of this work and have participated sufficiently to take public responsibility for the content. All authors read and approved the final manuscript.

## Authors' information
PH is a rhinologist and allergologist, working in the University Hospitals of Leuven, and Academic Medical Center, Amsterdam, and leading a research team on upper airways inflammation at the University of Leuven. He is the current Secretary-General of EAACI (2015–2017). AM is a Consultant Paediatric Allergist at the Department of Women and Child Health, Padua University Hospital, Italy and Professor of Paediatric Allergology at the Allergy and Clinical Immunology School, University of Padua. She was Secretary General of EAACI from 2013 to 2015 and is the current President of EAACI (2015–2017). WF is an otorhinolaryngologist and head of the department of Otorhinolaryngology of the Academic Medical Centre Amsterdam. JM is an ENT specialist and Director of the Rhinology Unit and Smell Clinic, ENT Department, Hospital Clínic de Barcelona; and Professor of Research and Head of the Laboratory Clinical and Experimental Respiratory Immunoallergy at IDIBAPS, Barcelona, Catalonia, Spain. CB is ENT specialist and allergologist at the Ghent University Hospital, and runs the Upper Airways Research Laboratory, Ghent University. He also is affiliated with the Karolinska Institute in Stockholm, Sweden. GWC is Professor of Respiratory Medicine and Director of Allergy & Respiratory Disease Clinic, Dept Internal Medicine, University of Genoa, IRCCS AOU San Martino, Genoa Italy. DP is Professor of Primary Care Respiratory Medicine at the University of Aberdeen, co-founder of the Respiratory Effectiveness Group (http://www.effectivenessevaluation.org) and Director of Observational and Pragmatic Research Institute, Singapore. NP is Professor of Allergy and Paediatric Allergy at the Universities of Manchester, UK and Athens, Greece. GS is Hon. Consultant Rhinologist and Allergist at the Royal National TNE Hospital, London and Hon. Senior Lecturer at University College, London. GR is Professor for Otorhinolaryngology and Chairman of the ORL-Department at the Paracelsus Medical University Salzburg, Austria. PD is a pulmonologist and allergist, Professor of Pulmonology and Head of Department at the University Hospital of Montpellier. He was the Vice-President for Education and Specialties of EAACI from 2011 to 2015 and President of the French Allergy Society from 2010 to 2012. In addition, PD is Associate Editor of the journal ALLERGY, is a member of the editorial board of several national and international medical allergy journals and is a member of the French National Academy of Medicine. RM is the director of a Medical and Scientific research consultancy. JB is a Professor Emeritus at the University of Montpellier in France. He is recognized as past chairman of the Global Initiative for Asthma (GINA) and as the founder and Chairman of ARIA (Allergic Rhinitis and its impact on Asthma), in collaboration with the World Health Organization. Prof Bousquet is also past Chairman of the WHO Global Alliance Against Chronic Respiratory Diseases (GARD), Director of the WHO Collaborating Centre for Asthma and Rhinitis in Montpellier, and coordinator of several projects of the European Union in research, health and ICT. Professor Bousquet's current interests lie with the European Innovation Partnership on Active and Health Aging, and updating how chronic diseases like allergic rhinitis are managed using an integrated care pathway.

## Author details
[1] Department of Otorhinolaryngology, University Hospitals Leuven, Leuven, Belgium. [2] Department of Otorhinolaryngology, Academic Medical Center (AMC), Amsterdam, The Netherlands. [3] Department of Women and Child Health, Food Allergy Referral Centre, Padua University Hospital, Veneto Region, Padua, Italy. [4] Hospital Clinic, IDIBAPS, CIBERES, Barcelona, Catalonia, Spain. [5] Upper Airways Research Laboratory (URL), University Hospital Ghent, Ghent, Belgium. [6] Allergy and Respiratory Diseases, Department of Internal Medicine, IRCCS S Martino, IST, University of Genoa, Genoa, Italy. [7] Centre of Academic Primary Care, University of Aberdeen, Aberdeen, UK. [8] Allergy Department, 2nd Pediatric Clinic, University of Athens, Athens, Greece. [9] RNTNE Hospital, London, UK. [10] Department of Otorhinolaryngology, Paracelsus Medical University, Salzburg, Austria. [11] Division of Allergy, Department of Pulmonology, Hôpital Arnaud de Villeneuve, University Hospital of Montpellier, Montpellier, France. [12] MedScript Ltd, Dundalk, Co. Louth, Ireland. [13] University Hospital, Montpellier, France. [14] MACVIA-LR, Contre les Maladies Chronique pour un Vieillissement Actif en Languedoc Roussilon, European Innovation Partnership on Active and Healthy Aging Reference Site, Montpellier, France. [15] INSERM, VIMA: Ageing and Chronic Diseases. Epidemiological and Public Health Approaches, U1168 Paris, France. [16] UVSQ UMR-S1168, Universite Versailles St-Quentin-en-Yvelines, Versailles, France.

## Acknowledgements
We thank EAACI for allowing this survey to be conducted during the 32nd annual meeting in Milan, 2013.

## Competing interests
PH has received research grants and/or has been lecturing for GSK, Merck, Stallergenes and ALK. AM has provided educational lectures for Meda and Allergopharma. WF has received an educational grant from Meda and research grants from GSK and Biopharma. JM is or has been member of national and international scientific advisory Boards (consulting), received fees for lectures, or grants for research projects from ALK-Abelló, Boeringer-Ingelheim, Crucell, Esteve, FAES, GSK, Hartington Pharmaceuticals, Johnson and Johnson, MEDA Pharma, MSD, Novartis, Pierre Fabre, Sanofi-Aventis, Schering Plough, UCB, Uriach Group, Zambon. CB on the speaker's bureau for Meda. GWC has received honoraria for lectures or scientific advisory boards: ALK, Allergy Therapeutics, AstraZeneca, Boston Scientific, Bruschettini, Chiesi, Circassia, Faes, GSK, Meda, Menarini, Mundifarma, Novartis, Recordati, Roche, Sanofi-Aventis, Uriach, Stallergènes, Thermo Fisher, Teva, Valeas. DP has Board Membership with Aerocrine, Almirall, Amgen, AstraZeneca, Boehringer Ingelheim, Chiesi, Meda, Mundipharma, Napp, Novartis, and Teva. Consultancy: A Almirall, Amgen, AstraZeneca, Boehringer Ingelheim, Chiesi, GlaxoSmithKline, Meda, Mundipharma, Napp, Novartis, Pfizer, and Teva; Grants and unrestricted funding for investigator-initiated studies from UK National Health Service, British Lung Foundation, Aerocrine, AKL Ltd, Almirall, AstraZeneca, Boehringer Ingelheim, Chiesi, Eli Lilly, GlaxoSmithKline, Meda, Merck, Mundipharma, Napp, Novartis, Orion, Pfizer, Respiratory Effectiveness Group, Takeda, Teva, and Zentiva; Payments for lectures/speaking: Almirall, AstraZeneca, Boehringer Ingelheim, Chiesi, Cipla, GlaxoSmithKline, Kyorin, Meda, Merck, Mundipharma, Novartis, Pfizer, SkyePharma, Takeda, and Teva; Payment for manuscript preparation: Mundipharma and Teva; Patents (planned, pending or issued): AKL Ltd.; Payment for the development of educational materials: GlaxoSmithKline, Novartis; Stock/Stock options: Shares in AKL Ltd which produces phytopharmaceuticals and owns 80 % of Research in Real Life Ltd and its subsidiary social enterprise Optimum Patient Care; received Payment for travel/accommodations/meeting expenses from Aerocrine, Boehringer Ingelheim, Mundipharma, Napp, Novartis, and Teva; Funding for patient enrolment or completion of research: Almirral, Chiesi, Teva, and Zentiva; and Peer reviewer for grant committees: Medical Research Council (2014), Efficacy and Mechanism Evaluation programme (2012), HTA (2014). NP has received grants from GSK, Nestle and Merck, provided consultancy to GSK, Abbvie, Novartis, Menarini, Meda, and Alk-Abello, is on the speakers bureau for Novartis, Allegopharma, Uriach, GSK, Stallergens and MSD and provided educational presentations for Abbvie, Sanofi and Meda. GS has received research grants from GSK and ALK as well as honoraria for articles, consulting, lectures/chairing and/or advisory boards from ALK, Bausch and Lomb, Church and Dwight, Circassia, GSK, Groupo Uriach, Meda, Merck, Ono, Shionogi and Stallergenes. GR has received honoraria for consulting/lectures/chairing/advisory boards from ALK, Allergopharma, GSK, Meda, MSD, Novartis, Stallergenes, Sanofi-Aventis. PD is a consultant (and a speaker) for Stallergenes, Circassia, ALK, DBV and Chiesi and was a speaker for Merck, Astra Zeneca, Pierre Fabre Médicaments, Menarini, Allergopharma, Allergy Therapeutics Ltd., ThermoFischer Scientific and GlaxoSmithKline. RM is the director of a Medical and Scientific Affairs consultancy which has provided consultancy services to Meda, MACVIA ARIA and RIRL. JB has received honoraria for: Scientific and advisory boards—Almirall, Meda, Merck, MSD, Novartis, Sanofi-Aventis, Takeda, Teva, Uriach. Lectures during meetings—Almirall, AstraZeneca, Chiesi, GSK, Meda, Menarini, Merck, MSD, Novartis, Sanofi-Aventis, Takeda, Teva, Uriach. Board of Directors—Stallergènes.

**References**

1.  Fullerton B, Jeitler K, Seitz M, Horvath K, Berghold A, Siebenhofer A. Intensive glucose control versus conventional glucose control for type 1 diabetes mellitus. Cochrane Database Syst Rev. 2014;2:CD009122.

2.  Hellings PW, Fokkens WJ, Akdis C, Bachert C, Cingi C, Dietz de Loos D, et al. Uncontrolled allergic rhinitis and chronic rhinosinusitis: where do we stand today? Allergy. 2013;68:1–7.

3.  Mullol J, Bartra J, Del CA, Izquierdo I, Munoz-Cano R, Valero A. Specialist-based treatment reduces the severity of allergic rhinitis. Clin Exp Allergy. 2013;43:723–9.

4.  Fonseca JA, Nogueira-Silva L, Morais-Almeida M, Sa-Sousa A, Azevedo LF, Ferreira J, et al. Control of Allergic Rhinitis and Asthma Test (CARAT) can be used to assess individual patients over time. Clin Transl Allergy. 2012;2:16.

5.  Linhares DV, da Fonseca JA, Borrego LM, Matos A, Pereira AM, Sa-Sousa A, et al. Validation of control of allergic rhinitis and asthma test for children (CARATKids)—a prospective multicenter study. Pediatr Allergy Immunol. 2014;25:173–9.

6.  Demoly P, Bousquet PJ, Mesbah K, Bousquet J, Devillier P. Visual analogue scale in patients treated for allergic rhinitis: an observational prospective study in primary care: asthma and rhinitis. Clin Exp Allergy. 2013;43:881–8.

7.  Bousquet PJ, Bachert C, Canonica GW, Casale TB, Mullol J, Klossek JM, et al. Uncontrolled allergic rhinitis during treatment and its impact on quality of life: a cluster randomized trial. J Allergy Clin Immunol. 2010;126:666–8.

8.  Demoly P, Calderon MA, Casale T, Scadding G, Annesi-Maesano I, Braun JJ, et al. Assessment of disease control in allergic rhinitis. Clin Transl Allergy. 2013;3:7.

9.  Bousquet J, Addis A, Adcock I, Agache I, Agusti A, Alonso A, et al. Integrated care pathways for airway diseases (AIRWAYS-ICPs). Eur Respir J. 2014;44:304–23.

10.  Bousquet PJ, Combescure C, Neukirch F, Klossek JM, Mechin H, Daures JP, et al. Visual analog scales can assess the severity of rhinitis graded according to ARIA guidelines. Allergy. 2007;62:367–72.

11.  Bousquet PJ, Combescure C, Klossek JM, Daures JP, Bousquet J. Change in visual analog scale score in a pragmatic randomized cluster trial of allergic rhinitis. J Allergy Clin Immunol. 2009;123:1349–54.

12.  Meltzer EO. Allergic rhinitis: the impact of discordant perspectives of patient and physician on treatment decisions. Clin Ther. 2007;29:1428–40.

13.  Canonica GW, Bousquet J, Mullol J, Scadding GK, Virchow JC. A survey of the burden of allergic rhinitis in Europe. Allergy. 2007;62(Suppl 85):17–25.

14.  Keith PK, Desrosiers M, Laister T, Schellenberg RR, Waserman S. The burden of allergic rhinitis (AR) in Canada: perspectives of physicians and patients. Allergy Asthma Clin Immunol. 2012;8:7.

15.  Fromer LM, Ortiz G, Ryan SF, Stoloff SW. Insights on allergic rhinitis from the patient perspective. J Fam Pract. 2012;61:S16–22.

16.  Bousquet J, Bachert C, Canonica GW, Mullol J, Van CP, Bindslev-Jensen C, et al. Efficacy of desloratadine in intermittent allergic rhinitis: a GA(2)LEN study. Allergy. 2009;64:1516–23.

17.  Bousquet J, Bachert C, Canonica GW, Mullol J, Van CP, Bindslev-Jensen C, et al. Efficacy of desloratadine in persistent allergic rhinitis—a GA(2)LEN study. Int Arch Allergy Immunol. 2010;153:395–402.

18.  Klimek L, Bachert C, Mosges R, Munzel U, Price D, Virchow JC, et al. Effectiveness of MP29-02 for the treatment of allergic rhinitis in real-life: results from a noninterventional study. Allergy Asthma Proc. 2015;36:40–7.

19.  Bousquet PJ, Demoly P, Devillier P, Mesbah K, Bousquet J. Impact of allergic rhinitis symptoms on quality of life in primary care. Int Arch Allergy Immunol. 2013;160:393–400.

# 12

# The impact of cold on the respiratory tract and its consequences to respiratory health

Maria D'Amato[1], Antonio Molino[1], Giovanna Calabrese[1], Lorenzo Cecchi[2], Isabella Annesi-Maesano[3] and Gennaro D'Amato[4*]

## Abstract

The increasing use, and sometimes the abuse, particularly in industrialized countries of air conditioning at home, in car, hotel and shopping centres has highlighted new emerging public health issues, resulting from exposure of the airways to cool air or, more properly, resulting from sudden temperature changes. This is part of a wider problem, relating to air quality in indoor environment, such as homes or offices, where people spend more than 90% of their time. In particular, if indoor exposure occurs quickly and without any gradual adaptation to a temperature 2°–3° lower than the external temperature and especially with a 5° difference (avoiding indoor temperature below 24°) and an humidity between 40 and 60%, there is a risk of negative consequences on the respiratory tract and the patient risks to be in a clinical condition characterized by an exacerbation of the respiratory symptoms of his chronic respiratory disease (asthma and COPD) within a few hours or days. Surprisingly, these effects of cold climate remain out of the focus of the media unless spells of unusually cold weather sweep through a local area or unstable weather conditions associated with extremely cold periods of increasing frequency and duration. Moreover, the energy consumed by air conditioning induces an increase of $CO_2$ in atmosphere with increase of global warming. There is a need to better define the consequences of repeated exposure to cold air and the mechanisms by which such exposure could modify airway function and affect the outcomes of patients with pre-existing airway disease. This could help to promote adequate policy and public health actions to face the incoming challenges induced by climate change and global warming.

**Keywords:** Bronchial asthma, Airway hyperreactivity in asthma and COPD, Cold induced respiratory diseases, Climate change, Global warming and health, Air conditioning and asthma and COPD

## Background

It is common knowledge that the winter season, especially in the higher latitudes, is the difficult part of year for patients with chronic respiratory diseases and that inhalation of cold air has negative effects on the lungs for people with respiratory diseases and in particular on asthma patients. However, surprisingly these effects of cold climate remain out of the focus of the media except in the case of unusually cold weather spells or unstable weather conditions associated with extremely cold periods of increasing frequency and duration.

During warmer months, cold air continues to be a problem with the overuse of air conditioning and a question is on the effects of its abuse, particularly when it is regulated at very cold temperature, which is a frequent event in some countries. The increasing use, in particular in industrialized countries, of air conditioners at home, in car, hotel and shopping centres has highlighted new emerging public health issues, resulting from exposure of the airways to cool air or, more properly, resulting from sudden temperature changes. This is part of a wider problem, relating to air quality in enclosed environments, in homes or offices, where people spend more than 90% of their time.

*Correspondence: gdamatomail@gmail.com
[4] Department of Respiratory Diseases, High Specialty Hospital 'A. Cardarelli' and University of Naples Federico II, School of Specialization in Respiratory Diseases, Rione Sirignano, 10, 80121 Naples, Italy
Full list of author information is available at the end of the article

In recent years more discussion has taken place on "Indoor Air Quality" and more attention is being paid to related pathologies, from simple thermal discomfort to real pathologies such as sickness building syndrome [1] or aggravation of asthma and COPD.

The purpose of the present work is to better understand the consequences of repeated exposure to cold air by exploring the mechanisms by which such exposure could modify airway function and affect health outcomes of patients with pre-existing airway disease. In regards to health, we will describe the effects of cold air at first in healthy people like athletes and successively in respiratory patients. In regards to exposure, we will take into account the various risk factors interacting with cold temperature and air conditioning such as other meteorological variables, air pollution, biocontaminants and tobacco smoking, and their impact on respiratory health. The final aim of our work is to contribute to the promotion of adequate policy and public health actions to face the incoming challenges induced by climate change and global warming.

## Cold and air conditioning impact on respiratory health

Clinical discomfort due to respiratory illnesses can be exacerbated by indoor cold temperatures due to air conditioning. For chronic patients with precarious respiratory balances there is a risk of worsening of symptoms. Respiratory infections can be caused by cold air through increased bronchial inflammation caused by association of trigger factors such as cold and infections are both able to destabilize the patient.

Other trigger factors to consider, associated with cold and infectious agents, are cigarette smoke, urban pollution, inhalation of pollutants and irritants present in the air and in the working environments.

Patients with bronchial hyperreactivity are at risk of bronchospasm as a result of suddenly breathing cold air due to a variation in the inner balance of lower airways.

When air temperature drops quickly without any gradual adaptation, even for changes as low as 2°–3°, but especially for changes greater than 5°, there are possible negative consequences on their respiratory system and the patient is at risk of severe exacerbation of the symptoms of their obstructive respiratory disease (asthma and COPD).

Cold-induced airway damage is not only due to the direct effect of temperature, but also depends on the hyperventilation. Cooling of the airways is enhanced by increasing the airflow within the airways. Breathing of +20 °C air at 15 l/min decreases the tracheal temperature to 34 °C whereas breathing similar air at 100 l/min decreases this temperature to 31 °C. Therefore,

hyperpnea of temperate air shares similar effects to the inhalation of cold air [2].

Airways are lined by a thin layer of liquid, the airway surface fluid (ASL). Hyperpnea of cold air may cause the ASL to evaporate more rapidly than it can be replaced [3, 4], leading to drying and hypertonicity of the ASL. Of note, the absolute water content of subfreezing air is always near zero regardless of the level of saturation [5–7]. Therefore, while the effect of cold air on the skin is mainly cooling, the effect on the airways is both cooling and drying.

Under normal conditions, nasal breathing compensates in part for the effects of the cold air, and therefore, at rest and during light exercise the possible trigger sites for cold air- provoked respiratory symptoms include the facial skin and the nasal mucosa but not the lower airways.

The response mechanisms of airway inhalation of cold air go beyond changes of the ASL and involve a complex integrated system including the ASL but also mucosa, smooth muscle and blood vessels. Alveolar air, under normal conditions, is at a temperature of 37 °C and alveolar gas is fully saturated with water vapor at this temperature, properly humidified and heated by the components of the upper respiratory tract walls [8]. The role of these walls is not only to allow gaseous exchange, but it provides a large contact surface with the outside, it must also ensure adequate protection, in particular from dehydration and cooling. Inhalation of cold air induces activation of the epithelium to generate proinflammatory substances and that epithelial injury, determines activation of any exposed peripheral nerves. Vasomotor control in the airways is mediated by parasympathetic and sympathetic nerves, that through the release of neuropeptides such as Substance P and Calcitonin Gene Related Peptide (CGRP) [9], which can induce powerful vasodilation. Substances used for inhalation tests such as histamine, methacholine or substances locally released such as prostaglandins, produced locally by cells such as mast cells or eosinophils act on bronchial blood flow. Vasodilatation of bronchial vessels has been shown to cause thickening of the airway mucosa and should antagonize the effects of hyperventilation, but also helps to stimulate bronchial hyperresponsiveness that can trigger asthma attacks in predisposed subjects.

## Mechanisms of cold air effects in athletes

The respiratory system may be particularly affected by cold air exposure as inspired air has to be conditioned before participating in peripheral lung gas exchange, with an associated loss of heat and water. During exercise, a shift from nose to combined nose-and-mouth breathing takes place when the ventilation level exceeds approximately 30 l/min [7]. In such conditions, the possible trigger sites provoking respiratory symptoms include nasal mucosa, pharynx, larynx and the lower airways [6].

During physical exercises, nasal breathing quickly switches to mouth breathing, particularly at minute ventilations above 40 l/min, with the involvement of intrathoracic airways in this conditioning process [10].

Although exercising in cold air has minimal influence on the airways of normal individuals, it can induce a bronchoconstriction in asthmatic subjects and worsen airway obstruction in those with obstructive pulmonary diseases [11–13]. Winter athletes can be particularly affected by these environmental conditions, and an increased prevalence of airway hyperresponsiveness, asthma and chronic cough has been described in this population [14–18]. Bronchial biopsies of winter athletes have shown evidence of airway remodelling, possibly due to repeated cold-air and hyperventilation damage to the airways, although more research is needed on this influence on airway function [19, 20]. The mechanism of bronchoconstriction as a response to exercise-induced hyperpnoea, particularly in cold air, has been studied and appears primarily related to an increase in airway fluid osmolarity following hyperpnoea, although heat loss may be a modulator of this response, as well as a possible post-exercise "rewarming" of the airways [21].

Even in subjects without respiratory diseases, cold air can induce changes in the airways. Exposure to cold air can increase the number of granulocytes and macrophages in the lower airways [22]. Furthermore, cold-related impairment of respiratory mucociliary function can inhibit the clearance of pollutants [23]. Finally, in extreme cold temperatures, people tend to gather indoors and crowding can promote the transmission of infectious agents with ensuing airway inflammatory events.

Repeated cooling and drying of the airways are likely to take place in endurance athletes who frequently exercise at elevated ventilation levels. Indeed, a high prevalence of respiratory symptoms and airway hyperresponsiveness has been found in skiers, swimmers and long-distance runners. Studying the inflammatory infiltrate of the mucosa of the athletes with long and repeated exposure to cold air, identified a cell population different from asthma, with a greater number of neutrophils and a lesser number of eosinophils, mast cells and macrophages [22]: this further confirms that asthma and cold related diseases are two different entities, which, however, can influence each other.

## Cold air alone or in combination with other factors
### Cold and meteorological variables
The effect of cold temperature is modulated by other ambient conditions, too. As an example, cold damp air was reported by asthmatic patients to cause more symptoms than cold dry air, while a control group reported very few respiratory symptoms [11]. However, we need to consider combinations of several meteorological variables able to act on airways. Such combinations are referred to as "synoptic air masses", where humidity, visibility, cloud cover, air pressure, wind speed and others are added into the equation and are known to influence mortality and morbidity [24–26].

### Cold and air pollution
Climate change and air pollution due to anthropogenic activities are intrinsically connected with many greenhouse gases and particulate air pollutants originate from the same source, such as fossil fuel combustion [1].

Nitrate particles and organic carbon aerosols have a cooling effect on the climate. Sulfur dioxide partly converts to sulfate particles, which also have cooling potential, so they partly react with black carbon, neutralizing its strong warming effect [27].

Some studies, including the paper of Carder et al. [28] highlight that cold temperature in conjunction with black smoke concentrations increase respiratory mortality. Since extremes of cold and particulate pollution may coexist, for example during temperature inversion during winter, these results may have important public health implications. Cold is related to various acute or long term airways diseases. General exposure to cold exacerbates chronic bronchitis and triggers Raynaud's phenomenon of the lung (constriction of the pulmonary arteries and reduction of pulmonary blood volume in subjects with primary Raynaud phenomenon). Moreover, breathing very cold air at very high ventilation levels can led to acute pulmonary oedema or to frozen lungs [8]. It was also shown that inhalation of cold air causes vasodilation and thus increasing blood flow to the central airways in contrast to vasoconstriction in the intraparenchymal area [29]. In subjects who repeatedly hyperventilate very cold air, repeated episodes of significant variations in bronchial blood flow can lead to alterations in walls of bronchi and of pulmonary arteries, leading to faster than average decrease of lung function and increased thickness of walls of pulmonary arteries (Eskimo lung) [29]. According to a more recent classification, it is possible to classify cold- related diseases of the airways into three types: the short term responses are those that develop within minutes in response to sudden cooling of the airways, subjects with asthma or rhinitis are especially prone to these response; the long-term responses are those that develop in response to repeated and longstanding cooling and drying of the airway, usually in endurance athletes; finally, there are the physiological, reflex-mediated lower airway responses to cooling of the skin or upper airways [2].

There is no "universal" numerical value of air temperature that can be accepted as cut-off point for "cold". It is rather the magnitude of downward temperature change below the mean seasonal range for a given area that challenges the adaptive ability of people. Mortality increased to a greater extent with given fall of temperature in regions with warm winters, in populations with cooler homes, and among people who wore fewer clothes and were less active outdoors. As adaptive capacity shrinks with age, it is the elderly who are mostly affected. Thus, it has been documented that cold temperatures are associated with a 3–4% increase in daily mortality and hospitalization for respiratory causes in the population over 75 years old for each degree Celsius decrease in minimum temperature or minimum apparent temperature (defined as a combined indicator of temperature and humidity above a city specific threshold level ranging from 23 to 29 °C) [30].

To obtain information on the extent and severity of asthmatic symptoms during daily life in winter, a simple questionnaire was sent to 57 asthmatic patients and a control group of 180 age-matched men and women in Göteborg (Sweden), where the average winter temperature is at about the freezing point. About two-thirds of the asthmatic patients reported cold to be a factor causing breathing difficulties. In 37%, these symptoms made the patients avoid going out during the winter [11].

### Air conditioning, cold and cigarette smoke

Pathophysiological aspects in which repeated exposure to cold stimuli determines anatomical and functional alterations of the respiratory tract have been also discussed in the literature [1]. Cold air, that is temporarily inhaled, induces excessive secretions of airway mucus and elicits ciliary ultrastructural anomalies. The only exposure to cold stimuli, can defect, turn on the cold-mediated activation of the TRPM8 channel and determine mucus hypersecretion with excessive MUC5AC secretion, and obstacle mucociliary clearance through numerical and structural anomalies of the ciliary apparatus. The inhalation of cold air, however, can only activate the TRPM8 receptor, but cannot determine the baseline overexpression of this receptor in patients with COPD. Probably cigarette smoke, that is also the main risk factor for COPD, is the etiological factor for the elevated expression of the TRPM8 channel in these patients, and so they are predisposed and hypersensitive to cold stimulus, even as air conditioning [30]. The synergistic effect between smoking and exposure to cold air was also observed in other studies, evaluating changes in impedance in the respiratory tract after exposure to cold in young smokers and nonsmokers: a broncho-constricting effect extending largely into the small peripheral airways can be demonstrated by impedance measurement in a group of asymptomatic young smokers which is not observed in normal subjects after cold-air challenge [31, 32].

### Role of the upper airways in health and asthma

Breathing cold air has been long recognized to trigger bronchoconstriction in asthmatics. In a classical experiment Shturman-Ellstein et al. [33] demonstrated that if subjects with asthma breathed only through the nose during the exercise challenge, an almost complete inhibition of the post exercise bronchoconstrictive airway response was observed [33, 34]. However, as the nose is serving as outermost filter for the inspired air, it is exposed to environmental hazards with consequent high frequency of morbidity. Adding to the atopic predisposition, it is likely that asthmatic subjects have concomitant rhinitis, which does not allow proper conditioning of the inspired air with negative impact on the asthmatic condition. The cross-talk and interplay between upper and lower airways has been a center point in the philosophy of the Allergic Rhinitis and its Impact on Asthma (ARIA) initiative and has been reconfirmed over the years [35, 36].

The upper airways mucosal structures are particularly sensitive to cold air influences. Challenges with cold dry air have been proposed to assess the state of nasal responsiveness in both allergic and non-allergic rhinitis. This line of research is substantiating the importance of cold weather as trigger in the pathogenesis of rhinitis, which in turn is a recognized risk factor for the development of asthma. Cold weather spells as a characteristic feature of changing climate will need to be considered in assessing the risk for asthma, especially since heterogeneous human populations may adapt differently to them [36].

The microclimate refers to the complex temperature parameters, relative humidity, and air velocity, which affect the heat exchange between the individual and the environment. The values of these parameters must be maintained within very narrow ranges to maintain the ideal environmental conditions so that the subject can perceive so-called thermal well-being [1]. In this context it is necessary that all the parameters of the microclimate are appropriately adjusted: The human body is equipped with sophisticated thermoregulatory systems which, however, can be altered by environmental conditions [1].

When it is too hot, the thermoregulation system triggers a number of mechanisms that can deliver heat to the outside, while when it is too cold, it works by limiting the heat dispersion. Microclimate can affect heat exchanges between individuals and the environment and in some situations hinder the thermoregulation mechanisms. For example, high humidity values in the summer can increase the heat-related discomfort: the high presence of water vapor in the air hampers the evaporation of the water contained in the sweat, which is the fundamental process for the human body to disperse excess heat. This explains why, in the presence of sultriness, a climatic situation characterized by a high relative humidity value, the human body tolerates less heat discomfort and the perceived temperature than the actual ambient temperature. The reason why the wind can increase the discomfort associated with a cold feeling is related to the fact that it increases the rate at which the body loses heat. The so-called perceived temperature, that is, the feeling of "hot" or "cold", is therefore tied not only to the actual temperature but also to the other environmental conditions [1].

In buildings with natural ventilation, the outside air penetrates through existing openings in the building enclosure, such as joints or cracks in the walls, intersect around the doors (infiltration) and through the opening of doors and windows. The outside air can be introduced in a closed environment through mechanical, or forced, ventilation system that can also perform the functions of heating or cooling the air inlet, depending on the season (thermal ventilation systems).

In recent years, driven by economic and environmental motivations, thermally insulated buildings, where indoor climate conditions are closely regulated by ventilation and air conditioning systems are most frequently built. Nevertheless, in many countries there are no rigid rules to regulate the construction of ventilation systems, and although there are many studies on the possibility of using sensors within indoor environments [6, 37], there are no defined values and no environments closed monitoring systems [37].

The Sick Building Syndrome (SBS): indicates a well-defined symptomatic picture, manifested in a large number of occupants of modern or recently renovated buildings, equipped with mechanical ventilation and global air conditioning systems (without supplying fresh air from the outside) and used in offices, schools, hospitals, homes for seniors, civilian homes; a still unknown, probably multifactorial etiology, linked to factors related to buildings, air conditioning and ventilation systems, maintenance programs, type and organization of work and personal factors [38].

Regarding the pathologies more specifically associated with the use of conditioning systems, they may be related to the failure to achieve microclimatic targets or because they can be dangerous sources of biological or chemical pollution, especially if they are badly designed, in poor state of cleaning and maintenance [39]. Nasal breathing of cold air induces an engorgement of the venous sinuses in the submucosa [5, 10],

which leads to congestion, sneezing and, especially, rhinorrhea both in healthy and rhinitic subjects [13]. However, these responses are greater in subjects with rhinitis than in healthy subjects [40] and greater in subjects with asthma and rhinitis than in subjects with rhinitis alone [41]. Yet in a short time, cold air hyperpnea provokes bronchoconstriction in asthmatic subjects [42], especially in children and young adults [43, 44]. The pathophysiological mechanism beyond this response has been a matter of considerable debate: studies on the effect of cooling on the airways smooth muscle have been conflicting results [45–48]. Certain lower airway sensory receptors can be sensitive to cold and capable of inducing bronchoconstriction in animals [49, 50]. A fundamental role is certainly played by vasoconstriction, as already described before. It does not seem to be involved in a response mediated by eosinophils [51]. Besides bronchoconstriction, cold air hyperventilation also provokes coughing in susceptible people. Coughing and bronchoconstriction seem to be independent responses since pre-treatment with salbutamol blocks cold air-provoked bronchoconstriction but has no effect on cold air provoked coughing [52].

The long-term responses to cold exposure, include all those airways alterations, also anatomical, in part already described previously, comprising an increase in bronchoalveolar lavage fluid granulocytes in healthy humans [22], loss of ciliated epithelium, thickening of the lamina propria with increased concentrations of inflammatory cells, hyperresponsiveness and airway obstruction [53–57].

The last group finally includes reflex bronchoconstriction due to cold trigger of the skin or upper airway. It seems that the reflex bronchoconstriction provoked by facial or upper airway cooling is too mild to cause breathing difficulties in a person with near normal lung function. However, for a subject with severely impaired lung function these responses may be of clinical significance [58].

We do not know much about the molecular mechanisms underlying respiratory cold-related symptoms, but a role appears played by the receptor TRPM8. The discovery of thermosensitive ion channels of the transient receptor potential (TRP) family has demonstrated an underlying molecular mechanism for temperature detection. Transient receptor potential melastatin 8 (TRPM8) is a non-selective calcium permeable cation channel, that seems overexpressed and upregulated on the epithelium of patients with chronic lung disease and therefore, probably, is involved on hypersensitivity of this population to cold-related triggers [59] in association with phosphorylation of MARCKS-PSD [60].

## Air conditioning and respiratory infections

Exposure to air conditioners with very cold air, induces alterations of the respiratory airways that, mostly with pre-existing respiratory conditions such as asthma and COPD, may form a susceptible group, also in young adults [14], which not only can determine cold-related symptoms, as shortness of breath, wheezing, phlegm production, but also a greater susceptibility to infections. Indoor air can be an important vehicle for a variety of human pathogens airborne spread, already in normal conditions, as vegetative bacteria (staphylococci and legionellae), fungi (*Aspergillus*, *Penicillium*, and *Cladosporium* spp and *Stachybotryschartarum*), enteric viruses (noro- and rotaviruses), respiratory viruses (influenza and coronaviruses), mycobacteria (tuberculous and nontuberculous), and bacterial spore formers (*Clostridium difficile* and *Bacillus anthracis*) which can have pathogenic action on human health, together with exposure to other agents as noxious chemicals, particulates, pollen and other allergens [61]. Because these agents can infect a susceptible host, they must survive the prevailing environmental conditions, determined by air temperature, relative humidity (RH), turbulence, that are just a few of the factors involved, since a generalization is difficult considering the biological diversity of microorganisms. So it is obvious the role played by air conditioning, cold or warm. Various studies have shown that among the viruses, for example, rotavirus survived best at midrange RH but not at high temperature; among bacteria, staphylococci has ability to survive over a wide range of temperatures, RH, and exposure to sunlight [61].

As ubiquitous microorganisms, fungi pose a health threat in indoor environments. Fungal infections can be particularly serious in immunocompromised patients, especially airborne spores of *Aspergillus* spp that are blown in from natural ventilation sources. Fungal spores are aerosolized from municipal water supplies and dust and can be effectively transported over long distances by wind and air currents. The evolution of the fungal spore has enabled them to travel long distances and be more capable of withstanding environmental insults. The most important factor for fungal growth in indoor environments is humidity. In fact, results of many studies, showed that airborne fungal concentrations were not correlated to the diseases or personnel density, but were related to seasons, temperature, and relative humidity. There were similar dominant genera in all wards. They were *Aspergillus* spp *Penicillium* spp and *Alternaria* spp. Therefore, attention should be paid to improve the filtration efficiency of particle size of 1.1-4.7 μm for air conditioning system of wards. It also should be targeted to choose appropriate antibacterial methods and equipment for daily hygiene and

air conditioning system operation management [62]. In fact, the risk of air conditioning-caused infections is increased when, to save on air cooling costs, especially with regard to the air conditioning of rooms with large volumes of air to cool (department stores, ships, airplanes, etc.), instead of cooling hot air coming from the outside, it is preferable to keep the air cooled previously cooled from the inside (recirculation function) cool. This, however, significantly reduces air exchange in the environments while increasing the concentration of pollutants (irritants, fumes, allergenic pollens, etc.) and infectious agents (viruses and bacteria) that can add to their pathogenic activity already in itself represented by the particular physical characteristics of an artificially cold and dry air. Much work is directed at the need to use air filters for the control of respiratory diseases, especially of an allergic type, by applying filtering systems that regulate the level of pollution [63].

## Conclusions

There is a need to better define the consequences of repeated exposure to cold air and the mechanisms by which such exposure could modify airway function and affect the outcomes of patients with pre-existing airway disease [1]. This could help to promote adequate policy and public health actions to face the incoming challenges. By all means distinction should be drawn between effects on individuals and effects on populations, as populations are heterogeneous in their susceptibility, for example, a different response to cold exposure was studied by race [63], but reversible and irreversible effects should be identified.

### Authors' contributions
All the authors have contributed to the drafting, writing and reviewing of the manuscript. All authors read and approved the final manuscript.

### Author details
[1] Respiratory Department, 'Federico II University' – Division of Respiratory Medicine and Allergy, Hospital Dei Colli, Naples, Italy. [2] Interdepartmental Center of Bioclimatology, University of Florence, Florence, Italy. [3] Epidemiology of Allergic and Respiratory Diseases Department, IPLESP, INSERM & Sorbonne Université, Medical School Saint-Antoine, Paris, France. [4] Department of Respiratory Diseases, High Specialty Hospital 'A. Cardarelli' and University of Naples Federico II, School of Specialization in Respiratory Diseases, Rione Sirignano, 10, 80121 Naples, Italy.

### Acknowledgements
"The authors are indebted to Amir Moustafa for having managed the manuscript and its submission".

### Competing interests
The authors declare that they have no competing interests.

## References

1. D'Amato G, Holgate ST, Pawankar R, Ledford DK, Cecchi L, Al-Ahmad M, Al-Enezi F, Al-Muhsen S, Ansotegui I, Baena-Cagnani CE, Baker DJ, Bayram H, Bergmann KC, Boulet LP, Buters JT, D'Amato M, Dorsano S, Douwes J, Finlay SE, Garrasi D, Gómez M, Haahtela T, Halwani R, Hassani Y, Mahboub B, Marks G, Michelozzi P, Montagni M, Nunes C, Oh JJ, Popov TA, Portnoy J, Ridolo E, Rosário N, Rottem M, Sánchez-Borges M, Sibanda E, Sienra-Monge JJ, Vitale C, Annesi-Maesano I. Meteorological conditions, climate change, new emerging factors, and asthma and related allergic disorders. A statement of the World Allergy Organization. World Allergy Organ J. 2015;8(1):25. https://doi.org/10.1186/s40413-015-0073-0.
2. Koskela HO. Cold air-provoked respiratory symptoms: the mechanism and management. Int J Circumpolar Health. 2007;66(2):91–100.
3. Daviskas E, Gonda I, Anderson SD. Mathematical modeling of heat and water transport in human respiratory tract. J Appl Physiol. 1990;69:362–72.
4. Freed AN, Davis MS. Hyperventilation with dry air increases airway surface fluid osmolality in canine peripheral airways. Am J Respir Crit Care Med. 1999;159:1101–7.
5. Cole P, Forsyth R, Haight JS. Effects of cold air and exercise on nasal patency. Ann Otol Rhinollaryngol. 1983;92:196–8.
6. Sundell J, Levi H. Ventilation rates and health: multidisciplinary review of the scientific literature. Indoor Air. 2011;21(6):442–53.
7. Anderson SD, Togias AG. Dry air and hyperosmolar challenge in asthma and rhinitis. In: Busse WW, Holgate ST, editors. Asthma and rhinitis. 1st ed. Boston: Blackwell Scientific Publications; 1995. p. 1178–95.
8. Regnard J. Cold and the Airways. Int J Sports Med. 1992;13:S182–4.
9. Matran R. Neural control of airway vasculature: involvement of classical transmitters and neuropeptides. Supplementum: Acta Physiol Scand; 1990.
10. McLane ML, Nelson JA, Lenner KA, Hejal R, Kotaru C, Skowronski M, et al. Integrated response of the upper and lower respiratory tract of asthmatic subjects to frigid air. J Appl Physiol. 2000;88:1043–50.
11. Millqvist E, Bengtsson U, Bake B. Occurrence of breathing problems induced by cold climate in asthmatics—a questionnaire survey. Eur Respir J. 1987;71:444–9.
12. Marino C, de Donato F, Michelozzi P, D'Ippoliti D, Katsouyanni K, Analitis A, et al. Effects of cold weather on hospital admissions: results from 12 European cities within the PHEWE project. Epidemiology. 2009;20:S67–8.
13. Driessen JM, van derPalen J, van Aalderen WW, de Jongh FH, Thio RJ. Inspiratory airflow limitation after exercise challenge in cold air in asthmatic children. Respir Med. 2012;106(10):1362–8.
14. Hyrkas H, Jaakkola MS, Ikaheimo TM, Hugg TT, Jaakkola JJK. Asthma and allergic rhinitis increase respiratory symptoms in cold weather among young adults. Res Med. 2014;108:63–70.
15. Karjalainen EM, Laitinen A, Sue-Chu M, Altraja A, Bjermer L, Laitinen LA. Evidence of airway inflammation and remodeling in ski athletes with and without bronchial hyperresponsiveness to methacholine. Am J RespirCrit Care Med. 2000;161:2086–91.
16. Carlsen KH. Sports in extreme conditions: the impact of exercise in cold temperatures on asthma and bronchial hyper-responsiveness in athletes. Br J Sports Med. 2012;46:796–9.
17. Turmel J, Poirier P, Bougault V, Blouin E, Belzile M, Boulet LP. Cardio respiratory screening in elite endurance sports athletes: the Quebec study. Phys Sports Med. 2012;40:55–65.
18. Langdeau J-B, Turcotte H, Thibault G, Boulet LP. Comparative prevalence of asthma in different groups of athletes: a survey. Can Respir J. 2004;11:402–6.
19. Koskela HO. Cold air-provoked respiratory symptoms: the mechanisms and management. Int J Circumpolar Health. 2007;66(2):91–100.
20. Bougault V, Turmel J, St-Laurent J, Bertrand M, Boulet PL. Asthma, airway inflammation and epithelial damage in swimmers and cold-air athletes. Eur Respir J. 2009;33:740–6.
21. Sue-Chu M. Winter sports athletes: long-term effects of cold air exposure. Br J Sports Med. 2012;46:397–401.
22. Larsson K, Tornling G, Gavhed D, Müller-Suur C, Palmberg L. Inhalation of cold air increases the number of inflammatory cells in the lungs in healthy subjects. Eur Respir J. 1998;12:825–30.
23. Clary-Meinesz CF, Cosson J, Huitorel P, Blaive B. Temperature effect on the ciliary beat frequency of human nasal and tracheal ciliated cells. Biol Cell. 1992;76:335–8.
24. World Health Organization and World Meteorological Organization. Global climate change and human health: from science to practice. Atlas of Climate Change and Health. 2012. http://www.who.int/globalchange/publications/atlas/report/en/index.html. Accessed 20 Oct 2016.
25. Health Protection Agency. Public health adaptation strategies to extreme weather events (PHASE). http://www.phaseclimatehealth.eu/. Accessed 16 June 2014.
26. Analitis A, Katsouyanni K, Biggeri A, Baccini M, Forsberg B, Bisanti L. Effects of cold weather on mortality: results from 15 European cities within the PHEWE project. Am J Epidemiol. 2008;168:1397–408.
27. https://earthobservatory.nasa.gov/Features/Aerosols/2010/page3.php. Accessed 10 Sept 2015.
28. Carder M, McNamee R, Beverland I, Elton R, Van Tongeren M, Cohen GR, et al. Interacting effects of particulate pollution and cold temperature on cardiorespiratory mortality in Scotland. Occup Environ Med. 2008;65:197–204.
29. Schaefer O, Eaton RD, Timmermans FJ, Hildes JA. Respiratory function impairment and cardiopulmonary consequences in long-term residents of Canadian Arctic. Can Med Ass J. 1980;123(10):997–1004.
30. Li MC. The pathophysiological mechanisms underlying mucus hypersecretion induced by cold temperatures in cigarette smoke-exposed rats. Int J Mol Med. 2014;33:83–90.
31. Quaedvlieg M, Wouters E, Verdana F. Early airway obstruction in young asymptomatic smokers after cold-air challenge. Respiration. 1990;57:299–303. https://doi.org/10.1159/000195860.
32. Decramer M, Demedts M, van de Woestijne KP. Isocapnic hyperventilation with cold air in healthy non-smokers, smokers and asthmatic subjects. Bull Eur Physiopathol Respir. 1984;20(3):237–43.
33. Shturman-Ellstein R, Zeballos RJ, Buckley JM, Souhrada JF. The beneficial effect of nasal breathing on exercise-induced bronchoconstriction. Am Rev Respir Dis. 1978;118:65–73.
34. Van Gerven L, Boeckxstaens G, Jorissen M, Fokkens W, Hellings PW. Short-time cold dry air exposure: a useful diagnostic tool for nasal hyperresponsiveness. Laryngoscope. 2012;122:2615–20.
35. Bousquet J, van Cauwenberge P, Khaltaev N, Aria Workshop Group, World Health Organization. Allergic rhinitis and its impact on asthma. J Allergy Clin Immunol. 2001;108:S147–334.
36. Cruz A, Popov TA, Pawankar R, Annesi-Maesano I, Fokkens W, Kemp J, et al. Interactions between the upper and lower airways in rhinitis and asthma: ARIA update, in collaboration with GA(2)LEN. Allergy. 2007;62(Suppl 84):1–41.
37. Marques G, Pitarma R. An indoor monitoring system for ambient assisted living based on internet of things architecture. Int J Environ Res Public Health. 2016;13(11):1152.
38. Hodgson M. The Sick building syndrome. Occup Med. 1995;10(1):167–75.
39. Seppänen O, Kurnitski J. WHO guidelines for indoor air quality: dampness and mould. WHO publication; 2009.
40. Braat JPM, Mulder PG, Fokkens WJ, van Wijk RG, Rijntjes E. Intranasal cold air is superior to histamine challenge in determining the presence and degree of nasal hyperreactivity in nonallergic noninfectious perennial rhinitis. Am J Respir Crit Care Med. 1998;157:1748–55.
41. Hanes LS, Issa E, Proud D, Togias A. Stronger nasal responsiveness to cold air in individuals with rhinitis and asthma, compared with rhinitis alone. Clin Exp Allergy. 2006;36:26–31.
42. Deal EC Jr, McFadden ER Jr, Ingram RH Jr, Breslin FJ, Jaeger JJ. Airway responsiveness to cold air and hyperpnea in normal subjects and in those with hay fever and asthma. Am Rev Respir Dis. 1980;121:621–8.
43. Koskela HO, Rasanen SH, Tukiainen HO. The diagnostic value of cold air hyperventilation in adults with suspected asthma. Respir Med. 1997;91:470–8.
44. Nielsen KG, Bisgaard H. Hyperventilation with cold versus dry air in 2- to 5-year-old children with asthma. Am J Respir Crit Care Med. 2005;171:238–41.
45. Souhrada M, Souhrada JF. The direct effect of temperature on airway smooth muscle. Respir Physiol. 1981;44:311–23.
46. Jongejang RC, De Jongste JC, Raatgeep RC, Bonta IL, Kerrebijn KF. Effect of cooling on responses of isolated human airways to pharmacologic and electrical stimulation. Am Rev Respir Dis. 1991;143:369–74.
47. Freed AN, Fuller SD, Stream CE. Transient airway cooling modulates dry-air-induced and hypertonic aerosol-induced bronchoconstriction. Am Rev Respir Dis. 1991;144:358–62.

48. Mustafa SM, Pilcher CW, Williams KI. Cooling-induced bronchoconstriction: the role of ion-pumps and ion-carrier systems. Pharmacol Res. 1999;39:125136.

49. Jammes Y, Barthelemy P, Delpierre S. Respiratory effects of cold air breathing in anesthetitzed cats. Respir Physiol. 1983;54:41–54.

50. Giesbrecht GG, Pisarri TE, Coleridge JCG, Coleridge HM. Cooling the pulmonary blood in dogs alters activity of pulmonary vagal afferents. J Appl Physiol. 1993;74:24–30.

51. Gauvreau GM, Ronnen GM, Watson RM, O'Byrne PM Exercise-induced bronchoconstriction does not cause eosinophilic airway inflammation or airway hyperresponsiveness in subjects with asthma. Am J Respir Crit Care Med. 2000;162:1302–7.

52. Banner AS, Chausow A, Green J. The tussive effect of hyperpnea with cold air. Am Rev Respir Dis. 1985;131:362–7.

53. Davis MS, Freed AN. Repeated hyperventilation causes peripheral airways inflammation, hyperreactivity, and impaired bronchodilation in dogs. Am J Respir Crit Care Med. 2001;164:785–9.

54. Davis MS, Schofield B, Freed AN. Repeated peripheral airway hyperpnea causes inflammation and remodeling in dogs. Med Sci Sports Exerc. 2003;35:608616.

55. Helenius I, Lumme A, Haahtela T. Asthma, airway inflammation and treatment in elite athletes. Sports Med. 2005;35:565–74.

56. Karjalainen EM, Laitinen A, Sue-Chu M, Altraja A, Bjermer L, Laitinen LA. Evidence of airway inflammation and remodeling in ski athletes with and without bronchial hyperresponsiveness to methacholine. Am J Respir Crit Care Med. 2000;161:2086–91.

57. Davis MS, Schofield B, Freed AN. Repeated peripheral airway hyperpnea causes inflammation and remodeling in dogs. Med Sci Sports Exerc. 2003;35:608616.

58. Koskela HO, Koskela AK, Tukiainen HO. Broncho constriction due to cold weather in COPD. The roles of direct airway effects and cutaneous reflex mechanisms. Chest. 1996;110:632–6.

59. Li M, Yang G, Kolosov VP, Perelman JM, Zhou XD. Cold temperature induced mucin hypersecretion from normal human bronchial epithelial cells in vitro through a transient receptor potential melastatin 8 (TRPM8)-mediated mechanism. J Allergy Clin Immunol. 2011;128(3):626–34. https://doi.org/10.1016/j.jaci.2011.04.032.

60. Li MC, Juliy M. Role of phosphorylation of MARCKS-PSD in the secretion of MUC5AC induced by cold temperatures in human airway epithelial cells National Natural Science Foundation of China (81070031) and China Cooperation Research Foundation 2012—(81011120108).

61. Khalid Ijaz M, Zargar B, Wright KE, Rubino JR, Sattar SA. Generic aspects of the airborne spread of human pathogens indoors and emerging air decontamination technologies. Am J Infect Control. 2016;44:S109–20.

62. Sublett JL. Effectiveness of air filters and air cleaners in allergic respiratory diseases: a review of the recent literature. Curr Allergy Asthma Rep. 2011;11:395–402.

63. Farnell GS, Pierce KE, Collinsworth TA, Murray LK, Demes RN, Juvancic-Heltzel JA. The influence of ethnicity on thermoregulation after acute cold exposure. Wilderness Environ Med. 2008;19:238–44.

# 13

# Endotype-driven treatment in chronic upper airway diseases

Glynnis De Greve[1], Peter W. Hellings[1,2,3], Wytske J. Fokkens[2], Benoit Pugin[4], Brecht Steelant[4] and Sven F. Seys[4*]

## Abstract

Rhinitis and rhinosinusitis are the two major clinical entities of chronic upper airway disease. Chronic rhinosinusitis (CRS) and allergic rhinitis (AR) affect respectively up to 10 and 30% of the total population, hence being associated with an important socio-economic burden. Different phenotypes of rhinitis and CRS have been described based on symptom severity and duration, atopy status, level of control, comorbidities and presence or absence of nasal polyps in CRS. The underlying pathophysiological mechanisms are diverse, with different, and sometimes overlapping, endotypes being recognized. Type 2 inflammation is well characterized in both AR and CRS with nasal polyps (CRSwNP), whereas type 1 inflammation is found in infectious rhinitis and CRS without nasal polyps (CRSsNP). The neurogenic endotype has been demonstrated in some forms of non-allergic rhinitis. Epithelial barrier dysfunction is shown in AR and CRSwNP. Emerging therapies are targeting one specific pathophysiological pathway or endotype. This endotype-driven treatment approach requires careful selection of the patient population who might benefit from a specific treatment. Personalized medicine is addressing the issue of providing targeted treatment for the right patient and should be seen as one aspect of the promising trend towards precision medicine. This review provides a comprehensive overview of the current state of endotypes, biomarkers and targeted treatments in chronic inflammatory conditions of the nose and paranasal sinuses.

**Keywords:** Rhinitis, Chronic rhinosinusitis, Phenotype, Biomarker, Biologicals, Precision medicine, Personalised medicine

## Background

Persistent rhinitis and chronic rhinosinusitis (CRS) are the two major clinical entities of chronic upper airway disease. Worldwide questionnaire-based surveys show that allergic rhinitis affects up to 30% of the global population, whereas CRS is present in over 10% of the European population [1, 2]. Upper airway diseases are often associated with comorbidities such as asthma or COPD [3, 4]. The upper and lower airways cannot be separated from each other and immune modulating drugs, such as allergen immunotherapy and biologicals, affect both airway compartments.

Uncontrolled disease has been reported in 35–40% of patients with chronic upper airway disease and has a substantial impact on the patient's social, physical and economic health. The reasons for an uncontrolled disease are related to disorder-, diagnosis-, treatment- or patient-associated factors. The relative importance of these factors is unclear, specialists agree that optimal disease management approaches are needed [5–7].

Precision medicine is proposed to address this global issue by providing customized and individualized care based on the unique immunologic, genetic and psychosocial profile of the patient [8]. The concept of precision medicine is based on four pillars: *personalized care* with tailored diagnostic and therapeutic approaches, *prediction* of disease progression and success of treatment, *prevention* of disease and *participation* of the patient to achieve good adherence and optimal efficacy of the given treatment.

To fully implement precision medicine into daily practice, disease management based on disease control and phenotyping needs to be complemented with disease

*Correspondence: sven.seys@kuleuven.be
[4] Laboratory of Clinical Immunology, Department of Immunology and Microbiology, KU Leuven, Herestraat 49/PB811, 3000 Louvain, Belgium
Full list of author information is available at the end of the article

endotyping. For decades, to determine the best-fit treatment, a phenotype is being assigned to the patient based on clinical symptoms, atopy status and the presence of nasal polyps (for CRS patients). This approach is generally carried out almost entirely regardless of the underlying pathophysiological mechanisms. In complex diseases with mixed pathophysiologies, a phenotype-driven treatment is not always sufficient to obtain optimal control. Endotype classification based on thorough investigation of the underlying pathophysiological mechanisms is therefore gaining more interest. Endotyping will provide more insight in the inter-individual variability of clinical presentation and treatment response in patients with identical phenotypes. In addition, endotyping might in the future guide the decision making process of targeted treatments [9]. In order to make endotype-driven treatment a clinical applicable approach in daily practice, identification of measurable biological indicators, or so called "biomarkers", is needed [10]. The ideal biomarker serves as a signature of a well-defined endotype and is easily measurable, reproducible and affordable [11].

Currently we are in the era of extensive research towards identification of biomarkers and endotype-driven treatments. Research on endotyping is also performed for asthma and cancer and is well ahead of endotyping in upper airway diseases. The aim of the current review is to provide a comprehensive overview of the current state of endotypes, biomarkers and biological treatment in rhinitis and CRS. Since biomarkers can be used for many applications, only those that are (potentially) of valuable for the diagnosis or prediction of treatment response will be reviewed. Subsequently, current or potential treatment strategies targeting specific endotypes will be discussed.

## Endotypes and biomarkers in upper airway diseases

Rhinitis is characterized by inflammation of the nasal mucosa causing nasal obstruction, rhinorrhoea, sneezing and pruritus [12]. Three main phenotypes of rhinitis are described: allergic rhinitis (AR), infectious rhinitis and non-allergic non-infectious rhinitis (NAR). The latter phenotype can be subdivided in many subphenotypes such as idiopathic rhinitis (IR), hormonal rhinitis, gustatory rhinitis, drug-induced rhinitis, rhinitis of the elderly, atrophic rhinitis and occupational rhinitis [13]. In CRS the mucosal inflammation affects the nose and paranasal sinuses and is characterized by nasal obstruction and discharge, loss of smell and/or facial pain, which lasts longer than 12 weeks [14]. Traditionally a phenotype is addressed to the patient according to the presence (CRSwNP) or absence (CRSsNP) of nasal polyps on nasal endoscopy or radiological imaging.

A specific phenotype can be indicative for the presence of one particular endotype. However, one or mixed endotype(s) can also underlie different phenotypes in upper airway diseases, hence making clear distinction of endotypes more complex. Since the underlying pathophysiological events of both rhinitis and CRS are located at the upper airway mucosal lining, they share common endotypes (Fig. 1).

### Type 2 inflammation

Type 2 inflammation is characterized by the presence of eosinophils and type 2 cytokines IL-4, IL-5, IL-9 and IL-13, derived from Th2 cells and type 2 innate lymphoid cells (ILC2), in peripheral blood or nasal mucosa [15]. IL-25, IL-31, IL-33 and thymic stromal lymphopoietin (TSLP) secreted by epithelial cells are known to induce or enhance type 2 driven inflammation [16]. In sensitized individuals, contact with allergens activates mast cells via immunoglobulin E (IgE) dependent mechanisms [9] (Fig. 2).

Type 2 inflammation is a major feature of AR, local allergic rhinitis (LAR) and CRSwNP, hence the most common and studied endotype in upper airway diseases (Table 1). Topical and/or oral corticosteroids are the first-line treatment for these patients and are shown to reduce eosinophils in nasal mucosa [17–19]. However, treatment with corticosteroid can be insufficient to fully control the inflammation.

AR is predominantly defined by the type 2 endotype. Allergen exposure through nasal mucosa triggers the type 2 inflammatory cascade leading to a Th2-dominant milieu with eosinophilia and specific IgE production [20]. The diagnosis of AR is based on clinical features and allergen sensitization. A positive skin prick test (SPT) or ImmunoCap test, using rather arbitrary cut-off values of wheal diameter $\geq 3$ mm and serum IgE $\geq 0.35$ KU/l, are used to confirm atopic sensitization [21]. A negative SPT however, does not exclude presence of type 2 inflammation, e.g. LAR. Additional nasal allergen provocation test and nasal secretion sampling for specific IgE detection can provide evidence of type 2 inflammation [22]. In addition, serum total IgE, eosinophilic cationic protein (ECP, activation marker of eosinophils) and eosinophils have been proposed as diagnostic biomarkers with corresponding cut-off values of 98.7 IU/mL, 24.7 µg/mL and 4.0%, respectively, with sensitivities ranging from 55.7 to 75.2% and specificities from 69.7 to 74.4% [23]. Type 2 cytokines IL-4, IL-5 and IL-13 are also detectable in nasal fluids [24]. So far, no validated diagnostic cut-off values are available.

Unlike AR, type 2 inflammation in CRSwNP is characterised by polyclonal IgE formation and is usually not linked to atopy [25]. This endotype is the most common

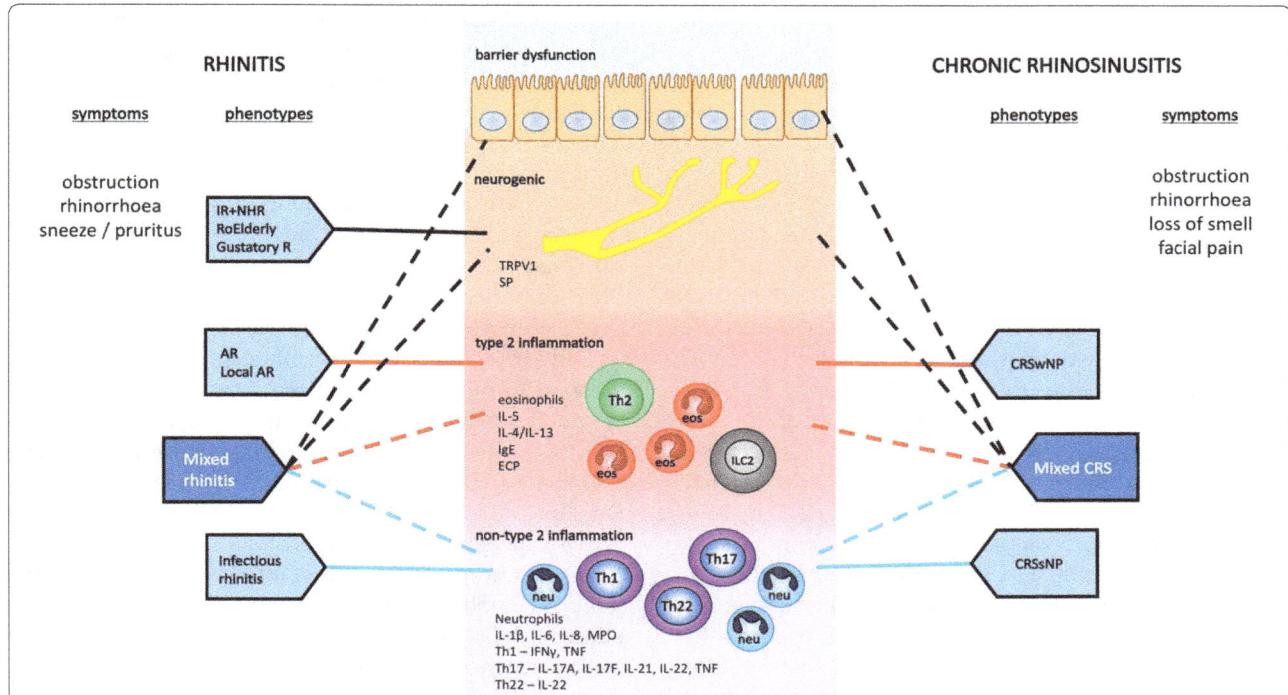

**Fig. 1** Overview of endotypes and phenotypes in rhinitis and chronic rhinosinusitis. Endotype predominantly underlying the phenotype, *solid lines*; endotype potentially contributing to the phenotype, *dashed lines*. *AR* allergic rhinitis; *CRSsNP* chronic rhinosinusitis without nasal polyps; *CRSwNP* chronic rhinosinusitis with nasal polyps; *IR* idiopathic rhinitis; *RoElderly* rhinitis of the elderly; *Gustatory R* gustatory rhinitis

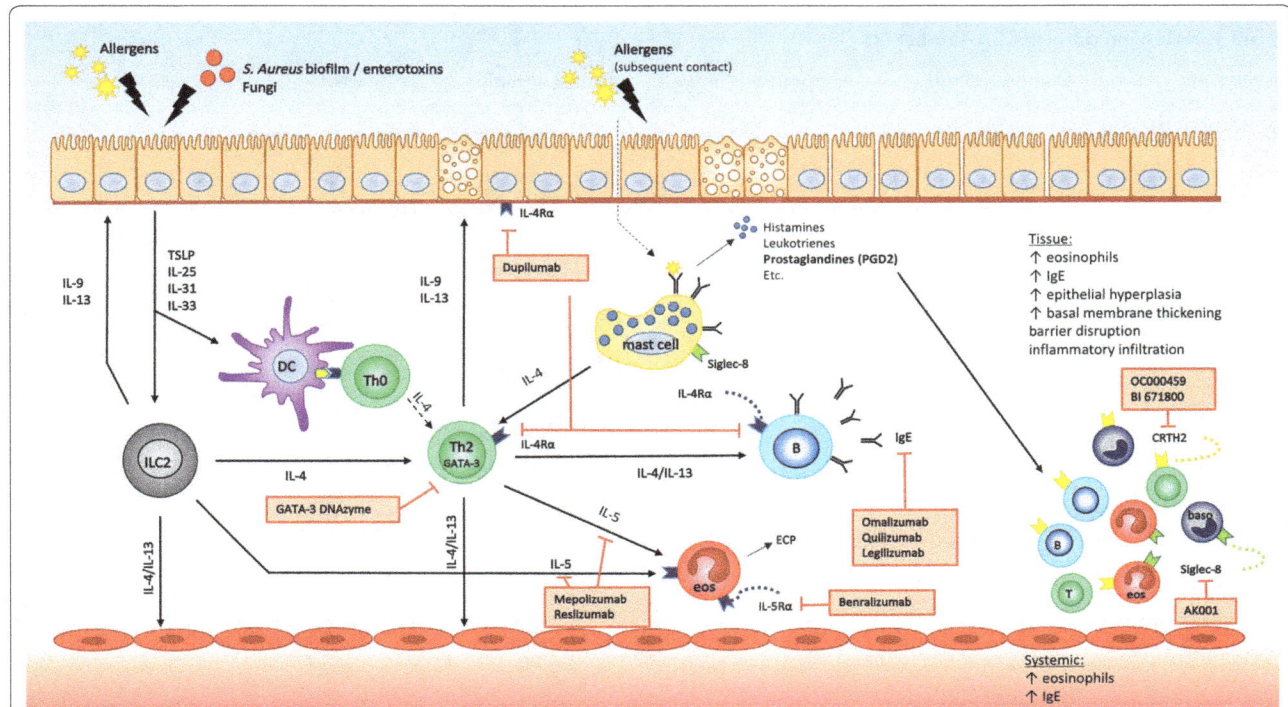

**Fig. 2** Type 2 inflammation and biologicals. *B* B cell; *baso* basophil; *DC* dendritic cell; *ECP* eosinophilic cationic protein; *eos* eosinophils; *ILC2* type 2 innate lymphoid cell; *Th* T helper cell

one in white people from Europe and US with eosinophilic CRSwNP [26–28].

In research setting, the diagnosis of eosinophilic CRSwNP is either based directly on tissue eosinophilia (>5 eosinophils/high power field or indirectly on ECP/myeloperoxidase (MPO) ratio (>1) determined on nasal biopsies [26, 27, 29]. A cut-off value of >10 eosinophil/HPF however is clinically more relevant to assess its impact on quality of life (QoL) [30]. One cross-sectional study with 51 patients shows that serum eosinophilia values of >0.3 × $10^9$ $L^{-1}$ or 4.4% of white blood cells have a positive predictive value and negative predictive value of 79 and 67%, respectively [31]. Furthermore, type 2 cytokines IL-4, IL-5 and IL-13 are detectable in nasal secretions. Surprisingly IL-13 levels were elevated in samples of healthy controls compared to those of patients with CRSsNP and CRSwNP, and IL-4 levels showed no significant raise. IL-5 was significantly higher in presence of nasal polyps compared to CRSsNP and healthy controls and might therefore be a useful biomarker to predict ongoing type 2 inflammation in CRSsNP patients [32]. Hence, all the above-mentioned markers, corresponding cut-off values and predictive values need to be validated in larger cohorts of patients.

Some studies evaluated the potential of type 2 inflammatory markers as prognostic biomarkers. Higher levels of mucosal and/or blood eosinophilia and presence of comorbid asthma are correlated with poor outcome in terms of QoL, recurrence of NP after sinus surgery and disease severity [29, 30, 33–35]. Other type 2 inflammation markers such as IgE, ECP and IL-5 are also predictive for recurrence of CRSwNP [28, 36].

*Staphylococcus aureus* is found in around 60% of CRS patients with eosinophilic inflammation and NP [37]. Whether *S. aureus* is an initiator or amplifier in CRS is a matter of debate. *S. aureus* biofilms are documented in CRS patients with more severe disease and worse postoperative outcome [38, 39]. Biofilms make bacteria more resistant to therapy with antibiotics, thus allowing them to penetrate submucosally and initiate type 2 inflammation. IL-4 and IL-13 may also compromise the immune response to *S. aureus* through the suppression of human β-defensin released in skin and mucosa [40, 41]. Importantly, *S. aureus* produces enterotoxins (SE) which can act as superantigens. These superantigens have the unique ability to amplify the type 2 inflammation through interaction with T-cells via the T cell receptors, as a result of their unrestricted antigen specificity, and in turn leading to the production of polyclonal IgE against SE (SE-IgE) [42]. Presence of SE-IgE itself is a risk factor for the development of comorbid asthma [26, 36, 37, 43, 44], and NP recurrence after surgery [28].

## Table 1  Potential diagnostic biomarkers

| Endotypes | Allergic rhinitis | Idiopathic rhinitis | Infectious rhinitis | CRSwNP | CRSsNP |
|---|---|---|---|---|---|
| **Type 2 inflammation** | | | | | |
| Serum | Eosinophils*<br>Total IgE<br>Specific IgE<br>ECP* | | | Eosinophils*<br>Total IgE*<br>IgE/SE-IgE*<br>ECP* | |
| Nasal fluids | Total/specific IgE*<br>IL-5*<br>IL-4, IL-13*<br>Eosinophils* | | | Total/specific IgE*<br>IL-5*<br>IL4, IL-13<br>ECP/MPO ratio*<br>ECP* | |
| **Non-type 2 inflammation** | | | | | |
| Nasal lavage/fluids | | | IL-1β, IL-6, IL-8, MPO<br>IFNγ<br>TNFα | | IL-1β, IL-6, IL-8, MPO*<br>IFNγ*<br>IL-17, IL-22, TNFα* |
| Nasal biopsy | | | Neutrophils | | Neutrophils |
| **Neurogenic endotype** | | | | | |
| Nasal fluids | | SP | | | |
| Nasal biopsy | | TRPV1 | | | |
| **Barrier dysfunction** | | | | | |
| Nasal biopsy | ↓TER | | ↓TER | ↓TER | |
| | ↓TJ | | ↓TJ | ↓TJ | ↓TJ |

*ECP* eosinophilic cationic protein; *MPO* myeloperoxidase; *TER* transepithelial resistance; *TJ* tight junctions; *TRPV1* transient receptor potential cation channel subfamily V receptor 1

* Also detectable in nasal biopsies

## Non-type 2 inflammation

Non-type 2 inflammation is mainly characterized by neutrophils in nasal mucosa [27, 44, 45]. Neutrophilic inflammation can be triggered by infections or chronic irritation, such as air pollution. This leads to dysregulation of the innate immune system and activation of the IL-17 pathway with recruitment of neutrophils to the nasal mucosa, which is known to be mediated via IL-8 [46–48]. In addition, type 1 immune response, metabolic and epigenetic factors, or the activation of the epithelial-mesenchymal trophic unit may lead to extensive remodeling without any inflammation, have been identified as modulating factors of the neutrophilic inflammation [49, 50] (Fig. 3).

Research on endotyping in non-type 2 inflammatory diseases lags well behind the type 2 inflammatory diseases, and so far no endotype-driven treatment has been proven to be effective. Since tissue neutrophilia is associated with reduced clinical response to corticosteroids, further exploration of none-type 2 is needed [18, 51].

Infectious rhinitis is associated with neutrophilic inflammation with increased pro-inflammatory cytokines IL-1β, IL-6, IL-8, interferon (IFN) γ, tumor necrosis factor (TNF)α and MPO [52, 53]. These cytokines can be detected in nasal lavage samples during acute upper respiratory tract infection.

CRSsNP is generally associated with neutrophilic inflammation and increased levels of IFNγ and IL-17, although it has also been documented in CRSwNP, especially in the Asian population [26]. Based on the study of Tomassen et al. three non-type 2 subendotypes were identified in patients with CRS: (1) neutrophilic inflammation characterized by pro-inflammatory cytokines IL-1β, IL-6, IL-8 and MPO; (2) Th17- or Th22- driven inflammation characterized by IL-17, IL-22 and TNFα; (3) Th1-driven inflammation characterized by IFNγ [44]. A combination of these subendotypes are often documented in both CRSsNP and CRSwNP, hence resulting in a mixed endotype [26]. During early stage CRSsNP, increased levels of transforming growth factor (TGF) β1 in sinus tissue compared to turbinate tissue from controls were reported, suggesting that TGFβ1 plays a pivotal role in initiating collagen production and remodelling process [54]. In CRSwNP patients with non-recurrent disease, higher levels of IFNγ indicative of Th1-driven inflammation were found compared to those with recurrent disease [28].

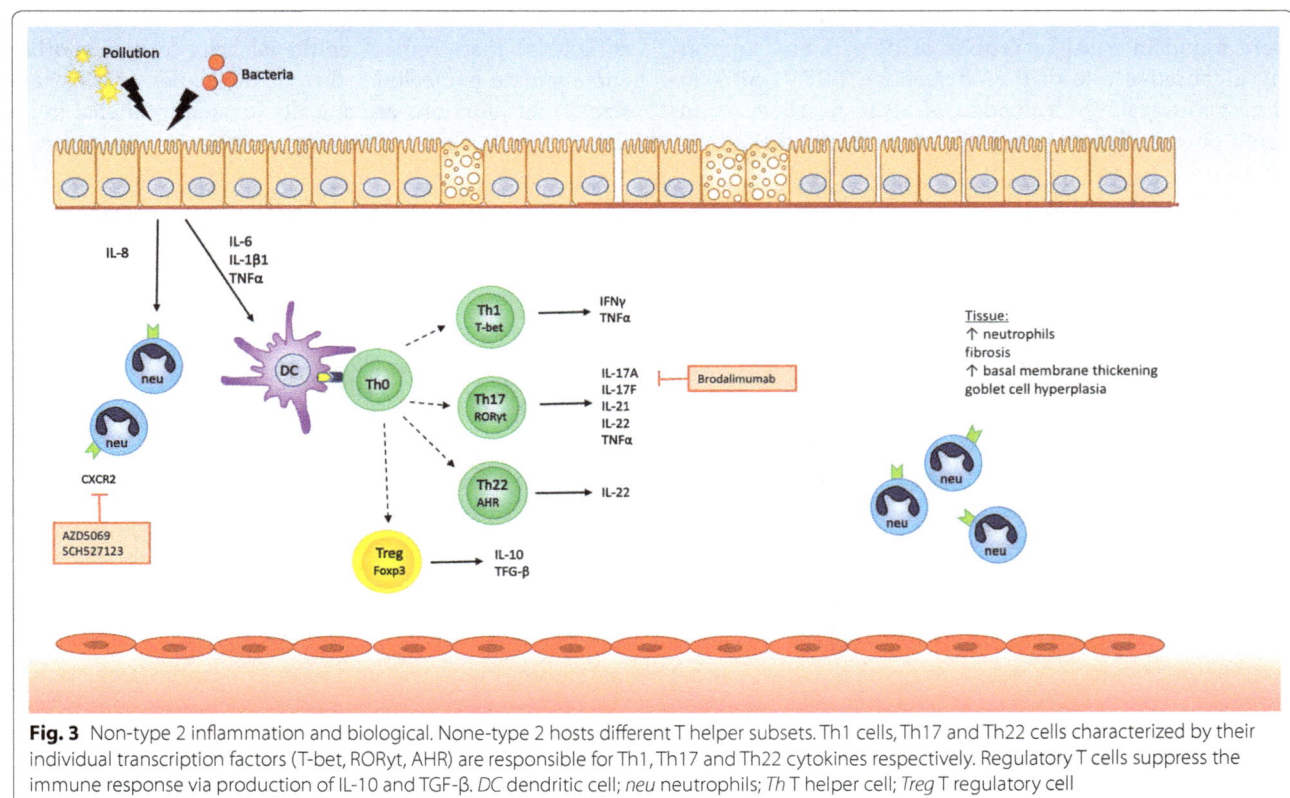

**Fig. 3** Non-type 2 inflammation and biological. None-type 2 hosts different T helper subsets. Th1 cells, Th17 and Th22 cells characterized by their individual transcription factors (T-bet, RORyt, AHR) are responsible for Th1, Th17 and Th22 cytokines respectively. Regulatory T cells suppress the immune response via production of IL-10 and TGF-β. *DC* dendritic cell; *neu* neutrophils; *Th* T helper cell; *Treg* T regulatory cell

### Neurogenic activation

Dysfunction of the neuronal system of the nose is underlying different subphenotypes of NAR such as idiopathic rhinitis (IR), gustatory rhinitis and rhinitis of the elderly [55]. Two pathophysiological mechanisms are proposed: 1/overexpression of transient receptor potential (TRP) channels and associated nasal hyperreactivity (NHR) and 2/imbalance of sympathetic and parasympathetic system [56] (Fig. 4).

NHR is present in two-thirds of patients with IR, i.e. aberrant reactivity of the nasal mucosa to common environmental stimuli such as smoke, chemical pollutants, strong odors and temperature and humidity alterations resulting in defensive responses such as sneezing, rhinorrhoea and nasal congestion [57]. The nasal mucosa is equipped with C-fibers, a specific type of sensory nerve, which express TRP channels on their endings. These nerves can be activated by non-allergic triggers, such as environmental irritants, alterations in temperature or osmolality, and can subsequently induce the release of neuropeptides like substance P (SP) and calcitonin G-related peptide (CGRP). These neuropeptides induce increased vascular permeability and glandular hypersecretion resulting in the above-mentioned rhinitis symptoms [56].

Van Gerven et al. demonstrated an association between IR and TRP subfamily V receptor 1 (TRPV1) overexpression in nasal mucosa. In addition, increased SP levels were found in nasal secretions of IR patients, supporting a causative role of the nociceptive TRPV1-SP signaling pathway [57]. Evaluation of SP in nasal secretions could potentially serve as a diagnostic biomarker for IR.

However, more easy and rapid tests are required to allow identification of IR patients in daily practice. The cold-dry air provocation test (CDA) is a diagnostic test for NHR with a high sensitivity and specificity, thus providing a reliable, easy, well-tolerated but most importantly non-invasive test using natural stimuli compared to a more labor intensive nasal sampling [58].

Moreover, the imbalance of the autonomous nervous system, also called "dysautonomia" might also contribute to the pathophysiological mechanism of NAR. Parasympathetic and sympathetic activity results in vasodilation and vasoconstriction, respectively. An imbalance of these components with loss of sympathetic tone and relative increased parasympathetic activity, results in vasodilation, increased mucosal blood flow and glandular hypersecretion [56]. Although the pathophysiology of rhinitis of the elderly is not clear, dysautonomia is thought to be the causative mechanisms leading to the typical clear rhinorrhea [13]. So far no biomarkers are evaluated to identify patients with dysautonomia.

### Epithelial barrier dysfunction

The epithelial lining forms the first barrier for exogenous pathogens or harmful particles. Besides being a physical barrier and maintaining mucociliary clearance, it modulates the innate immune response by through cytokine and chemokine production [59]. Proper functioning of the physical barrier is supported by dynamic junctional complexes that connect epithelial cells to one another and regulate paracellular flux of molecules of a certain size. Tight junctions are apically located epithelial junctions, consisting of different transmembrane proteins

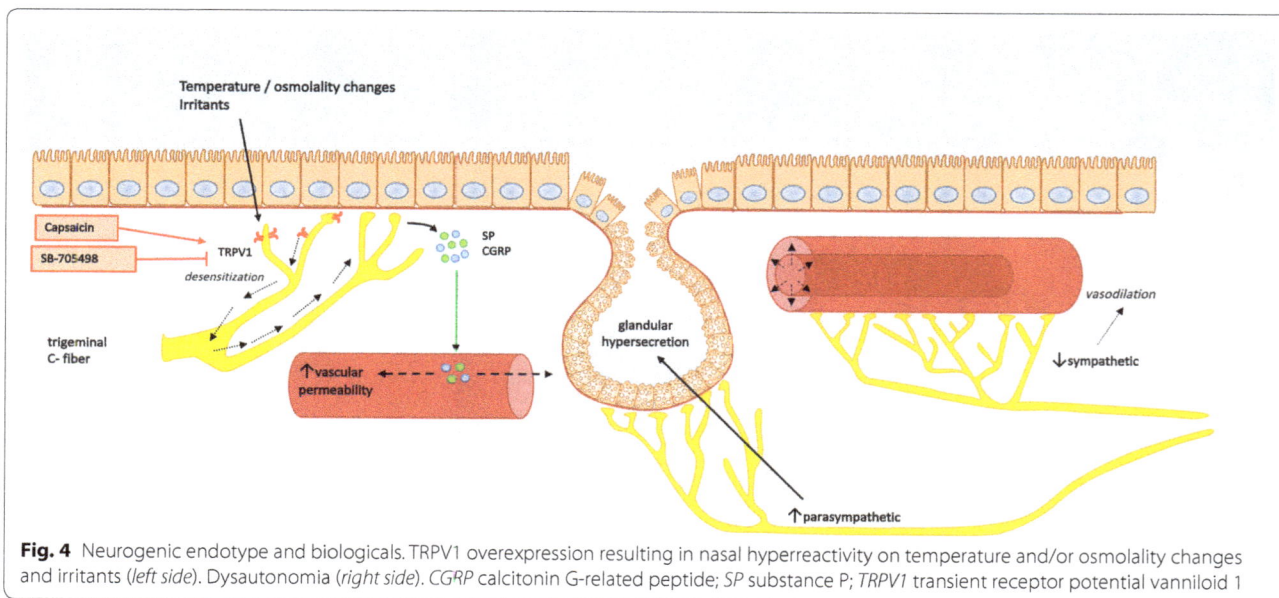

**Fig. 4** Neurogenic endotype and biologicals. TRPV1 overexpression resulting in nasal hyperreactivity on temperature and/or osmolality changes and irritants (*left side*). Dysautonomia (*right side*). *CGRP* calcitonin G-related peptide; *SP* substance P; *TRPV1* transient receptor potential vanniloid 1

such as claudin-1, claudin-4, occludin and junctional adhesion molecule A, which are connected to intracellular proteins like zonula occludens-1 (ZO-1) among others (Fig. 5).

A defective epithelial barrier has been documented in various chronic airway diseases, such as AR, CRS and asthma, and is associated with chronicity and severity of the inflammation [60–62]. A leaky epithelium was documented in CRSwNP due to decreased expression of occludin and claudin-4 on nasal biopsies [61]. Similarly a disrupted tight junction arrangement in AR was found to be due to decreased expression of occludin and ZO-1 [62].

Whether epithelial barrier dysfunction is a primary genetic event or a secondary phenomenon resulting from inflammation is not clear. A dysfunctional epithelial barrier results in increased permeability for foreign particles allowing them to migrate to the submucosal region, hence making it more vulnerable for inflammation. In addition, there is evidence that IL-4 disrupts epithelial integrity suggesting that type 2 inflammation can contribute to epithelial dysfunction [62]. Since epithelial barrier dysfunction is part of AR and CRS, restoring the barrier integrity may become a useful treatment approach. So far, no easy methods are available to evaluate barrier function in patients with upper airway disease.

## Treatment of chronic upper airway disease
### Therapies targeting type 2 inflammation
*Targeting IgE-pathway*
Omalizumab, a recombinant humanized anti-IgE monoclonal antibody (mAb), binds circulating IgE on its high-affinity receptor (FcεRI) preventing it to become cell-bound on effector cells such as mast cells, basophils, dendritic cells and eosinophils. Subsequently the expression of FcεRI reduces on the effector cells [63–65]. Omalizumab is approved by the European and US regulatory authorities for the treatment of severe allergic asthma and is currently under investigation for its use in the treatment of allergic rhinitis and CRS (Table 2).

Cumulative evidence exists that treatment with omalizumab is safe, well-tolerated and effective in reducing symptoms and rescue medication use in AR [66–73]. Adding omalizumab to allergen immunotherapy (AIT) for the treatment of allergic rhinitis with or without co-morbid allergic asthma appears to be superior to either treatments alone [72, 74, 75]. Combination therapy shows superiority in the treatment of polysensitized patients, due to its allergen-independent therapeutic

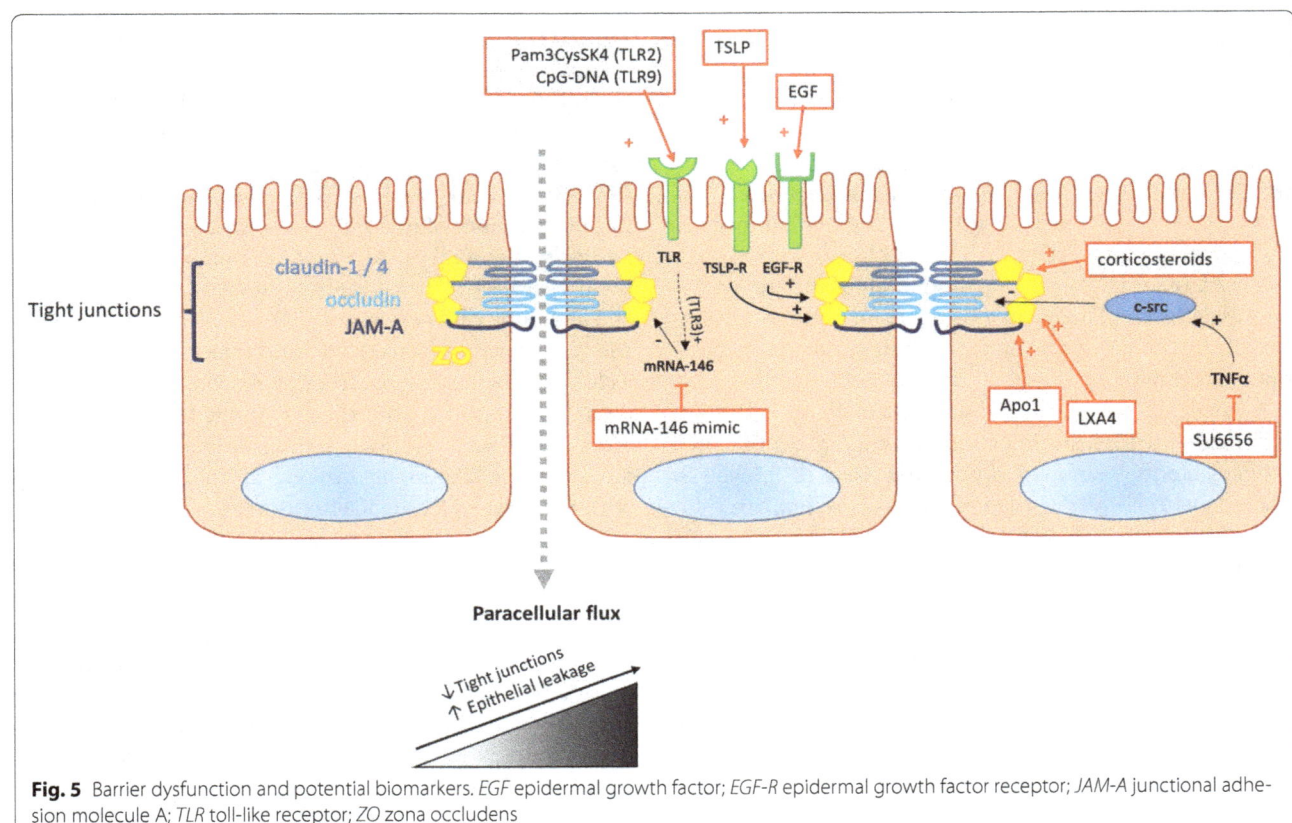

**Fig. 5** Barrier dysfunction and potential biomarkers. *EGF* epidermal growth factor; *EGF-R* epidermal growth factor receptor; *JAM-A* junctional adhesion molecule A; *TLR* toll-like receptor; *ZO* zona occludens

effect [76]. Furthermore, it has a protective effect on the development of adverse events of AIT, hence allowing rush-immunotherapy treatment with higher dose regimens and a shorter treatment course [72, 76, 77]. In patients with persistent AR and concomitant asthma, omalizumab is effective in preventing asthma exacerbation and improving quality of life [78, 79]. Unfortunately, omalizumab has no long-term effect [80, 81] unlike AIT, which remains the sole curative approach nowadays.

In CRSwNP patients and co-morbid asthma omalizumab showed reduced upper and lower airway symptoms, endoscopic nasal polyp score as well as less needs for further medical or surgical treatments [25, 82, 83]. On the other hand, one trial revealed that the molecule had a small and clinically irrelevant effect on CRS [84]. This trial however was underpowered and the presence of NPs was not taken into account. This emphasizes the importance of endotyping to properly select patients who will benefit most from anti-IgE treatment.

New promising biologicals targeting IgE are being developed with the aim of improving anti-IgE treatment. One such is ligelizumab, an anti-IgE mAb with greater affinity for IgE compared to omalizumab [85]. A second one is quilizumab, a mAb targeting the M1 epitope on membrane IgE [86]. Studies are currently running to assess their safety and efficacy in the treatment of asthma.

*Targeting IL5-pathway*

IL-5 is a key mediator in type 2 eosinophilic inflammation [26, 28, 36, 87]. It is responsible for survival, maturation and activation of eosinophils at the bone marrow and the site of inflammation [87–89]. To interfere with the IL-5 pathway, novel biologicals are developed targeting IL-5 or its receptor IL-5Rα on the effector cells. Mepolizumab and reslizumab are both humanized anti-IL5 mAb that neutralize IL-5. Both biologicals are already approved by the European and US Food and Drug Association (FDA) for its use in the treatment of severe eosinophilic asthma.

A phase II trial showed that reslizumab, at a dose of one single intravenous injection of 3 mg/kg, significantly reduces blood eosinophil counts and nasal IL-5 levels in patients with NP [88]. Individual NPs score improved for up to 4 weeks in only 50% of the patients. Additional post hoc analysis could identify a subpopulation of responders characterized by increased IL-5 levels in nasal secretions (i.e. >40 pg/mL).

A phase II trial with mepolizumab showed, similar to reslizumab, a reduction of blood eosinophil count paralleled by decreased levels of IL-5 in serum and nasal secretions of patients with CRSwNP [89]. However, nasal IL-5 and nasal total IgE were not significantly altered. More important, a reduction of the NP score was seen

in patients with severe and/or recurrent NP after treatment with two single intravenous injections of 750 mg of Mepolizumab with an interval of 4 weeks. This study could however not support the association between responders and increased IL-5 levels, which presumably is due to a small sample size. A sustained effect for up to 36 weeks after treatment with mepolizumab was seen in the responder group, suggesting its long-term effect.

Reslizumab and Mepolizumab are both safe and well-tolerated in patients with CRSwNP. After treatment cessation rebound eosinophilia was reported, but this phenomenon seemed to occur without major exacerbation symptoms [88]. Studies with larger sample size, long treatment duration and follow-up are needed to determine the optimal treatment scheme for clinical use [89].

Lastly, it is worth noting that benralizumab is a humanized mAb against the highly expressed IL-5Rα receptor on eosinophils [90]. Its efficacy and safety in uncontrolled asthma with eosinophilia has been demonstrated in a phase III trial. So far, no studies are published on its use in upper airway diseases.

*Targeting IL-4/IL-13 -pathway*

IL-4 and IL-13 can be seen as sibling cytokines as they share the IL-4Rα subunit to form a fully functional IL-4 (with common γC subunit) or IL-4 and IL-13 (with IL-13Rα subunit) receptor [91]. This explains their mutual and important role in the type 2 inflammation.

Dupilumab, a fully human anti-IL4Rα mAb, is designed to interfere with this pathway. It has been proven to be effective in the treatment of atopic dermatitis and asthma, in which it also improved sinonasal symptoms [92, 93]. Recently a phase II trial evaluating dupilumab in the treatment of uncontrolled CRSwNP was published by Bachert et al. [94]. Adding dupilumab subcutaneously once every week to intranasal corticosteroid treatment showed improved endoscopic NP score, CT score (Lund–Mackay scoring system), QoL and major symptoms such as loss of smell, nasal obstruction or congestion and nocturnal awakenings. This effect remained up to 16 weeks after treatment cessation. Further studies are needed to assess longer treatment duration and direct comparison with other type 2 biological treatments.

*Other type 2 directed therapies*

Chemoattractant receptor homologous molecule on Th2 cells CRTH2 is responsible for eosinophil, basophil and lymphocyte recruitment upon PGD2 release of activated mast cells. The CRTH2-antagonist, OC000459, showed improvement of nasal and ocular symptoms in grass pollen allergic patients after grass pollen provocation [95]. Another CRTH2 antagonist, BI 671800, reduced total nasal symptoms in patients with seasonal allergic rhinitis

**Table 2** Targets and potential treatments according to the specific endotypes and phenotypes

| Endotypes-targets | Allergic rhinitis | Idiopathic rhinitis | Infectious rhinitis | CRSwNP | CRSsNP |
|---|---|---|---|---|---|
| *Type 2 inflammation* | | | | | |
| IgE | Omalizumab (sc/iv) | | | Omalizumab (sc) | |
| | Legelizumab | | | Legelizumab | |
| MI prime mIgE | Quilizumab | | | Quilizumab | |
| IL-5 | Mepolizumab | | | Mepolizumab (iv) | |
| | Reslizumab | | | Reslizumab (sc) | |
| IL-5Ra | Benralizumab | | | Benralizumab | |
| IL-4/13 | Dupilumab | | | Dupilumab (sc) | |
| CRTH2 | OC000459 (po) | | | OC000459 | |
| | BI 671800 (po) | | | BI671800 | |
| GATA-3 | GATA-3 spec.DNAzyme | | | GATA-3 spec. DNAzyme | |
| Siglec-8 | AK001 | | | | |
| *Non-type 2 inflammation* | | | | | |
| Neutrophilic inflammation | | | | | |
| Th1 | | | | | |
| Th17/Th22 | | | Brodalumab | | Brodalumab |
| *Neurogenic endotype* | | | | | |
| TRPV1 | | Capsaicin (in) SB-705498 (IN) | | | |
| *Barrier dysfunction* | | | | | |
| None | | | | | |

*IN* intranasal; *IV* intravenous; *po* per os; *sc* subcutaneous

after grass pollen provocation [96]. A comparative study including 146 patients found that its efficacy on nasal symptoms score was superior to montelukast, but inferior to intranasal fluticasone furoate [96].

GATA-3 is an important transcription factor and considered to be a 'master switch' of type 2 inflammation. It is responsible for the differentiation of Th0 cells towards Th2 cells and promotes the production of IL-4, IL-5 and IL-9 [97]. Significantly higher levels of GATA-3 mRNA has been documented in eosinophilic NP [98]. The use of a GATA-3 specific DNAzyme in the treatment of allergic asthma has been investigated in a phase IIb study, which reported a significant attenuation of asthmatic responses after allergen provocation, together with an attenuation of Th2-regulated inflammation [99]. So far, these targeted treatments have not been investigated in rhinitis or in CRS.

Siglec-8 is a cell surface receptor selectively expressed on mast cells, eosinophils and basophils [100]. Currently, a phase II study is ongoing to evaluate the efficacy of AK001, a monoclonal antibody targeting siglec-8, in patients with CRSwNP.

*Allergen immunotherapy (AIT)*

AIT is the only potential curative treatment option for IgE-mediated allergic diseases. The mechanisms of action of AIT include very early desensitization of mast cells and basophils, early generation of allergen-specific regulatory T cells (Treg) and B cells (Breg), suppression of Th2 and Th1 cells and late decrease of IgE/IgG4 ratio, tissue mast cell count and eosinophil counts [101]. This results in a reduced type 1 hypersensitivity reaction upon specific allergen exposure.

Currently there are two types of AIT applied in clinical practice, i.e. subcutaneous and sublingual immunotherapy AIT (respectively SCIT and SLIT). Despite the fact that both types of AIT have proven efficacy for different types of allergens, it is difficult to predict response to this treatment. Nonetheless, different biomarkers have been evaluated to identify AIT-responsive endotypes.

Several studies have shown that increased IgG4 levels in serum are associated with clinical improvement [102, 103]. Determination of allergen-specific IgE and IgG4 antibody levels via microarrays has been proposed as a potential biomarker to monitor AIT. Wollman et al.

demonstrated that an IgG4 induced reduction of allergen-specific IgE binding has a high predictive value of 90% for clinical improvement. This assumption is based on the correlation between decreased allergen-specific IgE binding on Immuno Solid-phase Allergen Chip (ISAC) microarray and increased nasal tolerance in provocation tests [104]. Another clinical study performed by Schmid et al. showed that pre-treatment-specific IgE levels on ISAC microarray could predict the induction and magnitude of the IgG4 response during SCIT. Moreover, elevated IgE levels before treatment is thought to be a prerequisite for induction of IgG4 blocking antibodies. In addition IgE and IgG4 levels correlate with other functional immunological changes such as facilitated antigen binding, basophil sensitivity and clinical symptoms score [105].

Therefore, measuring IgE levels on serum samples before and after updosing could be used as a biomarker for early monitoring of AIT. This could be particularly useful in patients with uncertain clinical improvement upon AIT. For example, when IgE levels are decreased, AIT can be pursued aiming at further reduction of IgE. On the other hand, when no change or increase of the IgE levels or absence of IgG4 blocking antibodies is observed AIT should be modified or discontinued.

Another biomarker was proposed by Shamji et al. who demonstrated that ex vivo basophil hyporesponsiveness to allergen, confirmed with flow cytometry for intracellularly labelled diamine oxidase on blood samples, is useful to monitor efficacy and induction of allergen-specific tolerance during AIT [106]. Suppression of basophil responsiveness and subsequent histamine release was correlated with lower AR symptoms scores.

Several attempts are made to establish biomarkers for monitoring AIT. It appears essential that the proposed biomarkers should be compared with each other in regards to their predictive value as well as their reproducibility, complexity of measurement and cost-effectiveness. Further research towards biomarkers are needed and will generate essential information to create novel and improved AIT models.

**Therapies targeting non-type 2 inflammation**
Development of novel therapies targeting non-type 2 inflammation seems more challenging compared with type 2 inflammation. Different biologicals have been investigated but these showed only little or no improvement in clinically relevant asthma outcome parameters.

CXC chemokine 2 receptor (CXCR2) antagonists (e.g. AZD5069, SCH527123) target the CXCR2 receptors on neutrophils and prevent their activation through the chemokine IL-8. Their efficacy has been investigated in the treatment of severe asthma, in which no clinical improvement was seen, despite reduction of neutrophils in sputum and blood [107, 108].

Brodalumab is a human anti-IL17A mAb designed to target IL-17A, a cytokine that is associated with neutrophilic inflammation and corticosteroid resistance. A trial of brodalumab in patients with uncontrolled moderate to severe asthma, without being selected for neutrophilic inflammation, reported no improvement of symptoms or lung function [109].

So far, no trials evaluating targeted treatments of non-type 2 inflammation have been conducted in rhinitis or CRS. The relative poor evolution in the development of biologicals targeting non-type 2 inflammation indicates that the non-type 2 inflammation needs further research to identify distinct subendotypes.

**Therapies targeting neurogenic activation**
*Targeting TRPV1 pathway*
Capsaicin, the pungent substance in red pepper responsible for a burning sensation, has been proven to be effective in reducing NHR symptoms in IR [57, 110]. Capsaicin activates the TRPV1 channel which leads to influx of $Ca^{2+}$ resulting in neuronal excitation and release of neuropeptides, followed by a long-lasting refractory period, during which the neurons are not responsive anymore to a broad range of stimuli. Its therapeutic effect is thought to be due to the above-mentioned de-functionalization and/or degeneration of C-fibers by massive $Ca^{2+}$ influx [57]. Significant and long-term reduction (up to 9 months after treatment cessation) of NHR symptoms have been reported [111].

To optimize the treatment with capsaicin a study was performed comparing two regimens: application of five doses of capsaicin on one single day versus one dose of capsaicin every 2 days for 2 weeks. Both regimens seemed to be equally effective, but the former scheme is preferred as it is thought to enhance patient compliance [110].

An alternative therapeutic option is targeting the TRPV1 ion-channel with the selective TRPV1 antagonist SB-705498. Reduction of NHR symptoms due to intranasal application of SB-705498 has been documented [112] So far, no head-to-head trial has been performed comparing capsaicin and SB-705498.

**Therapies targeting epithelial barrier dysfunction**
Restoring epithelial barrier function might reduce excessive penetration of allergens and/or harmful particles into the submucosal space, ultimately impeding continuous activation of the immune system and subsequent symptoms. Interfering with Toll like receptor or epidermal growth factor receptor signaling has been demonstrated to have barrier modulating capacity in

different in vitro and murine studies (reviewed in Steelant et al.) [113]. Whether these treatments might also lead to clinical improvement of symptoms needs to be investigated.

Recent findings suggest that the therapeutic effect of locally applied corticosteroids might also result from their ability to enhance barrier integrity [62]. Since decades, corticosteroids are part of the standard treatment of the upper and lower airway diseases because of their anti-inflammatory properties [114, 115]. It was recently demonstrated that corticosteroids upregulate tight junction expression and thereby restore barrier function both in primary epithelial cell cultures and in a model of house dust mite (HDM)-induced allergic airway inflammation [62]. In addition, HDM AR patients taking inhaled steroids showed reduced epithelial permeability compared to steroid-naive patients [62].

## Current challenges in endotype-driven treatments

The recently gained insight into different pathophysiological mechanisms of rhinitis and CRS has been the driving force for the development of targeted therapies for patients with chronic upper airway disease. This evolution instigates the development of strategies to identify those patients who are most likely to benefit from these therapies. This so called endotype-driven treatment is one of the 4 pillars of precision medicine. Implementation of the principles of precision medicine into the management of airway diseases is a major challenge for the next decade [116].

Disease heterogeneity needs to be further explored and will lead to the discovery of new biomarkers that serve as a unique signature for a particular endotype. So far, important progresses have been made in identifying endotypes, of which type 2 inflammation is well ahead of other endotypes. Non-type 2 inflammation, the neurogenic endotype and barrier dysfunction needs further untangling and exploration.

So far, only a limited number of biomarkers are ready for use in clinical practice, such as blood eosinophils or serum specific and total IgE. Biomarkers should be pathway-specific, easy to measure, reproducible and affordable. The analysis of mediators in nasal secretions for endotyping is promising but requires further investigation. The biomarkers discussed in this article are mostly used in a research setting and represent potential biomarkers that need to be qualified and validated. An ideal strategy to reach biomarker identification, qualification and validation is through large-scale multi-center studies implying cooperation and standardization of laboratories and databanks all over the world. That way all efforts made towards precision medicine will be recognized more efficiently for implementation.

Besides ameliorating treatment approaches for the individual patients, precision medicine is thought to help in resolving the socio-economic burden of upper airway diseases [116]. It is believed that the reduction of the socio-economic burden due to endotype-driven treatment will outweigh the investments made in research of endotypes and development of novel treatment agents. Whilst the economic aspect is a motive for development of endotype-driven treatments, it is the main challenge at the same time. Considerable investments are required to conduct research on endotypes, biomarkers and biologicals. Raising political awareness about the allergy epidemics and its socio-economics costs is desired and will facilitate implementation in clinical practice. Because of the high cost associated with biological treatment, these molecules will in first place be retained for patients with severe and uncontrolled disease.

Three crucial prerequisites are identified to drive the next step in endotype-driven therapy:

- the demonstration of the predictive value of biomarkers in rhinitis and CRS, guiding the clinician in applying precision medicine in practise
- the recognition and better understanding of the contribution of one or more immunologic pathways or endotypes to the disease phenotype
- the demonstration of targeted treatment having superiority in clinically relevant outcomes and inferiority in cost over existing treatment options.

## Conclusion

This review provides an overview of the efforts made towards endotype-driven treatments in upper airway diseases. Current knowledge about type 2 inflammation is well ahead of other endotypes. Type 2 targeted treatments with monoclonal antibodies against IgE, IL5 and IL4Rα have been proven to be effective in chronic upper airway diseases supporting the importance of this endotype. Neurogenic inflammation as causative mechanism for nasal hyperreactivity is also well established and treatment with capsaicin is proven to be effective in IR with hyperreactivity. Barrier dysfunction and non-type 2 inflammation still need to be investigated more extensively to support its importance in upper airway diseases. Endotype-driven treatment still needs to face multiple challenges before its implementation in daily practice.

**Authors' contributions**
GDG, PWH, SFS conceived and designed the entire manuscript; wrote the manuscript: GDG, SFS; critically reviewed and revised the manuscript: PWH, WJF, BP, BS. All authors read and approved the final manuscript.

## Author details

[1] Department of Otorhinolaryngology-Head and Neck Surgery, UZ Leuven, Louvain, Belgium. [2] Department of Otorhinolaryngology, Academic Medical Center, Amsterdam, The Netherlands. [3] Upper Airways Research Laboratory, Department of Otorhinolaryngology-Head and Neck Surgery, Ghent University, Ghent, Belgium. [4] Laboratory of Clinical Immunology, Department of Immunology and Microbiology, KU Leuven, Herestraat 49/PB811, 3000 Louvain, Belgium.

## Acknowledgements

Not applicable.

## Competing interests

The authors declare that they have no competing interests.

## Funding

PWH is recipient of a senior clinical investigator grant from the Research Foundation - Flanders (FWO), Belgium. The author's laboratory is supported by the Interuniversity Attraction Pole (IUAP, P7/30), Belgium.

## References

1. Katelaris CH, Lee BW, Potter PC, Maspero JF, Cingi C, Lopatin A, et al. Prevalence and diversity of allergic rhinitis in regions of the world beyond Europe and North America. Clin Exp Allergy. 2012;42(2):186–207.
2. Hastan D, Fokkens WJ, Bachert C, Newson RB, Bislimovska J, Bockelbrink A, et al. Chronic rhinosinusitis in Europe–an underestimated disease. A GA²LEN study. Allergy. 2011;66(9):1216–23.
3. Bousquet J, Schünemann HJ, Samolinski B, Demoly P, Baena-Cagnani CE, Bachert C, et al. Allergic rhinitis and its impact on asthma (ARIA): achievements in 10 years and future needs. J Allergy Clin Immunol. 2012;130(5):1049–62.
4. Hens G, Vanaudenaerde BM, Bullens DM, Piessens M, Decramer M, Dupont LJ, et al. Sinonasal pathology in nonallergic asthma and COPD: 'united airway disease' beyond the scope of allergy. Allergy. 2008;63(3):261–7.
5. Muraro A, Fokkens WJ, Pietikainen S, Borrelli D, Agache I, Bousquet J, et al. European symposium on precision medicine in allergy and airways diseases: report of the European Union parliament symposium (October 14, 2015). Rhinology. 2015;53(4):303–7.
6. Hellings PW, Fokkens WJ, Akdis C, Bachert C, Cingi C, Dietz de Loos D, et al. Uncontrolled allergic rhinitis and chronic rhinosinusitis: where do we stand today? Allergy. 2013;68(1):1–7.
7. van der Veen J, Seys SF, Timmermans M, Levie P, Jorissen M, Fokkens WJ, et al. Real-life study showing uncontrolled rhinosinusitis after sinus surgery in a tertiary referral centre. Allergy. 2017;72(2):282–90.
8. Collins FS, Varmus H. A new initiative on precision medicine. N Engl J Med. 2015;372(9):793–5.
9. Tan HT, Sugita K, Akdis CA. Novel biologicals for the treatment of allergic diseases and asthma. Curr Allergy Asthma Rep. 2016;16(10):70.
10. Seys SF. Role of sputum biomarkers in the management of asthma. Curr Opin Pulm Med. 2017;23(1):34–40.
11. Agache I, Sugita K, Morita H, Akdis M, Akdis CA. The complex type 2 endotype in allergy and asthma: from laboratory to bedside. Curr Allergy Asthma Rep. 2015;15(6):29.
12. Bousquet J, Khaltaev N, Cruz AA, Denburg J, Fokkens WJ, Togias A, et al. Allergic rhinitis and its impact on asthma (ARIA) 2008 update (in collaboration with the World Health Organization, GA(2)LEN and AllerGen). Allergy. 2008;63(Suppl 86):8–160.
13. Papadopoulos NG, Bernstein JA, Demoly P, Dykewicz M, Fokkens W, Hellings PW, et al. Phenotypes and endotypes of rhinitis and their impact on management: a PRACTALL report. Allergy. 2015;70(5):474–94.

14. Fokkens WJ, Lund VJ, Mullol J, Bachert C, Alobid I, Baroody F, et al. EPOS 2012: European position paper on rhinosinusitis and nasal polyps 2012. A summary for otorhinolaryngologists. Rhinology. 2012;50(1):1–12.
15. Hammad H, Lambrecht BN. Barrier epithelial cells and the control of type 2 immunity. Immunity. 2015;43(1):29–40.
16. Divekar R, Kita H. Recent advances in epithelium-derived cytokines (IL-33, IL-25, and thymic stromal lymphopoietin) and allergic inflammation. Curr Opin Allergy Clin Immunol. 2015;15(1):98–103.
17. Walford HH, Lund SJ, Baum RE, White AA, Bergeron CM, Husseman J, et al. Increased ILC2s in the eosinophilic nasal polyp endotype are associated with corticosteroid responsiveness. Clin Immunol. 2014;155(1):126–35.
18. Venkatesan N, Lavigne P, Lavigne F, Hamid Q. Effects of fluticasone furoate on clinical and immunological outcomes (IL-17) for patients with nasal polyposis naive to steroid treatment. Ann Otol Rhinol Laryngol. 2016;125(3):213–8.
19. Wang C, Lou H, Wang X, Wang Y, Fan E, Li Y, et al. Effect of budesonide transnasal nebulization in patients with eosinophilic chronic rhinosinusitis with nasal polyps. J Allergy Clin Immunol. 2015;135(4):922. e926–929.e926.
20. Greiner AN, Hellings PW, Rotiroti G, Scadding GK. Allergic rhinitis. Lancet. 2011;378(9809):2112–22.
21. Del Giacco SR, Bakirtas A, Bel E, Custovic A, Diamant Z, Hamelmann E, et al. Allergy in severe asthma. Allergy 2016.
22. Rondón C, Bogas G, Barrionuevo E, Blanca M, Torres MJ, Campo P. Non-allergic rhinitis and lower airway disease. Allergy. 2017;72(1):24–34.
23. Jung YG, Kim KH, Kim HY, Dhong HJ, Chung SK. Predictive capabilities of serum eosinophil cationic protein, percentage of eosinophils and total immunoglobulin E in allergic rhinitis without bronchial asthma. J Int Med Res. 2011;39(6):2209–16.
24. Scadding G. Cytokine profiles in allergic rhinitis. Curr Allergy Asthma Rep. 2014;14(5):435.
25. Gevaert P, Calus L, Van Zele T, Blomme K, De Ruyck N, Bauters W, et al. Omalizumab is effective in allergic and nonallergic patients with nasal polyps and asthma. J Allergy Clin Immunol. 2013;131(1):110–116.e111.
26. Wang X, Zhang N, Bo Ms M, Holtappels G, Zheng M, Lou H, et al. Diversity of TH cytokine profiles in patients with chronic rhinosinusitis: a multicenter study in Europe, Asia, and Oceania. J Allergy Clin Immunol. 2016;138(5):1344–53.
27. Zhang N, Van Zele T, Perez-Novo C, Van Bruaene N, Holtappels G, DeRuyck N, et al. Different types of T-effector cells orchestrate mucosal inflammation in chronic sinus disease. J Allergy Clin Immunol. 2008;122(5):961–8.
28. Van Zele T, Holtappels G, Gevaert P, Bachert C. Differences in initial immunoprofiles between recurrent and nonrecurrent chronic rhinosinusitis with nasal polyps. Am J Rhinol Allergy. 2014;28(3):192–8.
29. Soler ZM, Sauer DA, Mace J, Smith TL. Relationship between clinical measures and histopathologic findings in chronic rhinosinusitis. Otolaryngol Head Neck Surg. 2009;141(4):454–61.
30. Soler ZM, Sauer D, Mace J, Smith TL. Impact of mucosal eosinophilia and nasal polyposis on quality-of-life outcomes after sinus surgery. Otolaryngol Head Neck Surg. 2010;142(1):64–71.
31. Snidvongs K, Lam M, Sacks R, Earls P, Kalish L, Phillips PS, et al. Structured histopathology profiling of chronic rhinosinusitis in routine practice. Int Forum Allergy Rhinol. 2012;2(5):376–85.
32. König K, Klemens C, Haack M, Nicoló MS, Becker S, Kramer MF, et al. Cytokine patterns in nasal secretion of non-atopic patients distinguish between chronic rhinosinusitis with or without nasal polys. Allergy Asthma Clin Immunol. 2016;12:19.
33. Matsuwaki Y, Ookushi T, Asaka D, Mori E, Nakajima T, Yoshida T, et al. Chronic rhinosinusitis: risk factors for the recurrence of chronic rhinosinusitis based on 5-year follow-up after endoscopic sinus surgery. Int Arch Allergy Immunol. 2008;146(Suppl 1):77–81.
34. Vlaminck S, Vauterin T, Hellings PW, Jorissen M, Acke F, Van Cauwenberge P, et al. The importance of local eosinophilia in the surgical outcome of chronic rhinosinusitis: a 3-year prospective observational study. Am J Rhinol Allergy. 2014;28(3):260–4.
35. Nakayama T, Yoshikawa M, Asaka D, Okushi T, Matsuwaki Y, Otori N, et al. Mucosal eosinophilia and recurrence of nasal polyps—new classification of chronic rhinosinusitis. Rhinology. 2011;49(4):392–6.

36. Bachert C, Zhang N, Holtappels G, De Lobel L, van Cauwenberge P, Liu S, et al. Presence of IL-5 protein and IgE antibodies to staphylococcal enterotoxins in nasal polyps is associated with comorbid asthma. J Allergy Clin Immunol. 2010;126(5):962–968, 968.e961–966.

37. Van Zele T, Gevaert P, Watelet JB, Claeys G, Holtappels G, Claeys C, et al. Staphylococcus aureus colonization and IgE antibody formation to enterotoxins is increased in nasal polyposis. J Allergy Clin Immunol. 2004;114(4):981–3.

38. Singhal D, Psaltis AJ, Foreman A, Wormald PJ. The impact of biofilms on outcomes after endoscopic sinus surgery. Am J Rhinol Allergy. 2010;24(3):169–74.

39. Singhal D, Foreman A, Jervis-Bardy J, Bardy JJ, Wormald PJ. Staphylococcus aureus biofilms: nemesis of endoscopic sinus surgery. Laryngoscope. 2011;121(7):1578–83.

40. Kisich KO, Carspecken CW, Fiéve S, Boguniewicz M, Leung DY. Defective killing of Staphylococcus aureus in atopic dermatitis is associated with reduced mobilization of human beta-defensin-3. J Allergy Clin Immunol. 2008;122(1):62–8.

41. Bogefors J, Kvarnhammar AM, Höckerfelt U, Cardell LO. Reduced tonsillar expression of human β-defensin 1, 2 and 3 in allergic rhinitis. FEMS Immunol Med Microbiol. 2012;65(3):431–8.

42. Huvenne W, Hellings PW, Bachert C. Role of staphylococcal superantigens in airway disease. Int Arch Allergy Immunol. 2013;161(4):304–14.

43. Bachert C, van Steen K, Zhang N, Holtappels G, Cattaert T, Maus B, et al. Specific IgE against Staphylococcus aureus enterotoxins: an independent risk factor for asthma. J Allergy Clin Immunol. 2012;130(2):376.e378–381.e378.

44. Tomassen P, Vandeplas G, Van Zele T, Cardell LO, Arebro J, Olze H, et al. Inflammatory endotypes of chronic rhinosinusitis based on cluster analysis of biomarkers. J Allergy Clin Immunol. 2016;137(5):1449.e1444–1456.e1444.

45. Cao PP, Li HB, Wang BF, Wang SB, You XJ, Cui YH, et al. Distinct immunopathologic characteristics of various types of chronic rhinosinusitis in adult Chinese. J Allergy Clin Immunol. 2009;124(3):478–484, 484.e471–472.

46. Bullens DM, Truyen E, Coteur L, Dilissen E, Hellings PW, Dupont LJ, et al. IL-17 mRNA in sputum of asthmatic patients: linking T cell driven inflammation and granulocytic influx? Respir Res. 2006;7:135.

47. Hellings PW, Kasran A, Liu Z, Vandekerckhove P, Wuyts A, Overbergh L, et al. Interleukin-17 orchestrates the granulocyte influx into airways after allergen inhalation in a mouse model of allergic asthma. Am J Respir Cell Mol Biol. 2003;28(1):42–50.

48. Lindén A, Dahlén B. Interleukin-17 cytokine signalling in patients with asthma. Eur Respir J. 2014;44(5):1319–31.

49. Agache I, Akdis CA. Endotypes of allergic diseases and asthma: an important step in building blocks for the future of precision medicine. Allergol Int. 2016;65(3):243–52.

50. Shi LL, Xiong P, Zhang L, Cao PP, Liao B, Lu X, et al. Features of airway remodeling in different types of Chinese chronic rhinosinusitis are associated with inflammation patterns. Allergy. 2013;68(1):101–9.

51. Wen W, Liu W, Zhang L, Bai J, Fan Y, Xia W, et al. Increased neutrophilia in nasal polyps reduces the response to oral corticosteroid therapy. J Allergy Clin Immunol. 2012;129(6):1522.e1525–1528.e1525.

52. van Kempen M, Bachert C, Van Cauwenberge P. An update on the pathophysiology of rhinovirus upper respiratory tract infections. Rhinology. 1999;37(3):97–103.

53. Bachert C, van Kempen MJ, Höpken K, Holtappels G, Wagenmann M. Elevated levels of myeloperoxidase, pro-inflammatory cytokines and chemokines in naturally acquired upper respiratory tract infections. Eur Arch Otorhinolaryngol. 2001;258(8):406–12.

54. Van Bruaene N, Perez-Novo C, Van Crombruggen K, De Ruyck N, Holtappels G, Van Cauwenberge P, et al. Inflammation and remodelling patterns in early stage chronic rhinosinusitis. Clin Exp Allergy. 2012;42(6):883–90.

55. Muraro A, Lemanske RF, Hellings PW, Akdis CA, Bieber T, Casale TB, et al. Precision medicine in patients with allergic diseases: airway diseases and atopic dermatitis-PRACTALL document of the European Academy of Allergy and Clinical Immunology and the American Academy of Allergy, Asthma & Immunology. J Allergy Clin Immunol. 2016;137(5):1347–58.

56. Bernstein JA, Singh U. Neural abnormalities in nonallergic rhinitis. Curr Allergy Asthma Rep. 2015;15(4):18.

57. Van Gerven L, Alpizar YA, Wouters MM, Hox V, Hauben E, Jorissen M, et al. Capsaicin treatment reduces nasal hyperreactivity and transient receptor potential cation channel subfamily V, receptor 1 (TRPV1) overexpression in patients with idiopathic rhinitis. J Allergy Clin Immunol. 2014;133(5):1332–1339, 1339.e1331–1333.

58. Van Gerven L, Boeckxstaens G, Jorissen M, Fokkens W, Hellings PW. Short-time cold dry air exposure: a useful diagnostic tool for nasal hyperresponsiveness. Laryngoscope. 2012;122(12):2615–20.

59. Parker D, Prince A. Innate immunity in the respiratory epithelium. Am J Respir Cell Mol Biol. 2011;45(2):189–201.

60. Xiao C, Puddicombe SM, Field S, Haywood J, Broughton-Head V, Puxeddu I, et al. Defective epithelial barrier function in asthma. J Allergy Clin Immunol. 2011;128(3):549–556.e541–512.

61. Soyka MB, Wawrzyniak P, Eiwegger T, Holzmann D, Treis A, Wanke K, et al. Defective epithelial barrier in chronic rhinosinusitis: the regulation of tight junctions by IFN-γ and IL-4. J Allergy Clin Immunol. 2012;130(5):1087.e1010–1096.e1010.

62. Steelant B, Farré R, Wawrzyniak P, Belmans J, Dekimpe E, Vanheel H, et al. Impaired barrier function in patients with house dust mite-induced allergic rhinitis is accompanied by decreased occludin and zonula occludens-1 expression. J Allergy Clin Immunol. 2016;137(4):1043–1053.e1041–1045.

63. MacGlashan DW, Bochner BS, Adelman DC, Jardieu PM, Togias A, McKenzie-White J, et al. Down-regulation of Fc(epsilon)RI expression on human basophils during in vivo treatment of atopic patients with anti-IgE antibody. J Immunol. 1997;158(3):1438–45.

64. Prussin C, Griffith DT, Boesel KM, Lin H, Foster B, Casale TB. Omalizumab treatment downregulates dendritic cell FcepsilonRI expression. J Allergy Clin Immunol. 2003;112(6):1147–54.

65. Lin H, Boesel KM, Griffith DT, Prussin C, Foster B, Romero FA, et al. Omalizumab rapidly decreases nasal allergic response and FcepsilonRI on basophils. J Allergy Clin Immunol. 2004;113(2):297–302.

66. Casale TB, Condemi J, LaForce C, Nayak A, Rowe M, Watrous M, et al. Effect of omalizumab on symptoms of seasonal allergic rhinitis: a randomized controlled trial. JAMA. 2001;286(23):2956–67.

67. Chervinsky P, Casale T, Townley R, Tripathy I, Hedgecock S, Fowler-Taylor A, et al. Omalizumab, an anti-IgE antibody, in the treatment of adults and adolescents with perennial allergic rhinitis. Ann Allergy Asthma Immunol. 2003;91(2):160–7.

68. Hanf G, Noga O, O'Connor A, Kunkel G. Omalizumab inhibits allergen challenge-induced nasal response. Eur Respir J. 2004;23(3):414–8.

69. Adelroth E, Rak S, Haahtela T, Aasand G, Rosenhall L, Zetterstrom O, et al. Recombinant humanized mAb-E25, an anti-IgE mAb, in birch pollen-induced seasonal allergic rhinitis. J Allergy Clin Immunol. 2000;106(2):253–9.

70. Bez C, Schubert R, Kopp M, Ersfeld Y, Rosewich M, Kuehr J, et al. Effect of anti-immunoglobulin E on nasal inflammation in patients with seasonal allergic rhinoconjunctivitis. Clin Exp Allergy. 2004;34(7):1079–85.

71. Okubo K, Ogino S, Nagakura T, Ishikawa T. Omalizumab is effective and safe in the treatment of Japanese cedar pollen-induced seasonal allergic rhinitis. Allergol Int. 2006;55(4):379–86.

72. Kamin W, Kopp MV, Erdnuess F, Schauer U, Zielen S, Wahn U. Safety of anti-IgE treatment with omalizumab in children with seasonal allergic rhinitis undergoing specific immunotherapy simultaneously. Pediatr Allergy Immunol. 2010;21(1 Pt 2):e160–5.

73. Ogino S, Nagakura T, Okubo K, Sato N, Takahashi M, Ishikawa T. Retreatment with omalizumab at one year interval for Japanese cedar pollen-induced seasonal allergic rhinitis is effective and well tolerated. Int Arch Allergy Immunol. 2009;149(3):239–45.

74. Rolinck-Werninghaus C, Hamelmann E, Keil T, Kulig M, Koetz K, Gerstner B, et al. The co-seasonal application of anti-IgE after preseasonal specific immunotherapy decreases ocular and nasal symptom scores and rescue medication use in grass pollen allergic children. Allergy. 2004;59(9):973–9.

75. Kopp MV, Hamelmann E, Zielen S, Kamin W, Bergmann KC, Sieder C, et al. Combination of omalizumab and specific immunotherapy is superior to immunotherapy in patients with seasonal allergic rhinoconjunctivitis and co-morbid seasonal allergic asthma. Clin Exp Allergy. 2009;39(2):271–9.

76. Kuehr J, Brauburger J, Zielen S, Schauer U, Kamin W, Von Berg A, et al. Efficacy of combination treatment with anti-IgE plus specific immunotherapy in polysensitized children and adolescents with seasonal allergic rhinitis. J Allergy Clin Immunol. 2002;109(2):274–80.

77. Casale TB, Busse WW, Kline JN, Ballas ZK, Moss MH, Townley RG, et al. Omalizumab pretreatment decreases acute reactions after rush immunotherapy for ragweed-induced seasonal allergic rhinitis. J Allergy Clin Immunol. 2006;117(1):134–40.

78. Vignola AM, Humbert M, Bousquet J, Boulet LP, Hedgecock S, Blogg M, et al. Efficacy and tolerability of anti-immunoglobulin E therapy with omalizumab in patients with concomitant allergic asthma and persistent allergic rhinitis: SOLAR. Allergy. 2004;59(7):709–17.

79. Humbert M, Boulet LP, Niven RM, Panahloo Z, Blogg M, Ayre G. Omalizumab therapy: patients who achieve greatest benefit for their asthma experience greatest benefit for rhinitis. Allergy. 2009;64(1):81–4.

80. Corren J, Shapiro G, Reimann J, Deniz Y, Wong D, Adelman D, et al. Allergen skin tests and free IgE levels during reduction and cessation of omalizumab therapy. J Allergy Clin Immunol. 2008;121(2):506–11.

81. Kopp MV, Hamelmann E, Bendiks M, Zielen S, Kamin W, Bergmann KC, et al. Transient impact of omalizumab in pollen allergic patients undergoing specific immunotherapy. Pediatr Allergy Immunol. 2013;24(5):427–33.

82. Vennera MeC, Picado C, Mullol J, Alobid I, Bernal-Sprekelsen M. Efficacy of omalizumab in the treatment of nasal polyps. Thorax. 2011;66(9):824–5.

83. Penn R, Mikula S. The role of anti-IgE immunoglobulin therapy in nasal polyposis: a pilot study. Am J Rhinol. 2007;21(4):428–32.

84. Pinto JM, Mehta N, DiTineo M, Wang J, Baroody FM, Naclerio RM. A randomized, double-blind, placebo-controlled trial of anti-IgE for chronic rhinosinusitis. Rhinology. 2010;48(3):318–24.

85. Arm JP, Bottoli I, Skerjanec A, Floch D, Groenewegen A, Maahs S, et al. Pharmacokinetics, pharmacodynamics and safety of QGE031 (ligelizumab), a novel high-affinity anti-IgE antibody, in atopic subjects. Clin Exp Allergy. 2014;44(11):1371–85.

86. Gauvreau GM, Harris JM, Boulet LP, Scheerens H, Fitzgerald JM, Putnam WS, et al. Targeting membrane-expressed IgE B cell receptor with an antibody to the M1 prime epitope reduces IgE production. Sci Transl Med. 2014;6(243):243–85.

87. Bachert C, Wagenmann M, Hauser U, Rudack C. IL-5 synthesis is upregulated in human nasal polyp tissue. J Allergy Clin Immunol. 1997;99(6 Pt 1):837–42.

88. Gevaert P, Lang-Loidolt D, Lackner A, Stammberger H, Staudinger H, Van Zele T, et al. Nasal IL-5 levels determine the response to anti-IL-5 treatment in patients with nasal polyps. J Allergy Clin Immunol. 2006;118(5):1133–41.

89. Gevaert P, Van Bruaene N, Cattaert T, Van Steen K, Van Zele T, Acke F, et al. Mepolizumab, a humanized anti-IL-5 mAb, as a treatment option for severe nasal polyposis. J Allergy Clin Immunol. 2011;128(5):989–995. e981–988.

90. Bleecker ER, FitzGerald JM, Chanez P, Papi A, Weinstein SF, Barker P, et al. Efficacy and safety of benralizumab for patients with severe asthma uncontrolled with high-dosage inhaled corticosteroids and long-acting β2-agonists (SIROCCO): a randomised, multicentre, placebo-controlled phase 3 trial. Lancet. 2016;388(10056):2115–27.

91. Ul-Haq Z, Naz S, Mesaik MA. Interleukin-4 receptor signaling and its binding mechanism: a therapeutic insight from inhibitors tool box. Cytokine Growth Factor Rev. 2016;32:3–15.

92. Wenzel SE, Jayawardena S, Graham NM, Pirozzi G, Teper A. Severe asthma and asthma-chronic obstructive pulmonary disease syndrome—Authors' reply. Lancet. 2016;388(10061):2742.

93. Simpson EL, Bieber T, Guttman-Yassky E, Beck LA, Blauvelt A, Cork MJ, et al. Two phase 3 trials of dupilumab versus placebo in atopic dermatitis. N Engl J Med. 2016;375(24):2335–48.

94. Bachert C, Mannent L, Naclerio RM, Mullol J, Ferguson BJ, Gevaert P, et al. Effect of subcutaneous dupilumab on nasal polyp burden in patients with chronic sinusitis and nasal polyposis a randomized clinical trial. JAMA. 2016;315(5):469–79.

95. Horak F, Zieglmayer P, Zieglmayer R, Lemell P, Collins LP, Hunter MG, et al. The CRTH2 antagonist OC000459 reduces nasal and ocular symptoms in allergic subjects exposed to grass pollen, a randomised, placebo-controlled, double-blind trial. Allergy. 2012;67(12):1572–9.

96. Krug N, Gupta A, Badorrek P, Koenen R, Mueller M, Pivovarova A, et al. Efficacy of the oral chemoattractant receptor homologous molecule on TH2 cells antagonist BI 671800 in patients with seasonal allergic rhinitis. J Allergy Clin Immunol. 2014;133(2):414–9.

97. Yagi R, Zhu J, Paul WE. An updated view on transcription factor GATA3-mediated regulation of Th1 and Th2 cell differentiation. Int Immunol. 2011;23(7):415–20.

98. Sun C, Ouyang H, Luo R. Distinct characteristics of nasal polyps with and without eosinophilia. Braz J Otorhinolaryngol. 2017;83(1):66–72.

99. Krug N, Hohlfeld JM, Kirsten AM, Kornmann O, Beeh KM, Kappeler D, et al. Allergen-induced asthmatic responses modified by a GATA3-specific DNAzyme. N Engl J Med. 2015;372(21):1987–95.

100. Macauley MS, Crocker PR, Paulson JC. Siglec-mediated regulation of immune cell function in disease. Nat Rev Immunol. 2014;14(10):653–66.

101. Akdis CA, Akdis M. Mechanisms of allergen-specific immunotherapy and immune tolerance to allergens. World Allergy Organ J. 2015;8(1):17.

102. Zhao D, Lai X, Tian M, Jiang Y, Zheng Y, Gjesing B, et al. The functional IgE-blocking factor induced by allergen-specific immunotherapy correlates with IgG4 antibodies and a decrease of symptoms in house dust mite-allergic children. Int Arch Allergy Immunol. 2016;169(2):113–20.

103. Nouri-Aria KT, Wachholz PA, Francis JN, Jacobson MR, Walker SM, Wilcock LK, et al. Grass pollen immunotherapy induces mucosal and peripheral IL-10 responses and blocking IgG activity. J Immunol. 2004;172(5):3252–9.

104. Wollmann E, Lupinek C, Kundi M, Selb R, Niederberger V, Valenta R. Reduction in allergen-specific IgE binding as measured by microarray: a possible surrogate marker for effects of specific immunotherapy. J Allergy Clin Immunol. 2015;136(3):806.e807–809.e807.

105. Schmid JM, Würtzen PA, Dahl R, Hoffmann HJ. Pretreatment IgE sensitization patterns determine the molecular profile of the IgG4 response during updosing of subcutaneous immunotherapy with timothy grass pollen extract. J Allergy Clin Immunol. 2016;137(2):562–70.

106. Shamji MH, Layhadi JA, Scadding GW, Cheung DK, Calderon MA, Turka LA, et al. Basophil expression of diamine oxidase: a novel biomarker of allergen immunotherapy response. J Allergy Clin Immunol. 2015;135(4):913.e919–921.e919.

107. Nair P, Gaga M, Zervas E, Alagha K, Hargreave FE, O'Byrne PM, et al. Safety and efficacy of a CXCR2 antagonist in patients with severe asthma and sputum neutrophils: a randomized, placebo-controlled clinical trial. Clin Exp Allergy. 2012;42(7):1097–103.

108. O'Byrne PM, Metev H, Puu M, Richter K, Keen C, Uddin M, et al. Efficacy and safety of a CXCR2 antagonist, AZD5069, in patients with uncontrolled persistent asthma: a randomised, double-blind, placebo-controlled trial. Lancet Respir Med. 2016;4(10):797–806.

109. Busse WW, Holgate S, Kerwin E, Chon Y, Feng J, Lin J, et al. Randomized, double-blind, placebo-controlled study of brodalumab, a human anti-IL-17 receptor monoclonal antibody, in moderate to severe asthma. Am J Respir Crit Care Med. 2013;188(11):1294–302.

110. Van Rijswijk JB, Boeke EL, Keizer JM, Mulder PG, Blom HM, Fokkens WJ. Intranasal capsaicin reduces nasal hyperreactivity in idiopathic rhinitis: a double-blind randomized application regimen study. Allergy. 2003;58(8):754–61.

111. Blom HM, Severijnen LA, Van Rijswijk JB, Mulder PG, Van Wijk RG, Fokkens WJ. The long-term effects of capsaicin aqueous spray on the nasal mucosa. Clin Exp Allergy. 1998;28(11):1351–8.

112. Holland C, van Drunen C, Denyer J, Smart K, Segboer C, Terreehorst I, et al. Inhibition of capsaicin-driven nasal hyper-reactivity by SB-705498, a TRPV1 antagonist. Br J Clin Pharmacol. 2014;77(5):777–88.

113. Steelant B, Seys SF, Boeckxstaens G, Akdis CA, Ceuppens JL, Hellings PW. Restoring airway epithelial barrier dysfunction: a new therapeutic challenge in allergic airway disease. Rhinology. 2016;54(3):195–205.

114. Schwiebert LM, Beck LA, Stellato C, Bickel CA, Bochner BS, Schleimer RP, et al. Glucocorticosteroid inhibition of cytokine production: relevance to antiallergic actions. J Allergy Clin Immunol. 1996;97(1 Pt 2):143–52.

115. Pundir V, Pundir J, Lancaster G, Baer S, Kirkland P, Cornet M, et al. Role of corticosteroids in functional endoscopic sinus surgery—a systematic review and meta-analysis. Rhinology. 2016;54(1):3–19.

116. Hellings PW, Fokkens WJ, Bachert C, Akdis CA, Bieber T, Agache I, et al. Positioning the principles of precision medicine in care pathways for allergic rhinitis and chronic rhinosinusitis—an EUFOREA-ARIA-EPOS-AIRWAYS ICP statement. Allergy. 2017. doi: 10.1111/all.13162.

# 14

# Expression profiling and functional analysis of Toll-like receptors in primary healthy human nasal epithelial cells shows no correlation and a refractory LPS response

J. van Tongeren[1†], K. I. L. Röschmann[1†], S. M. Reinartz[1], S. Luiten[1], W. J. Fokkens[1], E. C. de Jong[2] and C. M. van Drunen[1*]

## Abstract

**Background:** Innate immune recognition via Toll-like receptors (TLRs) on barrier cells like epithelial cells has been shown to influence the regulation of local immune responses. Here we determine expression level variations and functionality of TLRs in nasal epithelial cells from healthy donors.

**Methods:** Expression levels of the different TLRs on primary nasal epithelial cells from healthy donors derived from inferior turbinates was determined by RT-PCR. Functionality of the TLRs was determined by stimulation with the respective ligand and evaluation of released mediators by Luminex ELISA.

**Results:** Primary nasal epithelial cells express different levels of TLR1-6 and TLR9. We were unable to detect mRNA of TLR7, TLR8 and TLR10. Stimulation with Poly(I:C) resulted in a significant increased secretion of IL-4, IL-6, RANTES, IP-10, MIP-1β, VEGF, FGF, IL-1RA, IL-2R and G-CSF. Stimulation with PGN only resulted in significant increased production of IL-6, VEGF and IL-1RA. Although the expression of TLR4 and co-stimulatory molecules could be confirmed, primary nasal epithelial cells appeared to be unresponsive to stimulation with LPS. Furthermore, we observed huge individual differences in TLR agonist-induced mediator release, which did not correlate with the respective expression of TLRs.

**Conclusion:** Our data suggest that nasal epithelium seems to have developed a delicate system of discrimination and recognition of microbial patterns. Hypo-responsiveness to LPS could provide a mechanism to dampen the inflammatory response in the nasal mucosa in order to avoid a chronic inflammatory response. Individual, differential expression of TLRs on epithelial cells and functionality in terms of released mediators might be a crucial factor in explaining why some people develop allergies to common inhaled antigens, and others do not.

**Keywords:** Nasal epithelial cells, Pattern recognition receptors, Toll-like receptor, Chemokines, Cytokines

## Background

The mucosal barrier of the nose forms the first line of defence against air pollutants, airborne allergens, and (non-) pathogenic microorganisms. Epithelial cells are the outer lining of the mucosa of the nasal airway and play, besides their role as passive physical barrier, an important role in orchestrating innate and adaptive immune responses [1–3]. Epithelium can trigger antimicrobial responses by recognizing pathogen-associated molecular patterns (PAMPs) through the sentinel action of pattern recognition receptors (PRRs) like Toll-like receptors (TLRs).

Toll-like receptors are evolutionarily conserved pattern recognition receptors of the innate immune system [4]. Until now, 13 mammalian TLRs have been characterized and for most of the TLRs, except TLR10, TLR12

*Correspondence: C.M.vanDrunen@amc.uva.nl
[†]J. van Tongeren and K. I. L. Röschmann contributed equally to this work
[1] Department of Otorhinolaryngology, Academic Medical Center (AMC), Amsterdam, The Netherlands
Full list of author information is available at the end of the article

and TLR13, specific ligands have been identified [5, 6]. The first group of receptors recognize bacterial products. TLR2 is activated by a variety of bacterial lipoproteins, peptidoglycans (PGN), and lipoteichoic acids (LTA), by forming a heterodimer with TLR1 or TLR6 [7, 8]. TLR4 appears to form homodimers and under participation of adaptor molecules like MD-2 and CD14 this TLR recognizes lipopolysaccharide (LPS) from the outer membrane of gram-negative bacteria. Originally thought to be a receptor only for LPS, TLR4 now emerges as a molecule responsible for signalling induced by a broad variety of molecules such as respiratory syncytial virus protein F [9], fungal components [10], or endogenous ligands like heat shock proteins, lung surfactant protein A, and beta-defensin [11–13]. Lastly, TLR5 recognizes bacterial Flagellin. Viral compounds trigger endosome-associated receptors, such as TLR3 by double-stranded (ds) RNA or its synthetic analogon polyinosinic polycytidylic acid (Poly I:C) and viral single stranded (ss) RNA signals via TLR7 and TLR8. DNA-containing CpG motifs are recognized via TLR9 [14, 15].

Although TLRs can be involved in the initiation of adaptive immune responses through their presence on dendritic cells (DCs), they may also indirectly affect the adaptive immune response. Innate immune recognition via TLRs on barrier cells like epithelial cells has been shown to determine the functional properties of tissue-resident DCs, thereby instructing the outcome of antigen-specific immunity [16]. The overall complexity of the contribution of TLRs on immune responses can be influenced by several factors like their relative abundance, their individual expression pattern, or the timing of exposure. For example, stimulation of TLR2 and TLR4 signalling pathways has been shown to both drive [16, 17] and inhibit [18, 19] the development of Th2-mediated allergic inflammation in different experimental mouse models. Moreover, the impact of TLR4 stimulation on allergic inflammation is highly dependent upon the dose of the TLR4 agonist, with high LPS concentrations inducing Th1-responses and low concentrations inducing Th2-polarized inflammatory responses [20].

The LPS-induced pulmonary burden varies between different respiratory compartments and might therefore explain the functional differences between bronchial and alveolar epithelial cells with respect to LPS-dependent cytokine release. It is widely believed that alveolar epithelial cells are unresponsive to LPS due to low or absent expression of TLR4 and/or CD14 or MD-2 [21]. In contrast to this it has been reported that lung epithelial cells do express TLR 1–6, including adaptor molecules like CD14 and MD-2, with bronchial epithelial cells showing CD14-dependent activation of TLR4 and alveolar epithelial cells showing LPS-binding protein (LBP)-dependent

inhibition of TLR4 signalling [22, 23], confirming the relevance of co-factors for a proper TLR signalling. Small airway epithelial cells have been shown to express mRNA for the TLRs 1–6 and can respond to various stimuli such as viruses or bacteria resulting in the release of different pro- and anti-inflammatory cytokines and chemokines [24–26].

At present only limited data is available on the expression of TLRs by nasal epithelial cells. Claeys et al. showed constant expression of TLR2 and TLR4 in tissue biopsies from patients with nasal polyposis or chronic rhinosinusitis and in healthy individuals [27]. Isolated nasal epithelial cells from nasal polyps were shown to constitutively express mRNA of all 10 TLRs, with more pronounced expression of TLR 1–6 [28]. Primary nasal polyp epithelial cells express functional TLR3 and TLR4 and release high concentrations of proinflammatory chemokines and cytokines upon stimulation with dsRNA [29]. Until only one study investigated the expression and function of some but not all TLRs on primary nasal epithelial cells from non-allergic, non-diseased individuals specifically [30]. Given the role of TLRs expressed on epithelial cells within the induction of immune responses, the relatively limited knowledge on the expression of TLRs in nasal epithelium, and the protective effect of TLR polymorphism in childhood asthma [31], the aim of this study was to determine the expression and functionality of TLRs expressed in primary nasal epithelial cells from healthy donors.

## Methods

### Patient characteristics

Nasal tissue was obtained from 10 non-allergic ENT patients (defined by negative skin prick test or radioallergosorbent test (RAST)) with septum deviations that required inferior turbinectomy. Patients were between 18 and 65 years of age, were nonsmokers, had not received topical corticosteroids for at least 4 weeks before surgery, and were free of any respiratory tract infections. The study was reviewed and approved by the medical ethical committee of the Academic Medical Center Amsterdam and all patients gave their informed consent.

### Epithelial cell culture

Primary nasal epithelial cells were obtained by digesting nasal turbinates of non-allergic patients with 0.5 mg/ml collagenase 4 (Worthington Biochemical Corp., Lakewood, NJ) for 1 h in Hanks' balanced salt solution (HBSS; Sigma-Aldrich, Zwijndrecht, The Netherlands). Subsequently, epithelial cells were isolated by magnetic activated cell sorting (MACS), according to the manufacturers instruction (Miltenyi Biotec, Leiden, The Netherlands), resuspended in bronchial epithelial growth medium (BEGM) (Lonza Clonetics, Breda, The Netherlands), and seeded in a 75 ml flask. Culture medium was replaced every other day. Cells were grown to 80 % confluency in fully humidified air containing 5 % $CO_2$ at 37 °C.

NCI-H292 human airway epithelial cells (American Type Culture Collection, Mannassas, VA, USA) were cultured in RPMI 1640 medium (Invitrogen, Breda, The Netherland) supplemented with 1.25 mM L-glutamine, 100 U/ml penicillin, 100 µg/ml streptomycin and 10 % (v/v) fetal bovine serum (HyClone, Logan, UT, USA). Cells were grown in fully humidified air with 5 % $CO_2$ at 37 °C and sub cultured weekly.

### TLR stimulation experiment

Cells were cultured up to a confluence of 80 % in a six wells plate and incubated for 24 h in IMDM without supplements. Culture medium was removed and cells were stimulated with different TLR-agonists diluted in IMDM or with IMDM alone (control condition) for 24 h. Supernatants were removed after 1, 4, and 24 h and stored for further analysis; cells were used for RNA extraction. Each experiment was performed in triplicate. LPS (*Escherichia coli*), PGN (*Staphylococcus aureus*), and dsRNA (poly(deoxyinosinic-deoxycytidylic acid)) were from Sigma-Aldrich. ssRNA (LyoVec) and flagellin (*Salmonella typhimurium*) were from InvivoGen and the ligands were used at optimal concentrations as determined in a previous dose range finding experiment: PGN: 10 µg/mL, Poly(I:C): 20 µg/mL, LPS 1 µg/mL, Flagellin: 1 µg/mL, and CpG2216: 0.5 µM. As positive controls we used TNF-α (25 ng/mL) and IL-1β (10 ng/mL).

### RNA extraction and Real-time quantitative RT-PCR analysis

PCR was used to validate the differential expression of selected genes. Isolated mRNA (Kit from Macherey–Nagel, Düren, Germany) was transcribed into cDNA using the MBI Fermentas first strand cDNA kit. cDNA transcripts were quantified by real-time quantitative PCR (iCycler iQ MultiColor Real-Time PCR Detection System; Bio-Rad) with specific primers [32] and general SYBR green (Bio-Rad) fluorescence detection. mRNA expression of each sample was normalized to GAPDH. All PCRs have been performed for all participants on 3 biological replicates. Expression changes are presented as $2^{-\Delta Ct}$ indicating the difference in threshold cycle between the housekeeping gene GAPDH and the investigated TLR gene.

### FACS analysis

For flow cytometry analysis cells were stained with CD14-PE-Cy7 (1:20, BD Bioscience, Breda, the Netherland), TLR4-APC (1:10, ebioscience, San Diego, USA) or

left untreated. Cell numbers were quantified using the BD FACS Cantoll flowcytometer, histograms were generated using flowjo software version 7.6.2 (Treestar Inc, Ashland-OR, USA.

### Determining cytokine and chemokine production by ELISA

Cell free supernatants of stimulated and control treated cells were stored at −20 °C until analysis. Cytokine levels in supernatant of cells were determined by ELISA (IL-6 and IL8, BioSource International Camarillo-CA, USA) or using the xMAP technology (Luminex Corporation, Austin-TX, USA). A Bio-Plex Human Cytokine 17-Plex Panel kit (Bio-Rad, Veenendaal, The Netherlands). Concentrations were calculated from a dilution series of standards using the Luminex software. Lower detection limits are indicated per cytokine.

### Statistical analysis

Assessment of statistical significance for Luminex data was performed using two-tailed Student's t tests with GraphPad Prism. P values <0.05 were considered significant. Relationships between parameters were assessed using Pearson's correlation analysis.

### Results

### Baseline expression and functionality of TLR in human nasal epithelial cells

As shown in Figs. 1 and 2, primary nasal epithelial cells from healthy donors express TLR1 to TLR6 and TLR9, but not TLR7 and TLR8, and TLR10. Interestingly, we observed a huge individual variability spanning several 10 log-fold differences in the baseline expression of the TLRs to the extent that some healthy individuals do not express TLRs that are expressed by others.

In order to determine the functionality of the detected TLRs we stimulated primary nasal epithelial cells with their purified specific TLR ligands and used TNF-α and IL-1β as positive control to show the ability of our epithelial cells to respond to external triggers. As shown in Fig. 3, stimulation of primary heathy epithelial cells by PGN, Poly(I:C), and Flagellin resulted in increased release of IL-6 and IL-8 confirming the biological functionality of TLR2, TLR3, and TLR5 respectively. Remarkably, healthy primary nasal epithelial cells do not seem to respond to TLR4 ligation by LPS (Fig. 3) despite expressing the TLR4 gene and the use of a biological active LPS, as seen by the positive response in the epithelial cell line H292 (Fig. 4). Furthermore, we could show (Figs. 5, 6) surface expression of TLR4 and CD14, and co-expression of the adaptor MD-2 that are indispensable for proper TLR4 signalling [33, 34].

In a next step we analyzed, which additional cytokines and chemokines are released from primary nasal epithelial

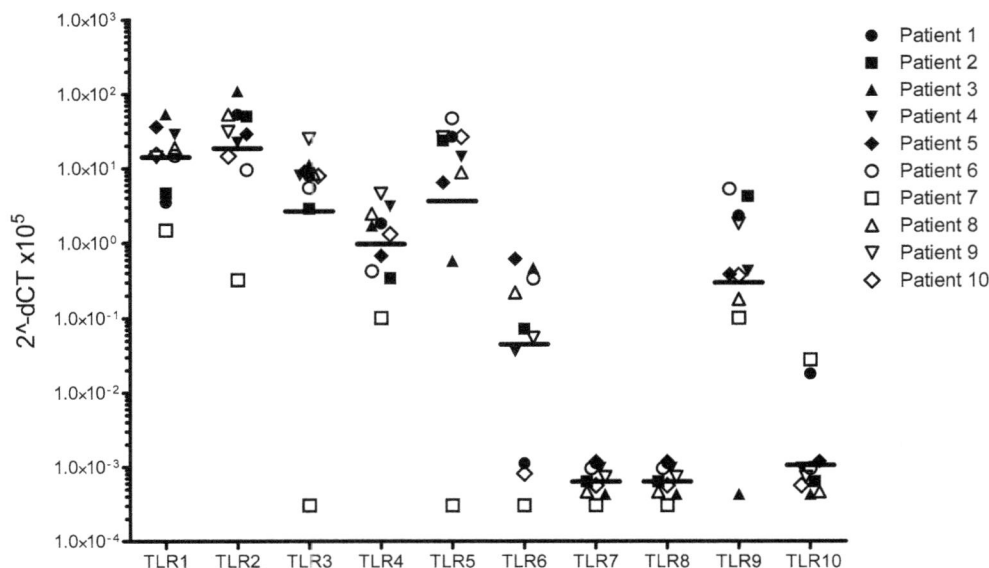

**Fig. 1** Toll-like Receptor (TLR) mRNA expression by primary nasal epithelial cells from 10 healthy patients undergoing turbinectomy (n = 10). TLR 1-10 mRNA expression was analyzed by quantitative RT-PCR. Results were normalized using GAPDH as endogenous control. Expression changes are presented as $2^{-\Delta Ct} \times 10^5$ indicating the difference in threshold cycle between the housekeeping gene GAPDH and the investigated TLR gene

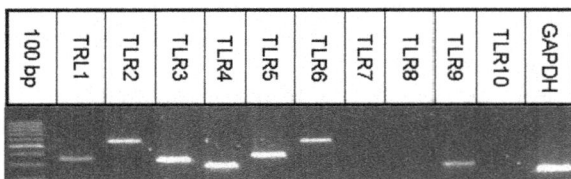

**Fig. 2** Toll-like Receptor (TLR) mRNA expression by primary nasal epithelial cells from one representative patient. Expression of TLRs was analyzed by quantitative RT-PCR. Products were visualized by agarose gel-electrophoresis in a 2 % agarose gel

cells in response to activation by different TLR ligands. As shown in Table 1 the multiplex ELISA showed that stimulation of primary nasal epithelial cells with Poly(I:C) resulted in a significant increased secretion of IL-4, IL-6, RANTES, IP-10, MIP-1β, VEGF, FGF, IL-1RA, IL-2R, and G-CSF. Furthermore, stimulation with PGN resulted in significantly increased production of IL-6, IL-1RA, and VEGF. In contrast to stimulation of epithelial TLR2 and TLR3, and confirming our previous observations, stimulation with a high concentration of LPS did not result in increased secretion of any cytokines or chemokines.

### No correlation between TLR expression levels and level of cytokine release

Strikingly, our data also revealed large individual differences in cytokine expression patterns. To investigate the functional consequences of this variation we first determined the individual mediator levels of all donors after stimulation with Poly(I:C). As shown in Fig. 7, some individuals seemed to be high responders (individual 3 and 9), while nasal epithelial cells from others (e.g. individual 11) hardly produced any significant levels of the mediators included in the assay used. Furthermore, these induction levels were not related to the expression levels of TLR3 (data not shown).

### Discussion

Epithelial cells are uniquely positioned at the interface between inside and outside of the organism, which makes them perfect candidates for initiating and orchestrating local immune responses. In addition to establishing which TLR receptors are expressed in primary nasal epithelial cells from healthy individuals, our data furthermore suggest that nasal epithelium has developed a delicate response system towards microbial exposures. Firstly, despite the presence of TLR4 and its prime co-stimulatory molecules CD14 and MD-2, nasal epithelium from healthy individuals does not respond to LPS. As the nasal mucosa is constantly exposed to high concentrations of endotoxin, this unresponsiveness could provide a mechanism to dampen the inflammatory response in the nasal mucosa in order to avoid a chronic inflammatory response. Secondly, levels of TLR expression in individuals varies strongly, to the extent that some individuals not express TLRs that others do. Thirdly, not only are the expression levels different between individuals,

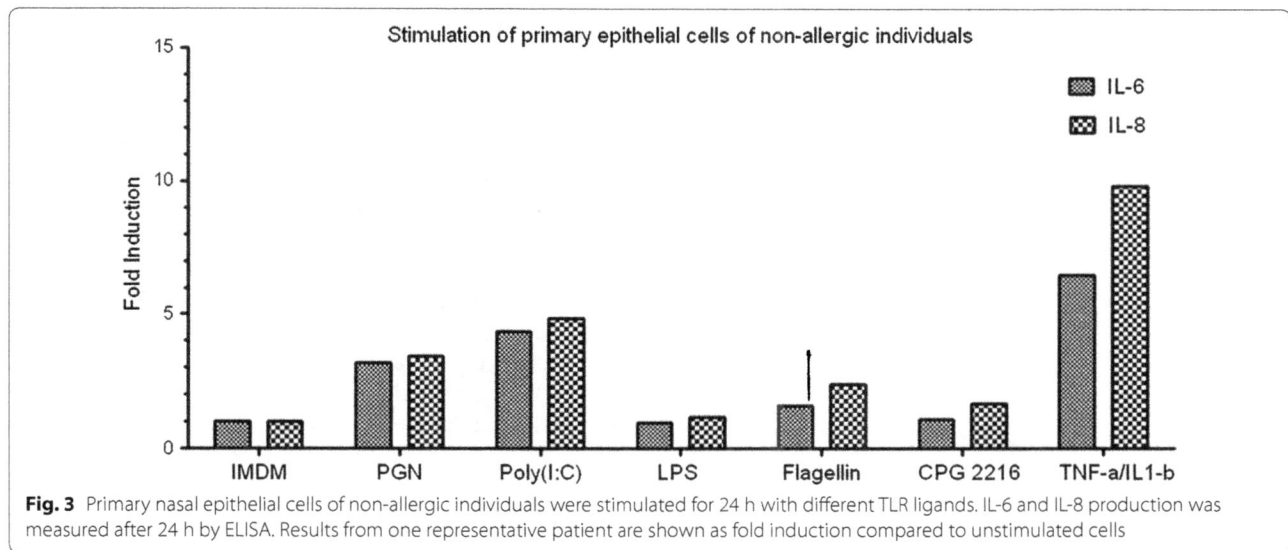

**Fig. 3** Primary nasal epithelial cells of non-allergic individuals were stimulated for 24 h with different TLR ligands. IL-6 and IL-8 production was measured after 24 h by ELISA. Results from one representative patient are shown as fold induction compared to unstimulated cells

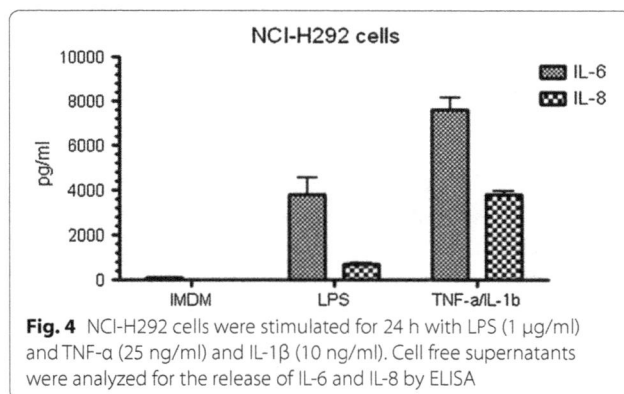

**Fig. 4** NCI-H292 cells were stimulated for 24 h with LPS (1 μg/ml) and TNF-α (25 ng/ml) and IL-1β (10 ng/ml). Cell free supernatants were analyzed for the release of IL-6 and IL-8 by ELISA

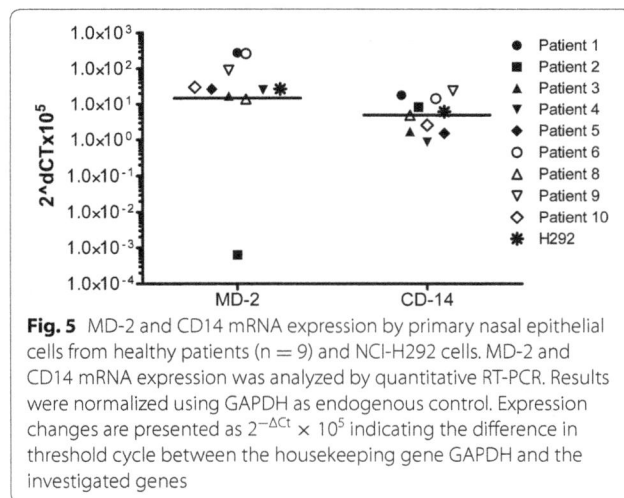

**Fig. 5** MD-2 and CD14 mRNA expression by primary nasal epithelial cells from healthy patients (n = 9) and NCI-H292 cells. MD-2 and CD14 mRNA expression was analyzed by quantitative RT-PCR. Results were normalized using GAPDH as endogenous control. Expression changes are presented as $2^{-\Delta Ct} \times 10^5$ indicating the difference in threshold cycle between the housekeeping gene GAPDH and the investigated genes

but independently of these differences, also the response induced by a specific TLR ligand varies strongly between individuals. And finally, the mediator response varies between different TLRs, even when they are thought to act through a common pathway. This complex level of variation in TLR signaling suggests that different healthy individuals may see different environments despite identical exposure. Although it should be noted that our sample size of 10 healthy individuals is relatively small, so that it would be difficult to generalize our conclusions for the general population

The expression of TLRs within the lower respiratory tract has been investigated intensively [22, 24, 25, 35], while data on TLR expression and functionality in nasal epithelial cells from healthy individuals is limited. Our experiments showed that primary nasal epithelial cells from most healthy donors express mRNA for TLR 1–6 and TLR9 and mainly respond to the TLR3 ligand Poly(I:C) and to the TLR2 and TLR5 agonists. The expression of TLR2, 3, and 4 has been shown in nasal epithelial cells derived from nasal polyps, with poly(I:C) inducing the secretion of RANTES, IP-10, IL-8 and GM-CSF [29]. We were able to confirm this outcome and in addition show a consistent and statistically significant up-regulation of IL-2R, VEGF, MIP-1β in all individuals. Closer inspection of our data shows strong up-regulation of other mediators as well (e.g. Mip-1α, MCP1, IL-7). However, as the induced expression of these mediators varies so strongly between individuals this up-regulation does not reach statistical significance. These observations show that healthy individuals differ strongly in their

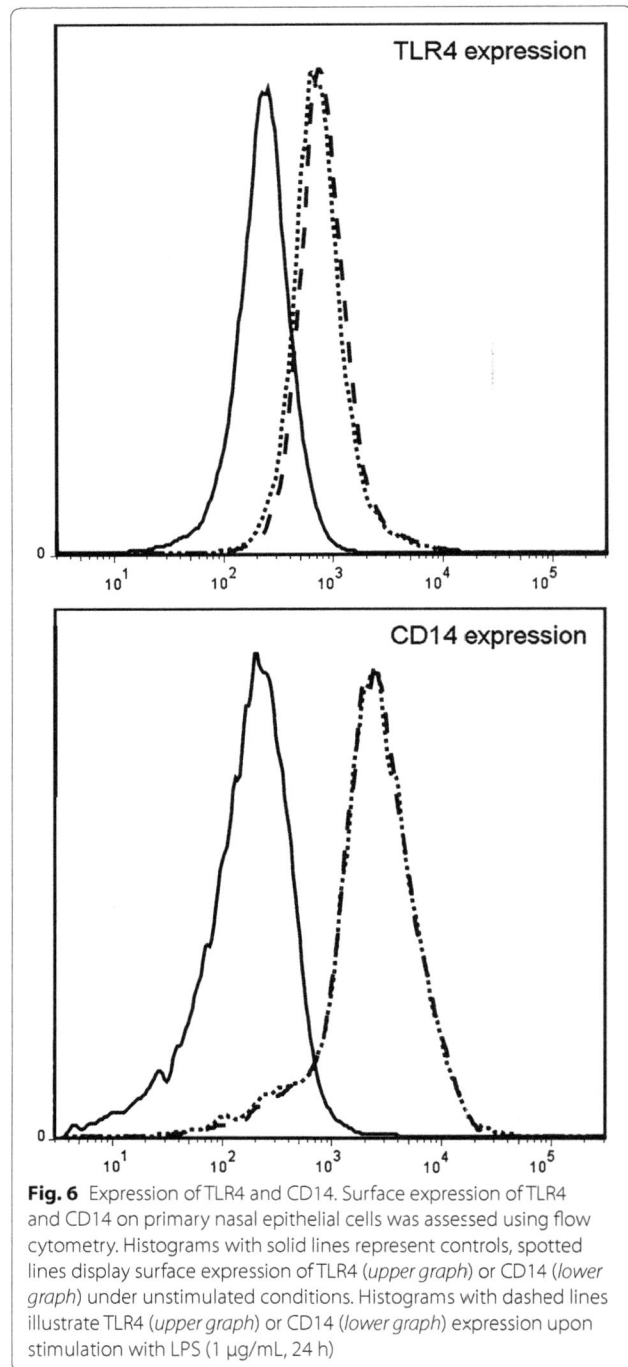

**Fig. 6** Expression of TLR4 and CD14. Surface expression of TLR4 and CD14 on primary nasal epithelial cells was assessed using flow cytometry. Histograms with solid lines represent controls, spotted lines display surface expression of TLR4 (*upper graph*) or CD14 (*lower graph*) under unstimulated conditions. Histograms with dashed lines illustrate TLR4 (*upper graph*) or CD14 (*lower graph*) expression upon stimulation with LPS (1 μg/mL, 24 h)

expression levels at the mRNA were low, so that differences in our detection technique (real time PCR) versus microarray [36] or differences in growth conditions [30, 36] may help to explain the observed expression differences for TLR7 and TLR10. Allowing for the specificity of TLR antibodies both TLR7 and TLR10 could be detected by immuno-histochemistry with moderate biological activity for the TLR7 agonist relative to TLR3 activation [30, 36].

The most striking discrepancy between TLR expression and responsiveness we observed for TLR4. Despite the presence of the receptor on the cell surface, the presence of key co-stimulatory molecules (CD14 and MD-2) and a seemingly intact downstream signaling cascade (the cells do response to other TLR stimulations), nasal epithelial cells do not respond to LPS. This unresponsiveness has also been observed in the epithelia of the gut where it was attributed to missing MD-2 expression [37] and in nasal epithelium from polyposis patients by Wang and co-workers [29]. Nasal polyposis epithelium showed a much weaker response to LPS than to polyIC stimulation, indicating that even in diseased tissue the nasal epithelial response to LPS is affected. In contrast, lung or renal epithelia are able to respond to LPS which suggests that the hypo-responsiveness could be an adaptation in epithelia that are exposed to high concentrations of LPS, whereas epithelia that are relative sterile do show a response to LPS.

The functional consequences of responding to TLR ligation are many. Expression of IP-10, MIP-1α, MIP-1β, IL-8 and G-CSF after TLR3 activation contribute to the recruitment and activation of neutrophils or macrophages. Furthermore, IL-8 and RANTES have been shown to be involved in the recruitment and survival of eosinophils [38]. These findings imply a role for TLR3 in the nasal immune response not only in Th1-mediated responses, but also in viral induced allergic exacerbations. This notion would also be in line with our recent observation that many aspects of TLR3 activation of nasal epithelial cells resemble that of activation by house dust mite allergen [39]. The inflammatory features of dsRNA mediated by TLR3 are also thought to contribute to the exacerbation of CRS and nasal polyps during viral infection [40]. TLR4 expression on lung epithelial cells has been shown to be required for DC activation in the lung and for priming of effector T helper response to HDM [16]. In the absence of TLR ligation, lung DCs are minimally active. Binding with the TLR4 ligand LPS leads to enhanced motility and sampling behavior. This response strictly depends on neighboring epithelial cells being triggered by TLR4. In addition, responses to allergens are substantially altered when epithelial cells cannot detect the endotoxin in the allergen,

response to external triggers, which will contribute to differences between the ability to fight off viral and bacterial infections. The absence of TLR7 and TLR10 mRNA expression differs from the previous observations of Renkonen [36] and Tengroth [30]. In both previous reports

**Table 1** Primary nasal epithelial cells of 5 non-allergic individuals were stimulated for 24 h with different TLR ligands: TLR2 (PGN: 10 μg/ml), TLR3 (Poly(I:C): 20 μg/ml), TLR4 (LPS 1 μg/ml)

| | Cut off value | IMDM | | Poly(I:C) | | LPS | | PGN | |
|---|---|---|---|---|---|---|---|---|---|
| | | Mean | SD | Mean | SD | Mean | SD | Mean | SD |
| IL-1β | 20 | BD | | 26 | 28 | BD | | BD | |
| IL1RA | 15 | 198 | 151 | 713** | 487 | 219 | 111 | 337** | 179 |
| IL-2 | 3 | BD | | 13 | 15 | BD | | BD | |
| IL-4 | 3 | BD | | 13** | 12 | BD | | BD | |
| IL-5 | 2 | BD | | BD | | BD | | BD | |
| IL-6 | 3 | 351 | 331 | 1793** | 1491 | 264 | 256 | 548** | 521 |
| IL-7 | 3 | 24 | 36 | 132 | 122 | 34 | 35 | 45 | 44 |
| IL-10 | 16 | BD | | BD | | BD | | BD | |
| IL-12 | 8 | BD | | 46 | 27 | BD | | BD | |
| IL-13 | 4 | BD | | BD | | BD | | BD | |
| IL-15 | 6 | BD | | 28 | 27 | BD | | BD | |
| IL-17 | 7 | 17 | 19 | 26 | 32 | 11 | 17 | 10 | 20 |
| Eotaxin | 6 | BD | | BD | | BD | | BD | |
| FGF basic | 15 | BD | | 40** | 40 | BD | | BD | |
| G-CSF | 2 | 72 | 95 | 655** | 700 | BD | | 132 | 179 |
| GMCSF | 4 | 36 | 74 | 58 | 148 | 18 | 47 | 20 | 48 |
| INF γ | 80 | BD | | BD | 16 | BD | | BD | |
| IP-10 | 24 | BD | | 1982** | 1666 | BD | | 29 | 27 |
| MCP 1 | 6 | 219 | 111 | 414 | 456 | 204 | 107 | 278 | 216 |
| MIP1α | 2 | 8 | 16 | 1122 | 2376 | 4 | 10 | 4 | 11 |
| MIP1β | 38 | BD | | 930** | 1321 | BD | | BD | |
| MIG | 4 | 5 | 11 | 23 | 22 | BD | | BD | |
| RANTES | 5 | 19 | 23 | 2120** | 1516 | 18 | 21 | 25 | 25 |
| TNFα | 10 | BD | | 43 | 68 | BD | | BD | |
| VEGF | 9 | 191 | 163 | 482** | 508 | 161 | 142 | 262** | 189 |
| EGF | 1 | BD | | 5 | 10 | BD | | 1 | 4 |
| HGF | 66 | BD | | 31 | 28 | BD | | BD | |
| IL-2R | 7 | 70 | 52 | 632** | 491 | 65 | 36 | 99 | 63 |
| IFNα | 2 | 14 | 21 | 39 | 39 | 10 | 18 | 22 | 20 |

Cell free supernatants were analysed using a Luminex array. Concentrations are presented as average of triplicates of 5 different patients in pg/ml. The detection limits are shown as cut off value

*SD* Standard deviation, *BD* below detection level

** $P < 0.05$

indicating that TLR4 signaling in epithelial cells is critical for the initiation of Th2 responses to inhaled allergens [41].

## Conclusions

Expression of TLRs on structural cells like epithelial cells and the respective functionality in terms of released mediators are important factors in the orchestration of local immune responses. We investigate the expression of all TLR receptors in primary nasal epithelial cells of healthy individuals and show an absence of TLR7 and TLR8 together with huge individual differences in mRNA expression level for TLR1-6 and TLR9. Although mRNA expression of TLRs of often taken as a measure of their

activity we show that this is should be done with caution. Specific TLR agonist-induced mediator release in nasal epithelial cells is very variable between different individuals and does not correlate with the expression levels of the respective TLRs, although we show this only for a relative small number of individuals. Most notably we show that despite the presence of TLR4, CD14, and MD2 in nasal epithelial cells, stimulation with LPS does not induce any mediator response. Supporting and strengthening previous observations in nasal polyposis patients that nasal epithelial cells seem to resemble gut epithelial cells where a yet unidentified mechanism prevents epithelia routinely exposed to bacterial flora from fortuitous

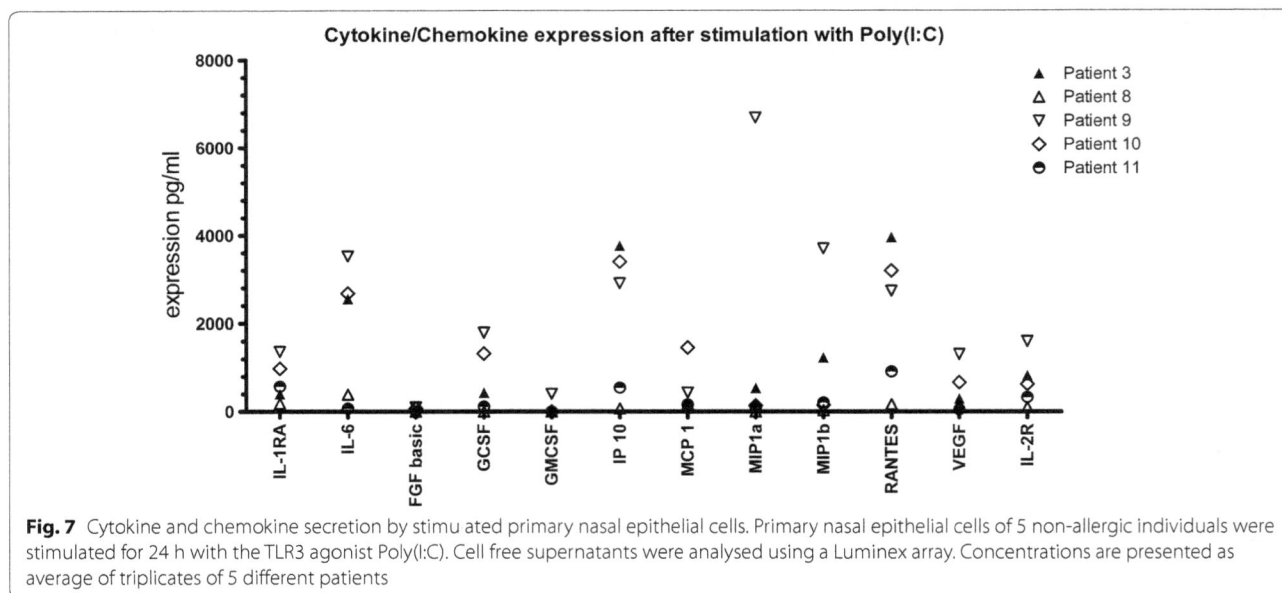

**Fig. 7** Cytokine and chemokine secretion by stimulated primary nasal epithelial cells. Primary nasal epithelial cells of 5 non-allergic individuals were stimulated for 24 h with the TLR3 agonist Poly(I:C). Cell free supernatants were analysed using a Luminex array. Concentrations are presented as average of triplicates of 5 different patients

activation. Our data suggest that we should probably consider individual expression and activation levels better as this would affect how individuals see their microbial environment.

### Abbreviations

TLR: Toll-like receptors; PAMP: pathogen-associated molecular patterns; PRR: pattern recognition receptors; LPS: lipopolysaccharide; Poly(I:C): poly(deoxyinosinic-deoxycytidylic) acid; PGN: peptidoglycan; CpG: cytosine—phosphate—guanine; TNF-α: tumor necrosis factor-alpha; IL: interleukin; RANTES: regulated upon activation, normal T cell Expressed, and Secreted; IP-10: interferon gamma-induced protein 10; MIP-1β: macrophage inflammatory protein 1 beta; VEGF: vascular endothelial growth factor; FGF: fibroblast growth factor; G-CSF: granulocyte colony-stimulating factor; RAST: radioallergosorbent test; DC: dendritic cells; RT-PCR: realtime PCR; HBSS: Hanks' balanced salt solution; MACS: magnetic activated cell sorting.

### Authors' contributions

JT and SR provided the clinical samples; JT, KR, SR, and SL did the experiments. JT, KR, and CvD performed the analysis, interpreted the data and have written the first draft of the manuscript. JvT, WF, EJ, and CD designed the experiments and helped interpreting the data. WF and EJ edited the manuscript. All authors read and approved the final manuscript.

### Author details

[1] Department of Otorhinolaryngology, Academic Medical Center (AMC), Amsterdam, The Netherlands. [2] Department of Cell Biology & Histology, Academic Medical Center (AMC), Amsterdam, The Netherlands.

### Acknowledgements

J van Tongeren received a ZonMw fellowship (92003459), furthermore this study was supported by the Interuniversity Attraction Poles programme (IUAP)—Belgian state—Belgian Science Policy P6/35.

### Competing interests

The authors declare that they have no competing interests.

### References

1. Toppila-Salmi S, van Drunen CM, Fokkens WJ, Golebski K, Mattila P, Joenvaara S, Renkonen J, Renkonen R. Molecular mechanisms of nasal epithelium in rhinitis and rhinosinusitis. Curr Allergy Asthma Rep. 2015;15(2):495.
2. van Tongeren J, Reinartz SM, Fokkens WJ, de Jong EC, van Drunen CM. Interactions between epithelial cells and dendritic cells in airway immune responses: lessons from allergic airway disease. Allergy. 2008;63(9):1124–35.
3. Vroling AB, Fokkens WJ, van Drunen CM. How epithelial cells detect danger: aiding the immune response. Allergy. 2008;63(9):1110–23.
4. Janeway CA Jr, Medzhitov R. Innate immune recognition. Annu Rev Immunol. 2002;20:197–216.
5. Akira S, Takeda K, Kaisho T. Toll-like receptors: critical proteins linking innate and acquired immunity. Nat Immunol. 2001;2(8):675–80.
6. Kaisho T, Akira S. Toll-like receptor function and signaling. J Allergy Clin Immunol. 2006;117(5):979–87.
7. Farhat K, Riekenberg S, Heine H, Debarry J, Lang R, Mages J, et al. Heterodimerization of TLR2 with TLR1 or TLR6 expands the ligand spectrum but does not lead to differential signaling. J Leukoc Biol. 2008;83(3):692–701.
8. Takeuchi O, Hoshino K, Akira S. Cutting edge: tLR2-deficient and MyD88-deficient mice are highly susceptible to Staphylococcus aureus infection. J Immunol. 2000;165(10):5392–6.
9. Kurt-Jones EA, Popova L, Kwinn L, Haynes LM, Jones LP, Tripp RA, et al. Pattern recognition receptors TLR4 and CD14 mediate response to respiratory syncytial virus. Nat Immunol. 2000;1(5):398–401.
10. Wang JE, Warris A, Ellingsen EA, Jorgensen PF, Flo TH, Espevik T, et al. Involvement of CD14 and toll-like receptors in activation of human monocytes by Aspergillus fumigatus hyphae. Infect Immun. 2001;69(4):2402–6.
11. Biragyn A, Ruffini PA, Leifer CA, Klyushnenkova E, Shakhov A, Chertov O, et al. Toll-like receptor 4-dependent activation of dendritic cells by beta-defensin 2. Science. 2002;298(5595):1025–9.
12. Guillot L, Balloy V, McCormack FX, Golenbock DT, Chignard M, Si-Tahar M. Cutting edge: the immunostimulatory activity of the lung surfactant protein-A involves Toll-like receptor 4. J Immunol. 2002;168(12):5989–92.
13. Vabulas RM, Ahmad-Nejad P, Ghose S, Kirschning CJ, Issels RD, Wagner H. HSP70 as endogenous stimulus of the Toll/interleukin-1 receptor signal pathway. J Biol Chem. 2002;277(17):15107–12.
14. Hemmi H, Takeuchi O, Kawai T, Kaisho T, Sato S, Sanjo H, et al. A Toll-like receptor recognizes bacterial DNA. Nature. 2000;408(6813):740–5.

15. Hemmi H, Kaisho T, Takeuchi O, Sato S, Sanjo H, Hoshino K, et al. Small anti-viral compounds activate immune cells via the TLR7 MyD88-dependent signaling pathway. Nat Immunol. 2002;3(2):196–200.
16. Hammad H, Chieppa M, Perros F, Willart MA, Germain RN, Lambrecht BN. House dust mite allergen induces asthma via Toll-like receptor 4 triggering of airway structural cells. Nat Med. 2009;15(4):410–6.
17. Redecke V, Hacker H, Datta SK, Fermin A, Pitha PM, Broide DH, et al. Cutting edge: activation of Toll-like receptor 2 induces a Th2 immune response and promotes experimental asthma. J Immunol. 2004;172(5):2739–43.
18. Hollingsworth JW, Whitehead GS, Lin KL, Nakano H, Gunn MD, Schwartz DA, et al. TLR4 signaling attenuates ongoing allergic inflammation. J Immunol. 2006;176(10):5856–62.
19. Page K, Ledford JR, Zhou P, Wills-Karp M. A TLR2 agonist in German cockroach frass activates MMP-9 release and is protective against allergic inflammation in mice. J Immunol. 2009;183(5):3400–8.
20. Eisenbarth SC, Piggott DA, Huleatt JW, Visintin I, Herrick CA, Bottomly K. Lipopolysaccharide-enhanced, toll-like receptor 4-dependent T helper cell type 2 responses to inhaled antigen. J Exp Med. 2002;196(12):1645–51.
21. Jia HP, Kline JN, Penisten A, Apicella MA, Gioannini TL, Weiss J, et al. Endotoxin responsiveness of human airway epithelia is limited by low expression of MD-2. Am J Physiol Lung Cell Mol Physiol. 2004;287(2):L428–37.
22. Schulz C, Farkas L, Wolf K, Kratzel K, Eissner G, Pfeifer M. Differences in LPS-induced activation of bronchial epithelial cells (BEAS-2B) and type II-like pneumocytes (A-549). Scand J Immunol. 2002;56(3):294–302.
23. Thorley AJ, Grandolfo D, Lim E, Goldstraw P, Young A, Tetley TD. Innate immune responses to bacterial ligands in the peripheral human lung—role of alveolar epithelial TLR expression and signalling. PLoS One. 2011;6(7):e21827.
24. Muir A, Soong G, Sokol S, Reddy B, Gomez MI, Van HA, et al. Toll-like receptors in normal and cystic fibrosis airway epithelial cells. Am J Respir Cell Mol Biol. 2004;30(6):777–83.
25. Ritter M, Mennerich D, Weith A, Seither P. Characterization of Toll-like receptors in primary lung epithelial cells: strong impact of the TLR3 ligand poly(I:C) on the regulation of Toll-like receptors, adaptor proteins and inflammatory response. J Inflamm (Lond). 2005;29(2):16.
26. Uehara A, Fujimoto Y, Fukase K, Takada H. Various human epithelial cells express functional Toll-like receptors, NOD1 and NOD2 to produce antimicrobial peptides, but not proinflammatory cytokines. Mol Immunol. 2007;44(12):3100–11.
27. Claeys S, de BT, Holtappels G, Gevaert P, Verhasselt B, van CP, et al. Human beta-defensins and toll-like receptors in the upper airway. Allergy. 2003;58(8):748–53.

28. Lin CF, Tsai CH, Cheng CH, Chen YS, Tournier F, Yeh TH. Expression of Toll-like receptors in cultured nasal epithelial cells. Acta Otolaryngol. 2007;127(4):395–402.
29. Wang J, Matsukura S, Watanabe S, Adachi M, Suzaki H. Involvement of Toll-like receptors in the immune response of nasal polyp epithelial cells. Clin Immunol. 2007;124(3):345–52.
30. Tengroth L, Millrud CR, Kvarnhammar AM, Kumlien Georén S, Latif L, Cardell LO. Functional effects of Toll-like receptor (TLR)3, 7, 9, RIG-I and MDA-5 stimulation in nasalepithelial cells. PLoS One. 2014;9(6):e98239.
31. Kormann MS, Depner M, Hartl D, Klopp N, Illig T, Adamski J, et al. Toll-like receptor heterodimer variants protect from childhood asthma. J Allergy Clin Immunol. 2008;122(1):86–92, 92.
32. Lebre MC, van der Aar AM, van BL, Van Capel TM, Schuitemaker JH, Kapsenberg ML, et al. Human keratinocytes express functional Toll-like receptor 3, 4, 5, and 9. J Invest Dermatol. 2007;127(2):331–41.
33. Hailman E, Lichenstein HS, Wurfel MM, Miller DS, Johnson DA, Kelley M, et al. Lipopolysaccharide (LPS)-binding protein accelerates the binding of LPS to CD14. J Exp Med. 1994;179(1):269–77.
34. Kennedy MN, Mullen GE, Leifer CA, Lee C, Mazzoni A, Dileepan KN, et al. A complex of soluble MD-2 and lipopolysaccharide serves as an activating ligand for Toll-like receptor 4. J Biol Chem. 2004;279(33):34698–704.
35. Sha Q, Truong-Tran AQ, Plitt JR, Beck LA, Schleimer RP. Activation of airway epithelial cells by toll-like receptor agonists. Am J Respir Cell Mol Biol. 2004;31(3):358–64.
36. Renkonen J, Toppila-Salmi S, Joenväärä S, Mattila P, Parviainen V, Hagström J, et al. Expression of Toll-like receptors in nasal epithelium in allergic rhinitis. APMIS. 2015;123(8):716–25.
37. Lenoir C, Sapin C, Broquet AH, Jouniaux AM, Bardin S, Gasnereau I, et al. MD-2 controls bacterial lipopolysaccharide hyporesponsiveness in human intestinal epithelial cells. Life Sci. 2008;82(9–10):519–28.
38. Lampinen M, Carlson M, Hakansson LD, Venge P. Cytokine-regulated accumulation of eosinophils in inflammatory disease. Allergy. 2004;59(8):793–805.
39. Golebski K, Luiten S, van Egmond D, de Groot E, Röschmann KI, Fokkens WJ, van Drunen CM. High degree of overlap between responses to a virus and to the house dust mite allergen in airway epithelial cells. PLoS One. 2014;9(2):e87768.
40. Fransson M, Adner M, Erjefalt J, Jansson L, Uddman R, Cardell LO. Up-regulation of Toll-like receptors 2, 3 and 4 in allergic rhinitis. Respir Res. 2005;6:100.
41. Tan AM, Chen HC, Pochard P, Eisenbarth SC, Herrick CA, Bottomly HK. TLR4 signaling in stromal cells is critical for the initiation of allergic Th2 responses to inhaled antigen. J Immunol. 2010;184(7):3535–44.

# 15

# The kinase LRRK2 is differently expressed in chronic rhinosinusitis with and without nasal polyps

Yue Ma[1,2], Chunquan Zheng[1]* [ID] and Le Shi[1,2]

## Abstract

**Background:** Chronic rhinosinusitis (CRS), commonly divided into CRS with nasal polyps (CRSwNP) and without nasal polyps (CRSsNP) is an inflammatory disease which mechanism remain unclear. Leucine-rich repeat kinase 2 (LRRK2) has been proved to be a negative regulator of inflammation response while its role in pathogenesis of CRS has yet to be revealed. This research study was designed to investigate the relationship between the expression level and biologic role of LRRK2 in CRS.

**Methods:** Expression of LRRK2 mRNA and noncoding repressor of NFAT (NRON) were examined by qRT-PCR. Protein levels of LRRK2 were performed by western blot and immunohistochemistry. Nuclear factor of activated T cells (NFAT) nuclear translocation was analyzed by immunohistochemistry. Additionally, LRRK2 mRNA and NRON expression in response to specific inflammatory stimulation was measured in human nasal epithelia cells (HNECs).

**Results:** The expression of LRRK2 was increased in CRSsNP patients ($p < 0.05$) and positively correlated with the expression levels of CD3 and Charot-Leyden crystal. Meanwhile, the NRON expression level is much lower in CRSsNP patients compared to both the control group and CRSwNP group ($p < 0.05$). Marked enhanced NFAT nuclear localization was observed in CRSwNP groups compared with the CRSsNP and control group ($p < 0.0001$). And the over-expression of LRRK2 was significantly regulated by lipopolysaccharide (LPS) in HNECs ($p < 0.05$). Moreover, IL-17A can increase LRRK2 expression and suppress NRON expression in vitro and dexamethasone can rescue the NRON inhibition.

**Conclusion:** LRRK2 and NRON may play different role in CRSsNP and CRSwNP. The molecular mechanisms identified here may aid in the design of novel therapeutic strategies to improve clinical outcomes.

**Keywords:** LRRK2, NRON, Long non-coding RNA, Chronic rhinosinusitis, Pro-inflammatory cytokine

## Background

In general, chronic rhinosinusitis (CRS) is an inflammatory disease that is composed of CRS with nasal polyps (CRSwNP) and without nasal polyps (CRSsNP). Although their pathogenesis is not yet clear, it is commonly acknowledged that the two types of CRS possess distinct inflammation and remodeling patterns [1, 2]. CRSsNP is characterized by Th1-biased inflammation and an elevated expression of transforming growth factor (TGF-β1), while CRSwNP is characterized by a Th2-biased inflammation [3]. Meanwhile, the dysregulation of innate immunity has been regarded as the key point for the initiation and perpetuation of inflammatory responses in CRS patients [4]. The toll-like receptor signaling pathway induced by lipopolysaccharide (LPS)has been reported as one of critical factors in the pathogenesis of CRS, but the mechanism remains unclear. Thus, there is an urgent need for a new biomarker that can further explain this mechanism.

Leucine-rich repeat kinase 2 (LRRK2), also known as Dardarin, is a large complex protein that contains several

*Correspondence: zheng_ent96@163.com
[1] Department of Otolaryngology-Head and Neck Surgery, Eye Ear Nose and Throat Hospital, Fudan University, 83 Fenyang Road, Xuhui District, Shanghai 200031, People's Republic of China
Full list of author information is available at the end of the article

domains [5–7]. Accumulating evidence has revealed that LRRK2 is involved in regulating inflammatory processes [8–10]. Participation in the signaling of IFN-γ [11, 12], enhancement of NF-kB-dependent transcription, and interference in reactive oxygen species (ROS) production all indicate that LRRK2 may play a pivotal role in the anti-microbial process [11].

It has already been identified that LRRK2 negatively regulates NFAT by interacting with NRON, a known repressor of NFAT. Long non-coding RNA (lncRNA) NRON and 11 additional proteins, including LRRK2, constitute a protein-RNA complex which could directly inhibit the translocation of NFAT to the nucleus [13, 14] such that cell activation and the proceeding immune reactivity are suppressed. For example, enhanced nuclear location of NFAT was associated with more severe colitis in LRRK2-deficient mice [14].

Therefore, LRRK2 is a negative regulator of this inflammation response. These findings implied that the changes in LRRK2 expression levels resulting from extrinsic signals may play a vital role in the regulation of immune responses. However, the role of LRRK2 in the pathogenesis of CRS has yet to be revealed. Our present study was designed to investigate the relationship between the expression level and biologic role of LRRK2 in CRS.

## Methods
### Subjects
The subjects (n = 74) were all recruited from the Department of Otolaryngology-Head and Neck Surgery, Eye, Ear, Nose, and Throat Hospital, Fudan University. All were CRS patients who had not taken oral and/or topical corticosteroids or any other sinonasal medications for at least 1 month prior to the study and were diagnosed

based on previously published criteria [15]. NPs were obtained from CRSwNP patients (n = 34), and nasal mucosa of middle turbinates were from CRSsNP patients (n = 23). At the same time, the nasal mucosa of inferior turbinates were collected from those patients (n = 17) who had no clinical symptoms or radiographic evidence of CRS and who underwent a septoturbinoplasty. Patients responding positively to a skin-prick test were diagnosed with an allergy. All of the patients' clinical data are presented in Table 1. The exclusion criteria for the study group ran as follow: age < 18 or > 80 years, a diagnosis of cystic fibrosis, Churg-Strauss syndrome, immunodeficiency, or autoimmune disease.

This study obtained permission from the local ethical committee of the Otolaryngology-Head and Neck Surgery, Eye, Ear, Nose, and Throat Hospital, Fudan University, and informed consent was signed by every subject.

### RNA extraction and real-time polymerase chain reaction
Total RNA was extracted using TRIzol reagent (Invitrogen) according to the manufacturer's instructions. Then, PrimeScript RT master mix (Takara) was used to synthesize complementary DNA (cDNA). An ABI 7900 Sequence Detection System (ABI) was used to perform qRT-PCR with SYBR Green chemistry. Table 2 showed the primers (Sangon Biotech). The expression of each gene was calculated using the comparative threshold cycle ($2^{-\Delta\Delta CT}$) method.

### Immunohistochemistry (IHC) staining
Immunohistochemistry was performed following the protocol for the streptavidin-biotin complex (SABC) kit (Weiao Biological Technology). The sections were incubated with primary antibody (polyclonal rabbit

## Table 1 Characteristics of included subjects

|  | Control subjects | Patients with CRSsNP | Patients with CRSwNP |
| --- | --- | --- | --- |
| No. of patients | 17 | 23 | 34 |
| Sex, male/female | 12/5 | 12/11 | 20/14 |
| Age (years), mean (SD) | 36 (8) | 52 (17) | 37 (13) |
| Atopy, no. | 0 | 4 | 6 |
| Asthma, no. | 0 | 0 | 2 |
| Aspirin intolerance, no. | 0 | 0 | 0 |
| Smoking, no. | 0 | 10 | 16 |
| Operation history, no. | 0 | 0 | 2 |
| Methodologies used |  |  |  |
| Tissue IHC | 10 | 16 | 25 |
| Tissue mRNA | 15 | 21 | 30 |
| Tissue western blot | 9 | 9 | 9 |

## Table 2 Primers

| Name | Sense | Antisense |
|---|---|---|
| GAPDH | CAAGGTCATCCATGACAACTTTG | GTCCACCACCCTGTTGCTGTAG |
| LRRK2 | GGATGTTGGTGATGGAGTT | GGCTGAGTGGAGGTATCT |
| NRON | AACAACCCAGCAAGGGAAGTAG | AAGAGCA TGAACGCACATCCTAG |
| CD3 | TAGAGGAACTTGAGGACAGA | GCAGAGTGGCAATGACAT |
| Tryptase | TCTGAAGCAGGTGAAGGT | AGTCCAAGTAGTAGGTGACA |
| CLC | TTGTCTACTGGTTCTACTGT | CAATGTCTGATTCCTCCTTC |
| CXCR1 | ATGCTGTTCTGCTATGGATT | CGATGAAGGCGTAGATGAT |
| CD68 | CTCCAGCAGAAGGTTGTC | TGATGAGAGGCAGCAAGA |

anti-human LRRK2; Abcam; 1:200 dilution; polyclonal goat anti-human NFAT1; Abcam; 1:100 dilution) at 4 °C overnight. 3′3-Diaminobenzidine (DAB) was used for the final visualization. To analyze LRRK2 expression, two pathologists scored the results independently according to the immunostaining intensity scale, which ran as follows: 0 = absent; 1 = mild; 2 = moderate; and 3 = marked. The numbers of immuno-positive cells within the samples were also counted in at least five random areas at a $400\times$ magnification, and at the same time, the percentage of immuno-positive cells was scored according to the standard scale as follows: 0 (0–9%); 1 (10–25%); 2 (26–50%); 3 (51–75%); and 4 (>76%). Multiplication of the two abovementioned scores provided the final score for each sample. The highest final score was 12 while the lowest was 0. To analyze NFAT nuclear translocation, the percentage of cells with NFAT1 nuclear staining in all immuno-positive cells were also counted in five random areas at a 400x magnification.

### Western blots

Protein samples (30 μg) were separated by electrophoresis using 10% sodium dodecyl sulfate polyacrylamide gels and then transferred to polyvinylidene difluoride (PVDF) membranes for incubation with anti-LRRK2 (Abcam; 1:1000) antibody. Image J (NIH) analysis and processing software was used to quantify data, which was expressed as densitometry units (DU). The expression of $\beta$-actin (Abcam; 1:1000) was regarded as an internal reference.

### Cell culture and stimulation

Following a previously established protocol, HNECs (Human Nasal Epithelia Cells) isolated from the middle turbinates of CRSsNP patients were cultured [16]. Briefly, nasal specimens were immersed in DMEM/F12 media (Hyclone) containing 1.4 mg/ml protease K and 0.1 mg/ml DNase for a 1.5 h incubation at 37 °C. Next, all cells were collected and immersed in DMEM/F12 (Hyclone)

containing 1% ITS for 2 h at 37 °C before being cultured in BEGM medium (Lonza).

When 80–90% confluence was reached, fresh media without hydrocortisone was added in the presence of the following stimulators or control PBS for 12 h: the recombinant cytokines human IFN-γ (100 ng/mL), IL-4 (100 ng/mL), IL-13 (100 ng/mL), IL-17A (100 ng/mL), TGF-β (10 ng/mL), and IL-1α (100 ng/mL; all purchased from Peprotech); the TLR agonists LPS (500 ng/mL, from *Escherichia coli* serotype 0111: B4; purchased from Sigma) and the glucocorticoid dexamethasone (Sigma; 10 μg/mL). After stimulation, HNECs were collected for qRT-PCR analysis.

### Statistical analysis

Statistical analyses were performed by SPSS v22.0 software (IBM Corporation). The data were presented as medians and interquartile ranges. Tests for Gaussian distribution were performed by Kolmogorov–Smirnov test. Differences between groups were evaluated by one-way analysis of variance and either by the two independent sample t test or the Mann–Whitney U test. The correlation analysis was performed to assess the correlation between two groups by Spearman's rank correlation. $p < 0.05$ was regarded as statistically significant.

### Results

#### NRON and LRRK2 mRNA levels in nasal tissues

As showed in Fig. 1a, significant upregulation of LRRK2 mRNA levels was found in CRSsNP groups but not in CRSwNP groups compared with the control group ($p < 0.0001$), and NRON levels were significantly higher in the inferior turbinate than in the middle turbinate of CRSsNP groups ($p < 0.0001$) and in NPs ($p < 0.01$) (Fig. 1b).

#### LRRK2 protein levels in nasal tissues

To verify the results at the protein level, western blots were performed. Strong bands for LRRK2 were observed in CRSsNP groups, whereas weak bands were found in the CRSwNP group and in the control group (Fig. 1c). The LRRK2 protein level was significantly higher in the CRSsNP group than in the CRSwNP group and the control group (Fig. 1d; $p < 0.0001$).

#### LRRK2 and NFAT immunoreactivity in nasal tissues

Immunohistochemistry was performed to further confirm the results pertaining to the protein levels of LRRK2 in the various samples. As depicted by immunohistochemistry staining (Fig. 2a–c), LRRK2 was significantly overexpressed in the CRSsNP group compared with the control group and CRSwNP group. The cytoplasmic or nuclear staining of LRRK2 was mainly located at the

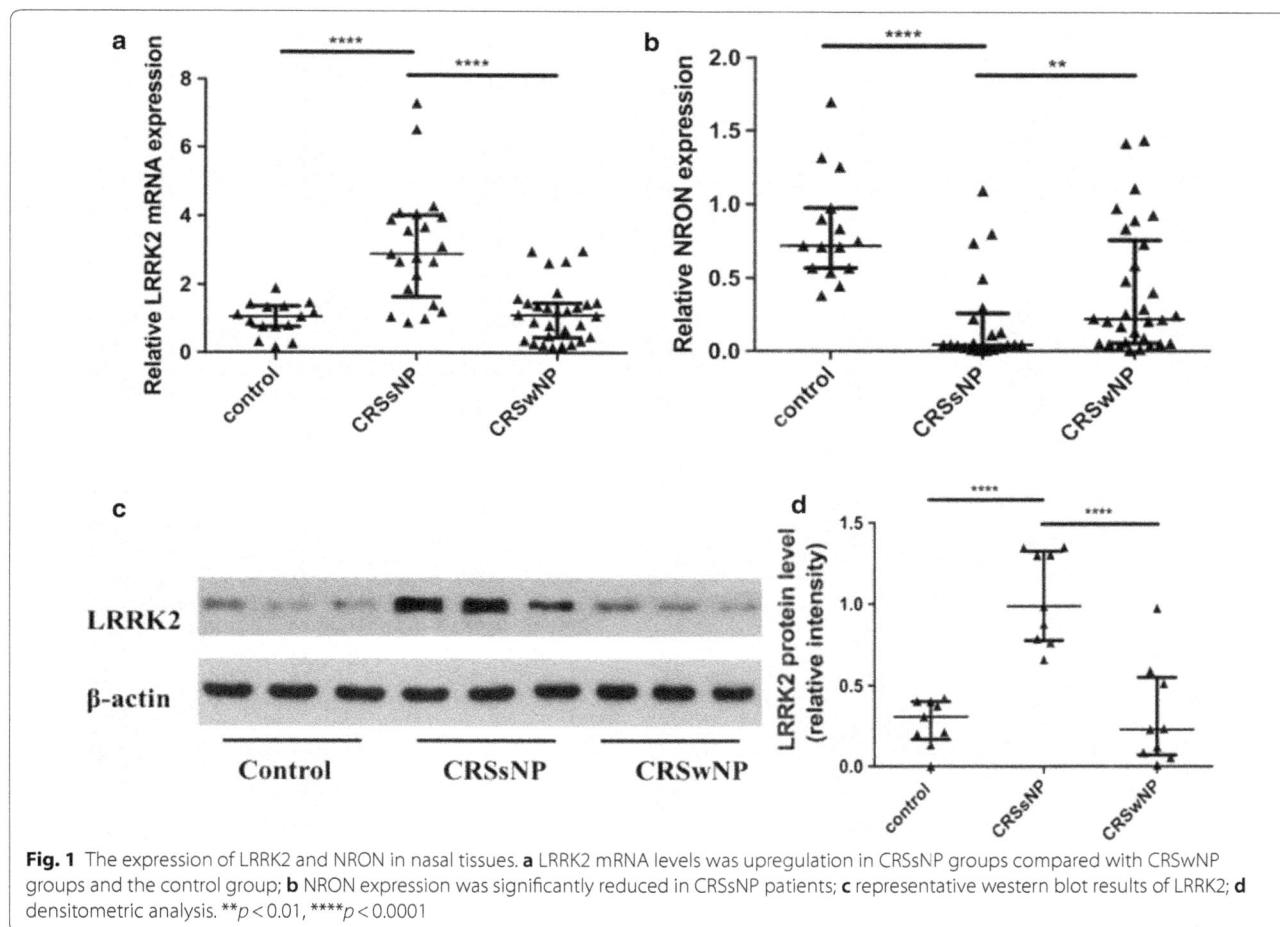

Fig. 1 The expression of LRRK2 and NRON in nasal tissues. **a** LRRK2 mRNA levels was upregulation in CRSsNP groups compared with CRSwNP groups and the control group; **b** NRON expression was significantly reduced in CRSsNP patients; **c** representative western blot results of LRRK2; **d** densitometric analysis. **$p < 0.01$, ****$p < 0.0001$

nasal epithelium and in submucosal inflammatory cells. In comparison with control groups and NPs, quantitative analysis of LRRK2 revealed an obvious elevation in immuno-labeling of LRRK2 in the CRSsNP group (Fig. 2d; $p < 0.01$). NFAT nuclear translocation was also detected by immunohistochemistry (Fig. 2e–g). Marked enhanced NFAT nuclear localization was observed in CRSwNP groups compared with the CRSsNP group and control group (Fig. 2h; $p < 0.0001$).

### Detection of LRRK2 producing cells in nasal mucosa

These results revealed that LRRK2+ cells were highly accumulated in the submucosal region of CRSsNP tissues and that the mRNA and protein expression levels of LRRK2 were also significantly higher in CRSsNP tissues (Fig. 2). Next, the expression of LRRK2 and the markers of inflammatory cells in CRSsNP were assessed by qRT-PCR and the relationship between these markers were analyzed by Spearman's rank correlation. The results demonstrated that the mRNA expression levels of LRRK2 in CRSsNP tissue were significantly and positively related to the expression of CD3 (r = 0.7286; $p = 0.0029$),

Charot–Leyden crystal (CLC; r = 0.5712; $p = 0.0284$), CD68 (r = 0.146; $p < 0.05$), but not CXCR1, tryptase and CD68, which indicated that the expression of LRRK2 may derive from T cells, eosinophils (Fig. 3).

### LPS and pro-inflammatory cytokines differentially regulate LRRK2 and NRON expression in human nasal epithelial cells (HNECs) in vitro

To further expose the role and mechanism of the LRRK2 signaling pathway in the nasal mucosa of CRS, the effects of TLR activation and pro-inflammatory cytokine stimulation were examined in cultured human nasal epithelial cells. As presented in Fig. 4a, mRNA expression levels of LRRK2 were significantly increased after stimulating the HNECs with LPS, the TLR agonists ($p < 0.001$). Meanwhile, stimulation with IL-17A increased very low LRRK2 mRNA expression ($p < 0.01$) compared with stimulation by the other pro-inflammatory cytokines, including IFN-γ, IL-4, IL-13, IL-1α, and TGF-β which also increased LRRK2 expression ($p < 0.01$). In contrast, NRON levels were significantly inhibited by stimulation with IL-17A ($p < 0.001$; Fig. 4b).

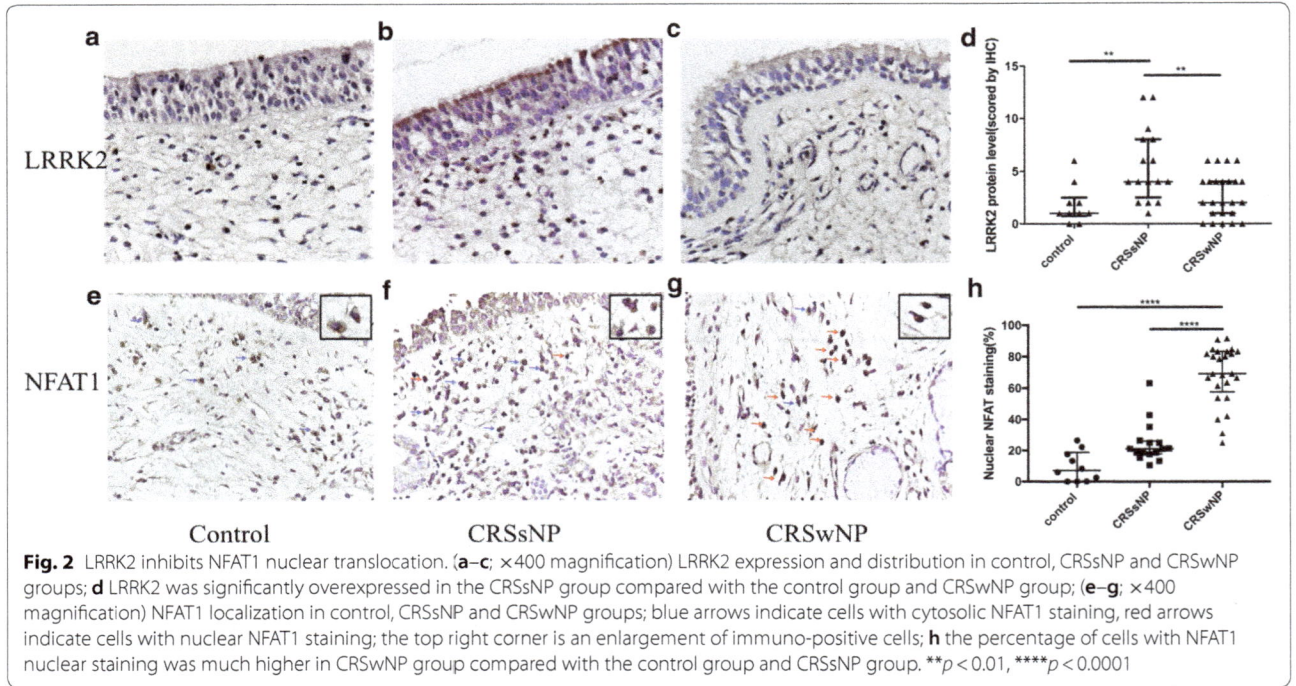

**Fig. 2** LRRK2 inhibits NFAT1 nuclear translocation. (**a–c**; ×400 magnification) LRRK2 expression and distribution in control, CRSsNP and CRSwNP groups; **d** LRRK2 was significantly overexpressed in the CRSsNP group compared with the control group and CRSwNP group; (**e–g**; ×400 magnification) NFAT1 localization in control, CRSsNP and CRSwNP groups; blue arrows indicate cells with cytosolic NFAT1 staining, red arrows indicate cells with nuclear NFAT1 staining; the top right corner is an enlargement of immuno-positive cells; **h** the percentage of cells with NFAT1 nuclear staining was much higher in CRSwNP group compared with the control group and CRSsNP group. **\*\***$p < 0.01$, **\*\*\*\***$p < 0.0001$

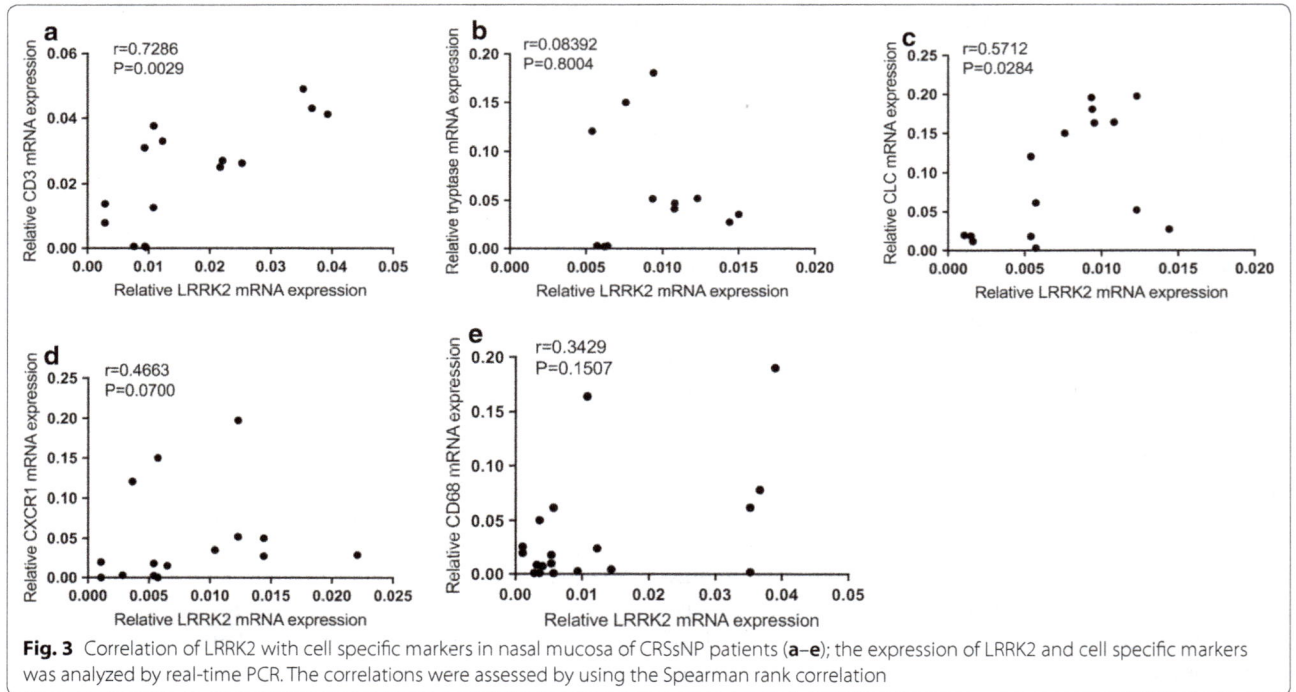

**Fig. 3** Correlation of LRRK2 with cell specific markers in nasal mucosa of CRSsNP patients (**a–e**); the expression of LRRK2 and cell specific markers was analyzed by real-time PCR. The correlations were assessed by using the Spearman rank correlation

## Glucocorticoid treatment increases LRRK2 expression in vitro

Because glucocorticoid treatment is recommended as one of the primary treatment of choice for patients with

CRS, the effect of glucocorticoids on LRRK2 mRNA and NRON expression in HNECs was examined. After incubating cells with dexamethasone, LRRK2 mRNA and NRON expression was more upregulated in the presence

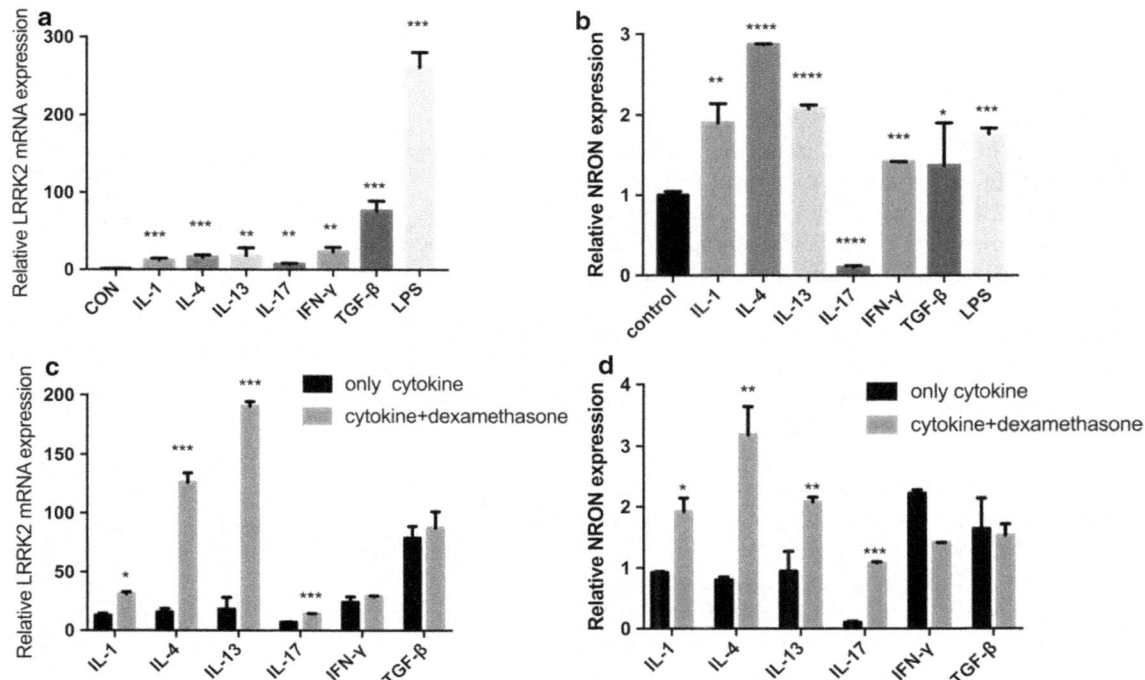

**Fig. 4** LRRK2 mRNA and NRON expression in cultured HNECs in response to pro-inflammatory cytokines, LPS and dexamethasone. **a** LRRK2 mRNA, **b** NORN expression after a 12 h stimulation; **c** LRRK2 mRNA, **d** NORN expression after pro-inflammatory cytokines stimulation with or without dexamethasone. Results represent mean values from 3 independent experiments. Data are expressed as means (SEMs). *$p < 0.05$, **$p < 0.01$, ***$p < 0.001$, ****$p < 0.0001$

of pro-inflammatory cytokines (IL-17A, IL-4, IL-13, IL-1α; $p < 0.05$) than without dexamethasone stimulation (Fig. 4c, d). In contrast, NRON expression was lower when the cells were stimulated with IFN-γ plus dexamethasone compared to only IFN-γ stimulation.

## Discussion

This study demonstrated that the expression of LRRK2 was increased in patients suffering from CRSsNP (Figs. 1, 2), and the over-expression of LRRK2 was regulated by LPS in HNECs (Fig. 4). Moreover, LRRK2 expression in CRSsNP tissues was correlated with the expression levels of CD3, CLC, and CD68, which suggested that T cells, eosinophils, and macrophages may be the main LRRK2-producing cells in nasal mucosa (Fig. 3). Meanwhile, NRON expression level is much lower in CRSsNP patients compared to both the control group and CRSwNP group (Fig. 1). Its expression can be strongly suppressed by stimulation with IL-17A in vitro, and dexamethasone can rescue this phenomenon.

CRS, commonly divided into CRSwNP and CRSsNP, is characterized by chronic inflammation of the paranasal sinuses. Due to the poor awareness of the initiation and progression of CRS, the development of effective treatments for this disease remains stagnant [17]. LRRK2 can

be physically associated with NRON and this protein-RNA complex has been proven to be a NFAT suppressor in many inflammatory diseases such as inflammatory bowel disease [18], and LRRK2 deficiency can lead to a more serious inflammation response. In the results presented herein, considerable data indicates that the up-regulation of LRRK2 expression in CRSsNP is obviously higher than in the CRSwNP group, and the percentage of cells with NFAT nuclear staining in CRSsNP is much lower in CRSwNP group (Fig. 2), which suggests that a lower expression of LRRK2 exhibits less of an inhibitory effect on NFAT. Moreover, this data supports that the idea that the defection of innate immunity may lead to a robust adaptive immune response, which triggers the generation of pro-inflammatory cytokines and the development of chronic inflammation [19].

NRON is a cytoplasmic lncRNA which has previously been reported to be highly expressed in human immune cells including macrophages, dendritic cells, and neutrophils along with its vital role in T cell cytokine production. NRON acts as a scaffold to maintain the structure of a ribonucleoprotein complex which can retain the transcription factor NFAT in the cytoplasm [13], meaning that NRON plays a significant role in the immune response. However, in this study, the expression level of

NRON is lower in CRSsNP group, which indicates that in the RNA-protein complex, LRRK2 may play a much more important role in the generation and the development of CRS than NRON.

Within the immune system, the expression of LRRK2 has been reported in lymphocytes, dendritic cells, and macrophages [11]. In this study, LRRK2-producing cells were identified in CRSsNP nasal mucosa. Considerable data had already shown that T cells and eosinophils may be the main LRRK2-producing cells in CRSsNP nasal mucosa, which was in line with the published reports.

It has also been reported that the induction of LRRK2 expression could be triggered in mouse bone marrow-derived macrophages under the stimulation of toll-like receptor 4 [20], whereas opposite findings were issued in another study [14]. Hence, to further explore the mechanism of LRRK2 and NRON expression in CRS, HNECs were incubated with LPS and pro-inflammatory cytokines (IFN-γ, TGF-β, IL-1α, IL-4, IL-13, IL-17A). The results showed that IL-17A can increase LRRK2 and suppress NRON expression which were coincidence with the expression of LRRK2 and NRON in nasal mucosa of CRSsNP patients, while other cytokines can induce both LRRK2 and NRON. The results indicate that IL-17A may play a significant role in the LRRK2 signaling pathway in CRSsNP patients, while both Th1 and Th2 cytokines participate in the inflammation activities of CRSsNP nasal mucosa. Further studies are urgently needed to confirm this theory.

Notably, this study found that dexamethasone universally enhanced the induced role of pro-inflammatory cytokines (IL-13, IL-1α, IL-4) in LRRK2 mRNA and NRON expression. What's more, it can rescue IL-17A cytokine-induced NRON suppression. Although the underlying molecular mechanisms require further characterization, this finding demonstrates that glucocorticoid treatment can make more LRRK2-NRON complex so that it can play a more significant role in the inhibition of NFAT translocation. Then, the inflammation response will be inhibited.

## Conclusions

In summary, it has been revealed here that LRRK2 is elevated in patients with CRSsNP, while NRON is lower in this group. LRRK2 can strongly inhibit the nuclear function of NFAT. IL-17A may play a significant role in the LRRK2 signaling pathway in CRSsNP patients. Further investigation will concentrate on the interaction of LRRK2 and NRON in CRS to reveal their effects on inflammation and the immune system. The molecular mechanisms identified here will help clarify the pathogenic processes involved in these two CRS subsets, as

well as aid in the design of novel therapeutic strategies to improve clinical outcomes.

**Abbreviations**
CRS: chronic rhinosinusitis; LPS: lipopolysaccharide; LRRK2: leucine-rich repeat kinase 2; NRON: noncoding repressor of NFAT; NFAT: nuclear factor of activated T cells; ROS: reactive oxygen species; lncRNA: long non-coding RNA; IHC: immunohistochemistry; SABC: streptavidin-biotin complex; PVDF: polyvinylidene difluoride; DU: densitometry units; HNECs: human nasal epithelia cells; CLC: Charot–Leyden crystal.

**Authors' contributions**
Yue Ma performed most of the experiment and was a major contributor in writing the manuscript. Chunquan Zheng designed the experiment and analyzed the results. Le Shi collected all the specimens and participant in the experiment. All authors read and approved the final manuscript.

**Author details**
[1] Department of Otolaryngology-Head and Neck Surgery, Eye Ear Nose and Throat Hospital, Fudan University, 83 Fenyang Road, Xuhui District, Shanghai 200031, People's Republic of China. [2] Shanghai Key Clinical Disciplines of Otorhinolaryngology, Shanghai, People's Republic of China.

**Acknowledgements**
Not applicable.

**Competing interests**
The authors declare that they have no competing interests.

**Funding**
This work was supported by grants from the National Natural Science Foundation of China (Nos.81470672).

**References**
1.  Stevens WW, Lee RJ, Schleimer RP, Cohen NA. Chronic rhinosinusitis pathogenesis. J Allergy Clin Immunol. 2015;136:1442–53. https://doi.org/10.1016/j.jaci.2015.10.009.
2.  Van Zele T, Claeys S, Gevaert P, Van Maele G, Holtappels G, Van Cauwenberge P, Bachert C. Differentiation of chronic sinus diseases by measurement of inflammatory mediators. Allergy. 2006;61:1280–9. https://doi.org/10.1111/j.1398-9995.2006.01225.x.
3.  Van Bruaene N, Derycke L, Perez-Novo CA, Gevaert P, Holtappels G, De Ruyck N, Cuvelier C, Van Cauwenberge P, Bachert C. TGF-beta signaling and collagen deposition in chronic rhinosinusitis. J Allergy Clin Immunol. 2009;124:253–9. https://doi.org/10.1016/j.jaci.2009.04.013.
4.  Kern RC, Conley DB, Walsh W, Chandra R, Kato A, Tripathi-Peters A, Grammer LC, Schleimer RP. Perspectives on the etiology of chronic rhinosinusitis: an immune barrier hypothesis. Am J Rhinol. 2008;22:549–59. https://doi.org/10.2500/ajr.2008.22.3228.
5.  Paisan-Ruiz C, Jain S, Evans EW, Gilks WP, Simon J, van der Brug M, Lopez de Munain A, Aparicio S, Gil AM, Khan N, Johnson J, Martinez JR, Nicholl D, et al. Cloning of the gene containing mutations that cause PARK8-linked Parkinson's disease. Neuron. 2004;44:595–600. https://doi.org/10.1016/j.neuron.2004.10.023.
6.  Zimprich A, Biskup S, Leitner P, Lichtner P, Farrer M, Lincoln S, Kachergus J, Hulihan M, Uitti RJ, Calne DB, Stoessl AJ, Pfeiffer RF, Patenge N, et al. Muta-

tions in LRRK2 cause autosomal-dominant parkinsonism with pleomorphic pathology. Neuron. 2004;44:601–7. https://doi.org/10.1016/j.neuron.2004.11.005.

7. Meylan E, Tschopp J. The RIP kinases: crucial integrators of cellular stress. Trends Biochem Sci. 2005;30:151–9. https://doi.org/10.1016/j.tibs.2005.01.003.

8. Russo I, Bubacco L, Greggio E. LRRK2 and neuroinflammation: Partners in crime in Parkinson's disease? J Neuroinflamm. 2014;11:52. https://doi.org/10.1186/1742-2094-11-52.

9. Dzamko N, Halliday GM. An emerging role for LRRK2 in the immune system. Biochem Soc Trans. 2012;40:1134–9. https://doi.org/10.1042/bst20120119.

10. Mamais A, Cookson MR. LRRK2: dropping (kinase) inhibitions and seeking an (immune) response. J Neurochem. 2014;129:895–7. https://doi.org/10.1111/jnc.12691.

11. Gardet A, Benita Y, Li C, Sands BE, Ballester I, Stevens C, Korzenik JR, Rioux JD, Daly MJ, Xavier RJ, Podolsky DK. LRRK2 is involved in the IFN-gamma response and host response to pathogens. J Immunol. 2010;185:5577–85. https://doi.org/10.4049/jimmunol.1000548.

12. Kuss M, Adamopoulou E, Kahle PJ. Interferon-gamma induces leucine-rich repeat kinase LRRK2 via extracellular signal-regulated kinase ERK5 in macrophages. J Neurochem. 2014;129:980–7. https://doi.org/10.1111/jnc.12668.

13. Willingham AT, Orth AP, Batalov S, Peters EC, Wen BG, Aza-Blanc P, Hogenesch JB, Schultz PG. A strategy for probing the function of noncoding RNAs finds a repressor of NFAT. Science. 2005;309:1570–3. https://doi.org/10.1126/science.1115901.

14. Liu Z, Lee J, Krummey S, Lu W, Cai H, Lenardo MJ. The kinase LRRK2 is a regulator of the transcription factor NFAT that modulates the severity of inflammatory bowel disease. Nat Immunol. 2011;12:1063–70. https://doi.org/10.1038/ni.2113.

15. Rosenfeld RM, Piccirillo JF, Chandrasekhar SS, Brook I, Kumar KA, Kramper M, Orlandi RR, Palmer JN, Patel ZM, Peters A, Walsh SA, Corrigan MD. Clinical practice guideline (update): adult sinusitis executive summary. Otolaryngol Head Neck Surg. 2015;152:598–609. https://doi.org/10.1177/0194599815574247.

16. Wang H, Bai J, Ding M, Liu W, Xu R, Zhang J, Shi J, Li H. Interleukin-17A contributes to the expression of serum amyloid A in chronic rhinosinusitis with nasal polyps. Eur Arch Otorhinolaryngol. 2013;270:1867–72. https://doi.org/10.1007/s00405-012-2295-x.

17. Fokkens WJ, Lund VJ, Mullol J, Bachert C, Alobid I, Baroody F, Cohen N, Cervin A, Douglas R, Gevaert P, Georgalas C, Goossens H, Harvey R, et al. EPOS 2012: European position paper on rhinosinusitis and nasal polyps 2012. A summary for otorhinolaryngologists. Rhinology. 2012;50:1–12. https://doi.org/10.4193/Rhino50E2.

18. Liu Z, Lenardo MJ. The role of LRRK2 in inflammatory bowel disease. Cell Res. 2012;22:1092–4. https://doi.org/10.1038/cr.2012.42.

19. Tieu DD, Kern RC, Schleimer RP. Alterations in epithelial barrier function and host defense responses in chronic rhinosinusitis. J Allergy Clin Immunol. 2009;124:37–42. https://doi.org/10.1016/j.jaci.2009.04.045.

20. Hakimi M, Selvanantham T, Swinton E, Padmore RF, Tong Y, Kabbach G, Venderova K, Girardin SE, Bulman DE, Scherzer CR, LaVoie MJ, Gris D, Park DS, et al. Parkinson's disease-linked LRRK2 is expressed in circulating and tissue immune cells and upregulated following recognition of microbial structures. J Neural Transm (Vienna). 2011;118:795–808. https://doi.org/10.1007/s00702-011-0653-2.

# 16

# Optimizing diagnostic tests for persulphate-induced respiratory diseases

M. H. Foss-Skiftesvik[1,2]*, L. Winther[3], H. F. Mosbech[3], P. S. Skov[5], M. S. Opstrup[1,3], H. Søsted[2], C. Zachariae[4], J. D. Johansen[2] and C. R. Johnsen[3]

## Abstract

**Background:** Persulphates from hair bleaching products are considered the major cause of occupational-rhinitis and asthma in hairdressers. The specific inhalation challenge (SIC) is considered 'reference standard' for diagnosing persulphate-induced asthma and rhinitis; however, the currently validated method of performing SIC with persulphate powder is time consuming with a duration of up to 4 days. The value of skin prick tests (SPTs) and histamine release tests (HRTs) with persulphates is unknown. The aim of this study was to establish a novel rapid SIC with persulphate powder to test for both rhinitis and asthma simultaneously in 1 day. In addition, we assessed the suitability of SPTs and HRTs for detecting persulphate-induced respiratory diseases.

**Methods:** The study population included 19 hairdressers with a history of work-related rhinitis and/or asthma symptoms, 12 symptomatic controls (10 with concurrent allergic asthma and rhinitis and two with non-allergic asthma), and 40 healthy controls. A previous severe asthmatic reaction and/or anaphylactic reaction to persulphates was considered an exclusion criterion for hairdressers. The 19 hairdressers and 12 symptomatic controls had SIC performed with $3 \times 5$ min exposures to potassium persulphate powder in a provocation chamber. All participants, including the 40 healthy controls, were subjected also to SPTs and HRTs with three persulphate salts at concentrations of 2–20 % and 0.03–1 %, respectively.

**Results:** None of the symptomatic controls had a nasal or bronchial response to SIC with potassium persulphate. Six hairdressers presented a nasal and two a bronchial response. No severe reactions occurred. No positive SPTs were recorded, neither among hairdressers, symptomatic controls, nor healthy controls. All three groups showed nonspecific non-IgE mediated histamine release to persulphates in HRT.

**Conclusions:** The proposed method for performing SIC showed a high specificity for detecting persulphate-induced asthma and rhinitis. The rapid SIC was able to produce positive nasal and bronchial responses in symptomatic hairdressers without any severe reactions occurring. SPTs and HRTs cannot predict asthma or rhinitis caused by persulphates.

**Keywords:** Specific inhalation challenge, Persulphates, Persulphate salts, Histamine release test, Skin prick tests, Occupational asthma, Occupational rhinitis

## Background

Persulphates are low-molecular weight chemicals (<10 kDA) with strong oxidizing properties and wide application in hair bleaching products. They are also found in dental prosthesis cleaners, food starch, paper and cellophane, as a reducing agent in photography, and as etching solution for printed circuit boards [1]. Persulphates can induce immediate and delayed reactions, such as contact dermatitis, contact urticaria, asthma, rhinitis, and anaphylaxis [2–6]. Reported cases of immediate type reaction caused by persulphates are predominantly among hairdressers, but also workers producing persulphates [7, 8] and consumers of hair bleaching products [3, 9] have been reported to react.

*Correspondence: majken.hougaard.foss-skiftesvik@reg onh.dk
[1] Department of Dermato-Allergology, National Allergy Research Centre, Copenhagen University Hospital Gentofte, Kildegårdsvej 28, 2900 Hellerup, Denmark
Full list of author information is available at the end of the article

As with most low-molecular weight agents, the mechanism by which persulphates induce immediate reactions is not fully understood. Immunoglobulin E (IgE) [4, 8, 10], T-cells [11, 12], and oxidative events have been proposed to contribute to the development of persulphate-induced asthma and rhinitis [13].

When assessing a patient with possible persulphate-induced rhinitis or asthma, various tests can be considered. Several studies describe the use of skin prick tests (SPTs) [10, 14, 15]; however, validation and standardization are lacking. Only one study addressed the use of histamine release test (HRT) [16] and results were inconclusive.

The specific inhalation challenge (SIC) is held as 'reference standard' for diagnosing occupational-rhinitis and asthma [17]. SIC with persulphate has been performed with a realistic approach attempting to reproduce conditions in the hairdressing salon [18–20]. Typically, mixtures of persulphate powder and lactose powder [20], or bleaching powder and hydrogen peroxide [21] are tipped from one tray to another inside a specially designed provocation chamber. The test has also been performed by administering an aqueous persulphate solution with a nebulizer and by spraying the solution directly into the nose when examining asthma [22, 23] and rhinitis [12], respectively. The SIC performed with persulphate in the realistic approach has previously been validated [20]. In this validated approach, the patient is exposed to a mixture of persulphate powder and lactose powder. The exposure is performed step-wise with increasing doses of persulphate during four consecutive days. The maximal exposure on the fourth day is 30 g of potassium persulphate for 10 min. A sensitivity of 100 % and a specificity of 87.5 % for diagnosing persulphate-induced asthma were reported. A disadvantage of this approach is, that it is very time consuming for both investigator and patient.

The aim of our study was, with a focus on Munoz' validated method, to establish a new realistic approach rapid SIC performed with potassium persulphate to test for both rhinitis and asthma simultaneously in 1 day. Instead of using the step-wise approach over several days, we exposed the patients to 30 g of potassium persulphate on the first day for $3 \times 5$ min. Instead of the typical tipping method, we used a new stirring method in order to obtain a more reproducible exposure. In addition, we assessed the potential for diagnosing persulphate-induced asthma and rhinitis by SPTs and HRTs using three different persulphates (ammonium persulphate, potassium persulphate and sodium persulphate) in concentrations from 2–20 and 0.03–1 %, respectively.

## Methods

The study was performed as a clinical single-blinded case–control study between February 2014 and May 2016.

### Hairdressers

Hairdressers with work-related respiratory symptoms who had either contacted the hot-line of the Research Center for Hairdressers and Beauticians or were refereed to our unit for suspected occupational asthma and/or rhinitis were eligible for inclusion in this study. Hairdressers with a history of severe asthmatic reactions and/or anaphylactic reactions to hair bleaching products were excluded. Standardized interviews were employed to obtain a detailed medical and occupational history, as well as records of atopic diseases and smoking. Respiratory symptoms suggestive of asthma and rhinitis were assessed and their association with exposure to persulphates and other hairdressing chemicals was explored. A positive stop/resume test was defined as respiratory symptoms improving after periods away from work and worsening at the workplace [24]. A physical examination that included rhinoscopy was performed to exclude nasal conditions mimicking rhinitis.

### Symptomatic controls

Individuals with a history of asthma and rhinitis without known sensitization or exposure to persulphates were recruited among patients in our unit and through an advertisement on a website for research subjects.

### Healthy controls

For the SPT and HRT with persulphates we recruited a group of healthy controls without known asthma, rhinitis, or urticaria.

Prior to any clinical tests, inhaled corticosteroids were discontinued for 2 weeks, oral antihistamine and nasal corticosteroids for 72 h, long-acting beta$_2$-agonist and leukotriene receptor antagonists for 48 h, and short-acting beta$_2$-agonist for 8 h. The following were considered exclusion criteria: unstable asthma during the last 3 months before inclusion, regular use of oral corticosteroids, baseline forced expiratory volume in 1 s (FEV$_1$) $\leq$70 % of predicted normal value, recent (<4 weeks) respiratory tract infection, chronic obstructive pulmonary disease, severe hypertension, immunological diseases, pregnancy or unstable cardiovascular diseases.

### Immunologic tests

SPTs were performed in duplicate with 10 common aeroallergens (Soluprick SQ®; ALK-Abelló, Hørsholm, Denmark), latex, and chlorhexidine digluconate (5 mg/mL). Negative (diluent) and positive (histamine 10 mg/mL) controls were also included. A positive reaction was defined by a wheal with a diameter $\geq$3 mm. The SPT was only considered to be valid when the positive control was positive and the negative control was negative. Atopy was defined as a positive SPT reaction to one or more of the common allergens.

In addition, SPTs were performed with freshly prepared solutions of ammonium persulphate (ACS reagent ≥98.0 %, CAS 7727-54.0), potassium persulphate (ACS reagent, ≥99.0 %, CAS 7727-21-1), and sodium persulphate (purum p.a., ≥99.0 %, CAS 7775-27-1); all Sigma-Aldrich, St. Louis, MO, USA. The persulphates were dissolved in physiologic saline solution. Ammonium and sodium persulphate were prepared at 2, 5, 7.5, 10 and 20 (wt/vol). Potassium persulphate was used at 2, 5, and 7.5 (wt/vol), as it was insoluble at higher concentrations. The solutions' pH ranged from 1.45 to 5. First, the lowest three concentrations of the persulphates solutions were applied. If no reaction occurred within 15 min, 10 % solution was applied. Finally, if no reaction occurred again, the test was performed with the 20 % solution. Reactions were recorded after 15 and 30 min.

Heparinized blood (5 mL) for HRT was collected at and sent to RefLab ApS (Copenhagen, Denmark) according to standard procedures. Blood samples were stored at room temperature for a maximum of 6 h prior to analysis. Persulphate solutions were prepared daily and tested at concentrations of 0.03, 0.06, 0.125, 0.25, 0.5 and 1.0 (wt/vol) in duplicates. Briefly, 25 µL aliquots were incubated with 25 µL persulphate dilutions at 37 °C for 1 h. During incubation, the released histamine bound to a glass fiber coated microtitre plate and was detected fluorometrically after coupling to o-phthaldialdehyde [25]. Positive reactions were categorized according to the lowest concentration producing significant histamine release (10 ng histamine/mL blood). If no histamine was released, the result was categorized as negative.

Finally, whole blood was collected, serum was separated and stored at −20 °C until total IgE was measured by the ImmunoCap® assay (Thermo Fisher Scientific, Waltham, MA, USA).

### Lung function tests

Hairdressers and symptomatic controls had relevant asthma medication discontinued prior to the performance of any lung function tests. Spirometry, including reversibility test and methacholine challenge was performed for each hairdresser and control 2–3 days before SIC.

Forced expiratory flow in the first second (FEV₁) and forced vital capacity (FVC) within 2 standard deviations (SD) of predicted normal values were considered normal. The reversibility test was deemed positive if FEV₁ increased by ≥12 % or >200 ml upon inhalation of

$\beta_2$-agonist. Bronchial hyperresponsiveness (BHR) was assessed by the bronchial provocation test with methacholine. The provocative dose of methacholine producing a 20 % fall in FEV₁ (PD20) was expressed in micrograms.

After spirometry, fractional exhaled nitric oxide (FeNO) was measured with a DENOX 88 analyzer (ECO MEDICS AG, Duernten Switzerland) and was considered elevated at ≥25 ppb [26].

### SIC with persulphate

SIC was performed on an outpatient basis. On a separate control day, SIC was performed with 50 g D-lactose monohydrate (Sigma-Aldrich). In the absence of a bronchial- and nasal response during the following 24 h, subjects were exposed to a mixture of 30 g potassium persulphate and 20 g lactose powder. The participants, but not the investigator, were blind to the nature of the challenges.

During exposure, participant sat at a table inside a provocation chamber (2.1 m × 2.2 m × 2.3 m) at ambient temperature and humidity. Fresh air was supplied at 0.5/h through a high efficiency particulate air and carbon filters. Test substances were contained in a 1-L Erlenmeyer flask (Schott, Mainz, Germany), placed 30 cm from the subjects' face on a magnetic stirrer (IKAMAG® RCT basic; IKA, Staufen, Germany), and swirled in the air by stirring the magnet (length: 7 cm) at 810 rpm. Maximal exposure consisted of 3 × 5 min, with 20-min intervals in between. During pauses and after maximal exposure was reached, participants were removed from the provocation chamber. Exposure was discontinued if the patient developed a significant bronchial response before maximal exposure was reached. Monitoring for a bronchial and nasal response was performed at baseline; in between each exposure; 15, 30, and 60 min after exposure; and hourly thereafter until sleep. Participants were monitored in the hospital during the first 8 h; thereafter, they performed self-measurements of FEV₁ and nasal symptoms at home until sleep and again the following morning when waking up.

### Quantification of potassium persulphate during SIC

To assess the reproducibility of the stirring method, the amount of potassium persulphate in the provocation chamber was quantified during three challenges on three separate days. Particles sized 10–300 nm and 0.1–10 µm were counted using a NanoTracer PNT800 (Philips Electronics, Eindhoven, The Netherlands) and a Dust Trak™ Aerosol Monitor Model 8520 (TSI, Shoreview, MN, USA), respectively, placed 30 cm away from the Erlenmeyer flask.

### Evaluation of bronchial response

Airway obstruction was assessed by $FEV_1$ using a portable asthma monitor (AM1; Jaeger, Hoechberg, Germany). A sustained $\geq 15$ % decrease in $FEV_1$ from baseline was considered a positive result for asthma, provided that fluctuations in $FEV_1$ were $\leq 10$ % on the control day [27].

### Evaluation of nasal response

Rhinitis was measured using three tests: Linder's symptoms score scale, changes in nasal cavity volume, and anterior rhinoscopy. SIC with persulphate was considered positive for rhinitis if $\geq 2$ tests were positive and the participant had <2 positive tests on the control day.

### Linder's symptoms score scale

Subjective symptoms of rhinoconjunctivitis were scored according to Linder's symptoms score scale [28, 29]. Participants rated sneezing, rhinorrhea, and nasal congestion from 0 to 3. Ocular symptoms scored 1 point, and itchiness of the nose, ears or palate scored 1 point for each location with itch. An increase of $\geq 3$ points from baseline was considered a positive result.

### Changes in nasal cavity volume

Swelling of the nasal mucosa was assessed by means of acoustic rhinometry using a Rhinoscan® SRE 2000 (RhinoMetrics A/S, Lynge, Denmark) as previously described [30]. Participant had acclimatized for 20 min before baseline measurements were performed. Total nasal volume (TNV) was measured at 2–6 cm from the nares. A $\geq 25$ % fall in TNV after exposure was considered a positive result [28].

### Scoring by anterior rhinoscopy

Anterior rhinoscopy was performed and rhinorrhea and nasal congestion were scored separately according to the method proposed by Hytonen [31]. A change in nasal status score of $\geq 4$ points between baseline and exposure was considered a positive response [31].

### Statistical analysis

Data were analyzed using SPSS 22.0 for Windows (SPSS Inc., Chicago, IL, USA). Results for categorical variables are presented as numbers and frequencies, and are compared by the Fischer's exact test. $P$ values $\leq 0.05$ were considered statistically significant (two-tailed tests). Continuous variables were compared with the Mann–Whitney U test and expressed as means ± SDs.

## Results

### Hairdressers

A total of 20 hairdressers were considered eligible for inclusion; one was excluded because of unstable asthma. All were female and the mean age was 31 years (Table 1). Six hairdressers were atopic and three had atopic dermatitis. FeNo was elevated in three, FEV1/FVC was reduced in three, and five showed bronchial hyperresponsiveness in the methacholine challenge. Seven hairdressers used asthma medication and six used rhinoconjunctivitis medication (Table 1). When asked about work-related symptoms, one hairdressers reported asthmatic symptoms ($\geq 2$ of the following: wheeze, cough, shortness of breath or hoarseness), one reported rhinitis symptoms ($\geq 1$ of the following: nasal itching, runny nose, blocked nose, itchy and watery eyes), and 17 reported both asthmatic and rhinitis symptoms. All 19 hairdressers reported symptoms in relation to hair bleaching and 11 (58 %) admitted that their symptoms could also be provoked by other hairdressing products such as hair dyes, hairsprays, permanent wave solutions, and perfume (Table 1).

### Symptomatic controls

A total of 14 symptomatic controls were eligible for inclusion; two had to be excluded due to unstable asthma leaving ten with concomitant allergic asthma and rhinitis and 2 with non-allergic asthma. The mean age was 21 years and 58 % were female (Table 1). Half had atopic dermatitis. Elevated FeNO was detected in 42 %, FEV1/FVC was reduced in three, and the methacholine challenge was positive in seven. All used asthma medication, whilst only the ten with concomitant allergic rhinitis used rhinitis medication (Table 1).

### Healthy controls

A total of 40 healthy participants had SPT and HRT with persulphates performed.

### Results of SIC

None of the participants reacted to placebo. None of the symptomatic controls developed a nasal or bronchial response when exposed to potassium persulphate in SIC. A total of six (32 %) hairdressers showed a positive reaction to SIC with persulphate; four had a nasal response, and two had a combined bronchial and nasal response (Table 2).

All hairdressers with a positive SIC, reported a positive stop/resume test, whereby their symptoms subsided in periods away from work and deteriorated again when returning to work. They had all been exposed to hairdressing for $\geq 6$ months before developing work-related respiratory symptoms. The typical time interval between initiating work with bleaching products and the appearance of symptoms, was minutes (n = 3), hours (n = 2), or it could not be defined (n = 1). Half of the hairdressers had discontinued their work, and hence were no longer exposed to persulphates on a

**Table 1  Main characteristics of participants**

| | Hairdressers (n = 19) | Symptomatic controls (n = 12) | Healthy controls (n = 40) | P value[α] |
|---|---|---|---|---|
| Mean age, years (SD) | 31 (10.5) | 21 (2.6) | 35 (12.9) | 0.002 |
| BMI, mean (SD) | 22.5 (3.8) | 22.4 (3.4) | 24.7 (4.3) | 1.000 |
| Sex (% female) | 19 (100) | 7 (58) | 43 | 0.02 |
| Smoking status, n (%) | | | | |
| Smoker | 7 (37) | 5 (42) | – | 0.79 |
| Never smoker | 12 (63) | 7 (58) | – | |
| Atopic dermatitis, n (%) | 3 (16) | 6 (50) | 0 (0) | 0.06 |
| Total IgE, mean (SD) | 58.3 (76) | 156.5 (202) | | 0.22 |
| Atopy[a] (%) | 6 (32) | 10 (83) | | 0.009 |
| FeNO ≥ 25 ppb, n (%) | 3 (16) | 5 (42) | | 0.20 |
| FeNO ≥ 50 ppb, n (%) | 1 (5.2) | 3 (25) | | |
| Lung function, mean (SD) | | | | |
| % FEV1 | 101.7 (9.7) | 106.6 (14.8) | | 0.48 |
| % FVC | 105.3 (8.7) | 116.8 (14.1) | | 0.025 |
| FEV1/FVC | 84.8 (7.6) | 78.9 (6.6) | | 0.43 |
| Methacholine test | | | | |
| BHR, n (%) | 5 (26) | 7 (58) | | 0.13 |
| Asthma medication, n (%) | | | | |
| None | 12 (63) | 0 (0) | | |
| SABA | 3 (16) | 7 (58) | | |
| SABA + low dose ICS | 1 (5) | 3 (25) | | |
| SABA + medium dose ICS | 1 (5) | 2 (17) | | |
| SABA + LABA/ICS | 1 (5) | 0 (0) | | |
| SABA + LTRA | 1 (5) | 0 (0) | | |
| Rhinitis medication, n (%) | | | | |
| None | 13 (68) | 2 (17) | | |
| OA | 2 (11) | 8 (67) | | |
| INS | 1 (5) | 1 (8) | | |
| OA + INS | 2 (11) | 1 (8) | | |
| OA + antihistamine eye drops | 1 (5) | 0 (0) | | |
| Work-related symptoms, n (%) | | | | |
| Rhinitis symptoms | 1 (5) | – | | |
| Asthma symptoms | 1 (5) | – | | |
| Both | 17 (90) | – | | |
| Trigger of symptoms, n (%) | | | | |
| Bleaching products | 19 (100) | – | | |
| Hair dye | 9 (49) | – | | |
| Hair spray | 4 (21) | – | | |
| Permanent solution | 3 (16) | – | | |
| Perfume | 3 (16) | – | | |
| Positive stop/resume test, n (%) | 16 (84) | – | | |

*SD* standard deviation, *BMI* body mass index, *SABA* short-acting beta$_2$-agonists, *LABA* long-acting beta$_2$-agonists, *ICS* inhaled corticosteroids, *LTRA* leukotriene receptor antagonists, *INS* intra-nasal steroid

[a] Defined as 1 ≥positive SPT or 1 ≥positive specific IgE to common inhalant allergens

[α] Comparing hairdressers with controls

daily basis. The nasal responses to SIC began within minutes (n = 2), after 1 h (n = 3), and after 3 h (n = 1). The two hairdressers reacting with bronchoconstriction did so after 3 h and 8 h, respectively. The characteristics of hairdressers with negative SICs are presented in Table 3.

**Table 2 Characteristics of hairdressers with a positive specific inhalation challenge**

| ID | Age (y) | WRAS | WRRS | Stop/ resume test | Duration of exposure before symptoms (y) | Time from exposure to symptom | Time since last exposure to persulphates (y) | Baseline FEV1/ FVC (% of pred.) | MCh PD20 (μg) |
|---|---|---|---|---|---|---|---|---|---|
| 2 | 21 | + | + | P | 5 | Within hours | CE | 87 (103 %) | 330 |
| 5 | 29 | + | + | P | 11 | Not definable | CE | 86.7 (104 %) | N |
| 8 | 32 | + | + | P | 1.5 | Within minutes | 8 | 85.5 (103 %) | 346 |
| 10 | 22 | + | + | P | 4–5 | Within hours | CE | 80.6 (96 %) | N |
| 16 | 23 | + | + | P | 0.5–1 | Within minutes | 2 | 85.4 (101 %) Rever: 12 % | N |
| 19 | 23 | + | + | P | 0.5–1 | Within minutes | 1/3 | 94.9 (113 %) | N |

| ID | Age (y) | FeNO (ppb) | T-IgE (kU/L) | Atopy[a] | HRT PP (mg/mL) | HRT SP (mg/mL) | HRT AP (mg/mL) | SIC response | Classification of SIC response |
|---|---|---|---|---|---|---|---|---|---|
| 2 | 21 | 6.3 | 73.2 | No | N | N | 2.5 | R A | 4 and 8 after 3rd exposure (late reaction) |
| 5 | 29 | 6.2 | 8.7 | Yes | N | 10.0 | 10.0 | R | 1 h after 3rd exposure (immediate reaction) |
| 8 | 32 | *31.2* | 46.4 | Yes | N | N | 5.0 | R | 1 h after 3rd exposure (immediate reaction) |
| 10 | 22 | 7.4 | 26.6 | No | N | N | 10.0 | R A | 1 and 3 h after 3rd exposure (immediate reaction/late reaction) |
| 16 | 23 | 13.0 | 39.8 | Yes | 10.0 | 2.5 | 1.25 | R | After 2nd exposure (immediate reaction) |
| 19 | 23 | 16.9 | 63.6 | Yes | 0.63 | – | 0.63 | R | After 3rd exposure (immediate reaction) |

*y* years, *WRAS* work-related asthma symptoms, *WRRS* work-related rhinitis symptoms, *MCh* methacholine challenge, *FeNO* fractional exhaled nitrogen oxide (increased values in italics), *T-IgE* total immunoglobulin E, *HRT* histamine release test, *PP* potassium persulphate, *AP* ammonium persulphate, *SP* sodium persulphate, *SIC* specific inhalation challenge, *N* negative, *P* positive, *CE* currently exposed, *R* rhinitis, *A* asthma

[a] Defined as ≥1 positive SPT to common inhalant allergens

## Quantification of potassium persulphate

Before exposure, the amount of particles sized 0.1–10 μm inside the provocation chamber ranged from 7 to 18 μg/m³ and the number of ultra-fine particles was 347–1260/cm³. No additional ultrafine particles were detected during a 3 × 5 min exposure to 50 g pure potassium persulphate in the Erlenmeyer flask.

The mean amount of particles sized 0.1–10 μm measured during a 5-min exposure to a mixture of 30 g potassium persulphate and 20 g lactose ranged from 0.25–0.57 mg/m³ and the proportion of potassium persulphate to lactose powder in the flask was 3:2. Thus, the estimated concentration of potassium persulphate in the air during a 5-min exposure was 150–340 μg/m³ with a mean of 240 μg/m³ and a standard deviation of 0.6 μg/m³. During the 20-min pause in between exposures, the amount of particles in the air returned to baseline values.

## SPT results

In two hairdressers, the negative control was positive due to dermographism and therefore their SPTs could not be evaluated (Table 4). All participants reacted to the positive control (histamine), whilst none were positive to latex, chlorhexidine, or any of the three tested persulphates (Table 4).

## Results of HRT with persulphates

Of the six hairdressers with a positive SIC, four (66.7 %) did not react to HRT with potassium persulphate or sodium persulphate at any of the tested concentrations. In contrast, all six hairdressers with positive SICs released histamine in response to ammonium persulphate at concentrations ranging from 0.063 to 1 %. So did also 96.2 % of symptomatic controls and healthy controls. For all three persulphates, the lowest concentration producing histamine release in the controls and healthy controls was 0.125 %, whilst some of the hairdressers reacted to concentrations of 0.06 %. None of the participants showed histamine release to any of the persulphates in concentration of 0.031 %.

## Discussion

### SIC

In this study, we aimed at improving the currently validated SIC with persulphate. The improvements consisted

**Table 3  Characteristics of hairdressers with a negative specific inhalation challenge**

| ID | Age (y) | WRAS | WRRS | Stop/resume test | Duration of exposure before symptoms (y) | Time from exposure to symptoms | Time since last exposure to persulphates (y) | Baseline FEV1/FVC (% of pred.) |
|---|---|---|---|---|---|---|---|---|
| 1 | 52 | + | + | N | 3 | Within hours | 5 | 86 (109 %) |
| 3 | 45 | + | + | P | 20 | Within hours | CE | 83 (104 %) |
| 4 | 49 | + | + | P | 28 | Within minutes | CE | 65 (81 %) Rever: 2.9 % |
| 6 | 30 | – | + | P | 10 | Within minutes | 3 | 81 (97 %) |
| 7 | 27 | + | + | P | 1 | Not definable | 1 | 84.9 (103.3 %) |
| 9 | 20 | + | + | P | 1 | Within minutes | CE | 98 (116 %) |
| 11 | 43 | + | + | P | 20 | Within hours | CE | 83 (103 %) |
| 12 | 23 | + | + | N | 3 | Within hours | CE | 74 (88 %) Rever: 12 % |
| 13 | 46 | + | – | N | 2 | Not definable | 3 | 83 (103 %) |
| 14 | 27 | + | + | P | 7 | Within minutes | CE | 83 (99 %) |
| 15 | 31 | + | + | P | 4 | Within minutes | 1/2 | 75 (90 %) Rever: 7.8 % |
| 17 | 20 | + | + | P | 4 | Not definable | 1/6 | 91 (108 %) |
| 18 | 29 | + | + | P | 8 | Within hours | CE | 91 (109 %) |

| ID | Age (y) | MCh PD20 (µg) | FeNO (ppb) | T-IgE (kU/L) | Atopy[a] | HRT PP (mg/mL) | HRT SP (mg/mL) | HRT AP (mg/mL) |
|---|---|---|---|---|---|---|---|---|
| 1 | 52 | N | 25 | 3.6 | No | 1.25 | 0.63 | 1.25 |
| 3 | 45 | N | 9.9 | 6.7 | No | N | 5.0 | 2.5 |
| 4 | 49 | N | 16.0 | 2.2 | No | 10.0 | 10.0 | 5.0 |
| 6 | 30 | 400 | 64.1 | 155 | No | N | 10.0 | 5.0 |
| 7 | 27 | N | 19.3 | 127 | D | N | 5.0 | 2.5 |
| 9 | 20 | N | 6.6 | <2 | No | N | 10.0 | 5.0 |
| 11 | 43 | N | 7.1 | 22.5 | No | N | 10.0 | 5.0 |
| 12 | 23 | N | 21.8 | 122 | No | 10.0 | 5.0 | 2.5 |
| 13 | 46 | 626 | 12.1 | 35.4 | No | N | 5.0 | 1.25 |
| 14 | 27 | N | 11.8 | 3.7 | No | N | 10.0 | 5.0 |
| 15 | 31 | 720 | 9.0 | 308 | D | 5.0 | 2.5 | 1.25 |
| 17 | 20 | N | 9.0 | 4.3 | No | 10.0 | 2.5 | 2.5 |
| 18 | 29 | N | 19.7 | 58.3 | No | N | N | N |

*y* years, *WRAS* work-related asthma symptoms, *WRRS* work-related rhinitis symptoms, *MCh* methacholine challenge, *FeNO* fractional exhaled nitrogen oxide (increased values in italics), *T-IgE* total immunoglobulin E, *HRT* histamine release test, *PP* potassium persulphate, *AP* ammonium persulphate, *SP* sodium persulphate, *SIC* specific inhalation challenge, *N* negative, *P* positive, *CE* currently exposed, *D* dermographism, *R* rhinitis, *A* asthma

[a] Defined as ≥1 positive SPT to common inhalant allergens

of: a more rapid approach; using the "stirring method" instead of the "tipping method"; and assessing not only asthma but also rhinitis.

When Munoz et al. validated the realistic method [20], repeated exposures on consecutive days were performed with a mixture of potassium persulphate and 150 g lactose using the tipping method. The duration of the exposure was 10 min each day, and the dose of potassium persulphate was increased from 5 to 30 g over 4 days until a positive reaction occurred. The patient was hospitalized during the entire procedure. The method proved safe and a sensitivity of 100 % and a specificity of 87.5 % for diagnosing occupational asthma were reported.

In our method, we skipped the first 3 days with low exposure, and went straight to exposing the patient to 30 g of potassium persulphate. Instead of 10 min exposure we performed 15 min exposure. To reduce the risk of adverse reaction, exposure was performed step-wise; 5 min at a time with 20 min pauses in between, and severe asthmatic reactions and/or anaphylactic reactions to bleaching products were considered exclusion criteria.

**Table 4 Results from skin prick tests**

| | Hairdressers (n = 19) | Symptomatic controls (n = 12) | Healthy controls (n = 40) |
|---|---|---|---|
| Positive control (p/n) | 19/0 | 12/0 | 40/0 |
| Negative control (p/n) | 2/17 | 0/12 | 0/40 |
| Potassium persulphate (p/n) Conc. (%) | 0/17 | 0/12 | 0/40 |
| 2 | – | – | – |
| 5 | – | – | – |
| 7.5 | – | – | – |
| Ammonium persulphate (p/n) Conc. (%) | 0/17 | 0/12 | 0/40 |
| 2 | – | – | – |
| 5 | – | – | – |
| 7.5 | – | – | – |
| 10 | – | – | – |
| 20 | – | – | – |
| Sodium persulphate (p/n) Conc. (%) | 0/17 | 0/12 | 0/40 |
| 2 | – | – | – |
| 5 | – | – | – |
| 7.5 | – | – | – |
| 10 | – | – | – |
| 20 | – | – | – |

p positive, n negative

Given that none of the symptomatic controls with allergic asthma and rhinitis reacted to SIC, it seems that the proposed method has a high specificity for persulphate-induced asthma and rhinitis. In this group of hairdressers, SIC produced a nasal response in 33 % (6/18 with work-related rhinitis symptoms) and a bronchial response in 11 % (2/18 with work-related asthma symptoms).

We registered no adverse events or severe asthmatic reactions although our exposure was higher than Munoz' on the fourth day. Hence, it seems that the rapid method is safe when tested in patients without a history of severe asthmatic reactions or anaphylactic reactions to bleaching products.

We have several reasons for using the level of exposure we did. Firstly, we chose 3 × 5 min exposure to better mimic the hairdressers' exposure during a typical working day. Since hairdressers are mainly exposed to persulphates when they mix bleaching powder with hydrogen peroxide [32], we wanted to mimic this process. We estimated that a typical hairdressers performs this process three times a day. Secondly, the ratio of persulphate to lactose powder was changed as to better mimic the level hairdressers are exposed to in their daily practice. During

mixing of the paste that is applied to the clients hair, 20–80 g bleaching powder [33], containing up to 60 % persulphate (12–48 g) [1], is typically used. We therefore used a ratio of persulphate to lactose powder of 3:2 (30 g persulphate:20 g lactose powder). To obtain a more uniform and reproducible exposure, we used a magnetic stirrer. In our study, the participants were exposed to levels of up to 0.34 mg/m$^3$ for 3 × 5 min during SIC. The permissible threshold limit value of exposure to potassium persulphate, as defined by the Occupational Safety and Health Administration in the United States, is a time weighted average (TWA) of 0.1 mg/m$^3$ during a typical working day of 8 h. According to the excursion limit of potassium persulphate, the TWA should not be exceeded more than 3 times for no longer than 30 min during a working day. Hence, the TWA was exceeded during our exposure, but the excursion limit was respected.

A limitation of our approach is that the patients were sent home after 8 h of observation in the clinic. This is convenient for the patient, but it introduces a potential bias. If the patient develops a positive nasal or bronchial response during this period at home, it is difficult to interpret whether the response was caused by exposure to persulphates or by exposure to other allergens encountered outside the hospital. However, in our study, all hairdressers reacted whilst being monitored in our department, so it is unlikely that this is a problem in our results.

Another limitation of our study is that the included hairdressers were merely under suspicion of having occupational asthma and rhinitis, but they were not clearcut cases, which explains why only some hairdressers had a positive reaction to SIC. Firstly, they did not have serial peak flow measurement at and away from work performed prior to inclusion. If we had included only patient with a peak flow pattern suggestive of occupational asthma it might have improved the sensitivity of the test for detecting persulphate-induced asthma. Secondly, many had normal findings in spirometry, FeNO, and the methacholine challenge suggesting that they did not in fact have asthma although they reported asthmatic symptoms. Third, although persulphates are considered the major cause of occupational asthma and rhinitis in hairdressers [34] more than half reported that their work-related respiratory symptoms could also be provoked by other hairdressing products suggesting that their respiratory symptoms were not merely caused by persulphates. Also, some of the hairdressers had not been active hairdressers for several years and therefore were not still exposed to persulphates meaning that they could have lost airway responsiveness. Taken together, several factors exist that could explain why not all hairdressers reacted to the SIC and consequently the sensitivity of our approach cannot be determined.

### HRT and SPTs with persulphate salts

This is the first study, to the best of our knowledge, to report results of HRT with persulphates. We found that persulphates, especially ammonium persulphate, induced non-IgE-mediated histamine release in both hairdressers and controls. Additionally, most of the SIC-positive hairdressers did not show histamine release. Ammonium persulphate has recently shown to have oxidative activity capable of promoting degranulation of human mast cells and basophils [13]. Thus, persulphates stimulate nonspecific non-IgE-mediated histamine release even in individuals without symptoms of persulphate-induced respiratory diseases, voiding the use of HRT to document asthma or rhinitis caused by persulphates.

We performed SPTs in duplicate with all three persulphates simultaneously, at concentrations as high as 20 %. To our knowledge, this has not been done before. We did not register any positive SPTs with persulphates in any of the participants, although all responded positively to the histamine control. Given the high persulphate concentrations applied, lack of positive reactions does not seem to be caused by using excessively low dosage. In addition, by testing all three persulphates, we ensured that we would not miss any patient sensitized to only one of the three persulphates [35].

Although several reports of positive SPTs with persulphates exist [8, 19, 21, 23], an equal amount of studies have failed to produce positive reactions [7, 14, 30, 31]. Moreover, in some patients, positive reactions are not reproducible over time [36].

The fact that specific IgEs to persulphates have been detected in only three [10, 37], out of more than 40 reported positive SPT cases, indicates that positive SPT reactions are caused by nonspecific non-IgE medi-ated histamine release. Indeed, when researchers with a method capable of detecting specific IgE to persulphates tested five patients with positive SPT reactions, they found that only two had demonstrable specific IgE [10], suggesting that the remaining positive SPT reactions were not mediated by IgE.

All in all, the majority of positive SPT reactions appear to be caused by direct histamine release rather than IgE-mediated mechanisms. Moreover, they have been reported by only a fraction of investigators, and are not always reproducible. Taken together, this indicates that SPTs cannot be applied to testing for persulphate-induced asthma and rhinitis.

## Conclusions

The new rapid SIC with potassium persulphate proved safe when tested in hairdressers without a history of previous serious asthmatic reactions and had a high specificity for diagnosing persulphate-induced asthma and rhinitis. Based on our results, neither histamine release nor SPTs with persulphates appear adequate in predicting asthma and rhinitis caused by persulphates.

### Abbreviations

ACS: American Chemical Society; BHR: bronchial hyperresponsiveness; CAS: Chemical Abstract Service; FeNO: fractional exhaled nitric oxide; $FEV_1$: forced expiratory volume in 1 s; HRT: histamine release test; IgE: immunoglobulin E; rpm: revolutions per minute; SIC: specific inhalation challenge; SPT: skin prick test; TNV: total nasal volume.

### Authors' contributions

MHF-S, LW, HFM, PSS, MSO, HS, CZ, JDJ, CRJ participated in the study design. Drs. MHF-S and CRJ were responsible for conduction of the clinical investigations. Dr. PSS was responsible for performing the HRTs. Dr. MHF-S conceived the manuscript, drafted the initial version, and revised the final edition, whilst the remaining co-authors revised the initial and final manuscript. All authors read and approved the final manuscript.

### Author details

[1] Department of Dermato-Allergology, National Allergy Research Centre, Copenhagen University Hospital Gentofte, Kildegårdsvej 28, 2900 Hellerup, Denmark. [2] Department of Dermato-Allergology, Research Centre for Hairdressers and Beauticians, Copenhagen University Hospital Gentofte, Hellerup, Denmark. [3] Allergy Clinic, Department of Dermato-Allergology, Copenhagen University Hospital Gentofte, Hellerup, Denmark. [4] Department of Dermato-Allergology, Copenhagen University Hospital Gentofte, Hellerup, Denmark. [5] Reflab ApS, Copenhagen, Denmark.

### Acknowledgements

We wish to thank the nurses at the Allergy Clinic for their help with practicalities and Professor Geo Clausen (Technical University of Denmark) for kindly lending us equipment for particle quantification.

### Competing interests

The authors declare that they have no competing interests.

### Funding

The funding for this study was provided by The Health Foundation, Danish Hairdressers' and Beauticians' Union, Danish Hairdressers Association, The Beckett Fund, Torben and Alice Frimodt's Fund, Director Jacob Madsen and wife Olga Madsen's Fund, Carl and Ellen Hertz' Grant for Danish medical- and natural science.

### References

1. Pang S, Zondlo M. Final report on the safety assessment of ammonium, potassium, and sodium persulfate. Int J Toxicol. 2001;20(4):7–21.
2. Schwensen JF, Johansen JD, Veien NK, Funding AT, Avnstorp C, Østerballe M, et al. Occupational contact dermatitis in hairdressers: an analysis of patch test data from the Danish Contact Dermatitis Group, 2002–2011. Contact Dermat. 2014;70(4):233–7.

3. Hoekstra M, van der Heide S, Coenraads PJ, Schuttelaar ML. Anaphylaxis and severe systemic reactions caused by skin contact with persulfates in hair-bleaching products. Contact Dermat. 2012;66:317–22.

4. Munoz X, Cruz M-J, Orriols R, Bravo C, Espuga M, Morell F. Occupational asthma due to persulfate salts—diagnosis and follow-up. Chest. 2003;123(6):2124–9.

5. Hougaard MG, Menne T, Sosted H. Occupational eczema and asthma in a hairdresser caused by hair-bleaching products. Dermatitis. 2012;23:284–7.

6. Bonnevie P. Aetologie und Pathogenese der Eczemkrankheit. Kopenhagen: Nyt Nordisk Forlag; 1939.

7. Merget R, Buenemann A, Kulzer R, Rueckmann A, Breitstadt R, Kniffka A, et al. A cross sectional study of chemical industry workers with occupational exposure to persulphates. Occup Environ Med. 1996;53:422–6.

8. Wrbitzky R, Drexler H, Letzel S. Early reaction type allergies and diseases of the respiratory passages in employees from persulphate production. Int Arch Occup Environ Health. 1995;67:413–7.

9. Fisher AA. Persulfate hair bleach reactions. Arch Dermatol. 1976;112(10):1407–9.

10. Aalto-Korte K, Makinen-Kiljunen S. Specific immunoglobulin E in patients with immediate persulfate hypersensitivity. Contact Dermat. 2003;49:22–5.

11. Yawalkar N, Helbling A, Pichler CE, Zala L, Pichler WJ. T cell involvement in persulfate triggered occupational contact dermatitis and asthma. Ann Allergy Asthma Immunol. 1999;82:401–4.

12. Diab KK, Truedsson L, Albin M, Nielsen J. Persulphate challenge in female hairdressers with nasal hyperreactivity suggests immune cell, but no IgE reaction. Int Arch Occup Environ Health. 2009;82(6):771–7.

13. Pignatti P, Frossi B, Pala G, Negri S, Oman H, Perfetti L, et al. Oxidative activity of ammonium persulfate salt on mast cells and basophils: implication in hairdressers' asthma. Int Arch Allergy Immunol. 2013;160(4):409–19.

14. Hytonen M, Leino T, Sala E, Kanerva L, Tupasela O, Malmberg H. Nasal provocation test in the diagnostics of hairdressers' occupational rhinitis. Acta Otolaryngol Suppl. 1997;529(0365–5237):133–6.

15. Moscato G, Pala G, Perfetti L, Frascaroli M, Pignatti P. Clinical and inflammatory features of occupational asthma caused by persulphate salts in comparison with asthma associated with occupational rhinitis. Allergy. 2010;1(65):784–90.

16. Parra FM, Igea JM, Quirce S, Ferrando MC, Martin JA, Losada E. Occupational asthma in a hairdresser caused by persulphate salts. Allergy. 1992;47(6):656–60.

17. Moscato G, Vandenplas O, Van Wijk RG, Malo JL, Perfetti L, Quirce S, et al. EAACI position paper on occupational rhinitis. Respir Res. 2009;10:16.

18. Pepys J, Hutchcroft BJ, Breslin AB. Asthma due to inhaled chemical agents—persulphate salts and henna in hairdressers. Clin Allergy. 1976;6:399–404.

19. Blainey AD, Ollier S, Cundell D, Smith RE, Davies RJ. Occupational asthma in a hairdressing salon. Thorax. 1986;41:42–50.

20. Munoz X, Cruz M, Orriols R, Torres F, Espuga M, Morell F. Validation of specific inhalation challenge for the diagnosis of occupational asthma due to persulphate salts. Occup Environ Med. 2004;61(10):861–6.

21. Schwaiblmair M, Vogelmeier C, Fruhmann G. Occupational asthma in hairdressers: results of inhalation tests with bleaching powder. Int Arch Occup Environ Health. 1997;70:419–23.

22. Moscato G, Pignatti P, Yacoub M-R, Romano C, Spezia S, Perfetti L. Occupational asthma and occupational rhinitis in hairdressers. Chest. 2005;128(5):3590–8.

23. Hagemeyer O, Marek E, van Kampen V, Sander I, Raulf M, Merget R, et al. Specific inhalation challenge in persulfate asthma. Advs Exp Med Biol Respir. 2015;85–91.

24. Moscato G, Pala G, Barnig C, De BF, Del Giacco SR, Folletti I, et al. EAACI consensus statement for investigation of work-related asthma in non-specialized centres. Allergy. 2012;67:491–501.

25. Vissers YM, Iwan M, Adele-Patient K, Skov PS, Rigby NM, Johnsen PE, et al. Effect of roasting on the allergenicity of major peanut allergens Ara h 1 and Ara h 2/6: the necessity of degranulation assays. Clin Exp Allergy. 2011;41(11):1631–42.

26. Dweik R, Boggs P, Erzurum S, Irvin C. American Thoracic Society documents. An official ATS clinical practice guideline: interpretation of exhaled nitric oxide levels (FENO) for clinical application. Am J Respir Crit Care Med. 2011;184(1):602–15.

27. Vandenplas O, Suojalehto H, Aasen TB, Baur X, Burge PS, de Blay F, et al. Specific inhalation challenge in the diagnosis of occupational asthma: consensus statement. Eur Respir J. 2014;43(6):1573–87.

28. Dordal MT, Lluch-Bernal M, Sánchez MC, Rondón C, Navarro A, Montoro J, et al. Allergen-specific nasal provocation testing: review by the rhino-conjunctivitis committee of the Spanish society of allergy and clinical immunology. J Investig Allergol Clin Immunol. 2011;21(1):1–12.

29. Linder A. Symptom scores as measures of the severity of rhinitis. Clin Allergy. 1988;18(1):29–37.

30. Hilberg O, Pedersen OF. Acoustic rhinometry: recommendations for technical specifications and standard operating procedures. Rhinology. 2000;16:3–17.

31. Hytonen M, Sala E. Nasal provocation test in the diagnostics of occupational allergic rhinitis. Rhinology. 1996;34:86–90.

32. Nilsson PT, Marini S, Wierzbicka A, Kåredal M, Blomgren E, Nielsen J, et al. Characterization of hairdresser exposure to airborne particles during hair bleaching. Ann Occup Hyg. 2015;1–11.

33. National Industrial Chemical Notification and Assessment Scheme (NICNAS). Ammonium, potassium and sodium persulfate. Priority existing chemical assessment report no. 18. 2001.

34. Moscato G, Galdi E. Asthma and hairdressers. Curr Opin Allergy Clin Immunol. 2006;6:91–5.

35. Bregnhøj A, Søsted H. Type I ammonium persulfate allergy with no cross reactivity to potassium persulfate. Contact Dermat. 2009;61(6):356–7.

36. Muñoz X, Gómez-Ollés S, Cruz MJ, Untoria MD, Orriols R, Morell F. Course of bronchial hyperresponsiveness in patients with occupational asthma caused by exposure to persulfate salts. Arch Bronconeumol. 2008;44(3):140–5.

37. Brauel R, Brauel P, Stresemann E. Kontakturticaria, rhinopathie und allergishes bronchialasthma durch ammoniumpersulfat in blondiermittel. Allergologie. 1995;18:438–40.

# 17

# Epidemiology of spider mite sensitivity: a meta-analysis and systematic review

Ying Zhou[1†], Haoyuan Jia[2†], Xuming Zhou[2], Yubao Cui[2*] and Jun Qian[3*]

## Abstract

**Background:** Spider mites, including *Tetranychus urticae*, *Panonychus citri*, and *Panonychus ulmi*, are common pests in gardens, greenhouses, and orchards. Exposure, particularly occupational exposure, to these organisms may lead to the development of respiratory or contact allergies. However, the prevalence of sensitivity to spider mites is unclear.

**Methods:** We examined the literature to generate an estimate of the global prevalence of allergies to spider mites.

**Results:** Electronic databases were searched and twenty-three studies reporting the prevalence of sensitivity to spider mites (based on skin prick tests or IgE-based detection systems) in an aggregate total of 40,908 subjects were selected for analysis. The estimated overall rate of spider mite sensitivity was 22.9% (95% CI 19–26.8%). Heterogeneity was high and meta-regression analysis considering variables such as published year, country, number of study subjects, methods for allergen detection (skin prick test, ImmunoCAP, RAST testing, or intradermal test), and mite species revealed no single significant source. Twelve of the 23 studies reported rates of monosensitization (i.e., patients responsive to spider mites but no other tested allergen), yielding a global average of 7% (95% CI 5–9%), hence spider mites represent a unique source of allergens.

**Conclusions:** Spider mites are an important cause of allergic symptoms. However, the publication bias and heterogeneity evident in this study indicate that further trials using standardized detection methods are needed to determine the association of exposure and symptoms as well as the specific patient characteristics that influence developing spider mite sensitivity.

**Keywords:** Allergy, Spider mites, *Tetranychus urticae*, *Panonychus citri*, *Panonychus ulmi*

## Background

The allergenic role of mites of the genus *Dermatophagoides* in indoor floor and mattress dust was discovered in 1967 [1, 2]. Since then, numerous species have been described as the source of allergens capable of sensitizing and inducing allergic symptoms in susceptible and genetically predisposed individuals [3]. The major mites in indoor house dust, *D. pteronyssinus*, *D. farinae*, *Blomia tropicalis*, and *Euroglyphus maynei*, account for 80% of the total allergenic species, with storage mites making up

the remainder [4, 5]. Domestic mites, including all indoor mites, belong to the subphylum Chelirata, class Arachnida, subclass Acari, superorder Acariformes, and order Astigmata [6].

Spider mites, also called webspinning mites [7], are common pests in landscapes and gardens and feed on many fruit trees, vines, berries, vegetables, and ornamental plants. All spider mites, belonging to the suborder Prostigmata of the subclass Acari, are outdoor phytophagous mites which cause significant damage to fruit trees throughout the world, causing a considerable economic burden on agriculture [8]. In a Korean study of 2412 patients, 9.8% were sensitized to spider mites [8]. An online search revealed that spider mites are important outdoor allergens that may contribute to work-related asthma and rhinitis in fruit farmers and children living in rural areas and produce a set of allergens that differ

*Correspondence: ybcui1975@hotmail.com; qian@wuxiph.com
†Ying Zhou and Haoyuan Jia have contributed equally to this work
2 Department of Clinical Laboratory, Wuxi People's Hospital Affiliated to Nanjing Medical University, No. 299 at Qingyang Road, Wuxi 214023, Jiangsu Province, People's Republic of China
3 Department of Pediatrics, Wuxi Children's Hospital, Wuxi 214023, People's Republic of China
Full list of author information is available at the end of the article

from those generated by indoor mites [9]. The aim of our present study was to analyze existing information on the prevalence of spider mite sensitization.

### Search strategy

We have used a search and analysis strategy based on the PRISMA system [10]. To identify related studies published through June 1st, 2017, we performed systematic literature searches of electronic databases including Pub-Med, the Cochrane Library, EMBASE, Medion, and Web of Science. Search terms were applied by various combinations of Medical Subject Headings (MeSH) and non-MeSH terms as follows: [(spider mite or *Tetranychus* or *Panonychus*) AND (sensitization or allergy or hypersensitivity or specific IgE positive or skin test positive or RAST positive)]. Titles and abstracts identified by electronic searches were examined independently and on screen by two researchers to select potentially relevant studies. Eligibility criteria are given below. Differences were resolved by consensus. A full text paper was obtained wherever possible.

### Eligibility criteria

Studies that investigated the prevalence of sensitivity to spider mites (family Tetranychidae) in full journal articles were selected for review, including cross-sectional, cohort studies, controlled clinical trials and other types. Studies published in conference proceedings, books, book chapters, or research not published in English were excluded.

Eligible studies focused on individuals with allergic disorders defined by in vivo or in vitro tests with mite extract made from *Tetranychus* or *Panonychus* mites. Thus, inclusion into the meta-analysis was restricted to those studies that reported prevalence data for sensitivity to spider mites.

### Data extraction

The following specific information relating to data collection and results was extracted individually from each identified article and entered into a pre-designed Excel spread sheet: data and geographical location, study design, participant inclusion and exclusion criteria, recruitment procedures, number of investigated subjects, age and gender of investigated subjects, occupations or characteristics of the patients, number sensitized to spider mites, detection methods, and mite species. To ensure accuracy, two researchers extracted the data and then compared the results of their extractions.

### Meta-analysis according to the studied population groups

For meta-analysis, the prevalence rates of spider mite sensitization were pooled using the random effects model [11]. Heterogeneity was calculated via Cochran's Q and $\tau^2$ tests, and inconsistency is presented as $I^2$, which describes the percentage of variability that is due to heterogeneity rather than chance [11].

### Meta-regression analysis

To identify the sources of heterogeneity among studies, meta-regression analysis was carried out [12]. Possible sources of heterogeneity, including published year, country, number of study subjects, methods for allergen detection (skin prick test, ImmunoCAP, RAST testing, or intradermal test), and mite species (*Tetranychus urticae*, *Panonychus ulmi*, or *Panonychus citri*), were included in the analysis.

### Publication bias and meta-analysis

The possibility of publication bias was assessed by graphical analysis of funnel plots. Deeks' funnel plot asymmetry analysis was performed to identify publication bias [13]. In Deeks' funnel plots, each data point represents a study, its effect size or prevalence, and the standard error. The meta-analysis was conducted using the Stata v12 software package (Stata Corporation, College Station, TX, USA) and the graphical representation was conducted using forest plots.

## Results
### Characteristics of included studies

Our searches initially retrieved 48 journal article references from electronic databases. Twenty-four of these were subsequently removed due to either duplication or a failure to meet the inclusion criteria. The remaining twenty-four full text articles were then retrieved and critically appraised [8, 9, 14–35]. Of these, the Gargano study [30] was subsequently deleted from the analysis, because this study selected only patients that were SPT+ and tested them to see what percentage had spider mite reactive IgEs. This does not represent an unbiased patient population (since all patients were known to be SPT+). The remaining 23 studies were found to be eligible and were entered into our review and meta-analysis (Fig. 1). Among the 23 included papers, 13 were conducted in Korea, three were conducted in Italy, one was conducted in Japan, two were conducted in Spain, two were conducted in South Africa, and two were conducted in Sweden (Table 1). The sample sizes of the studies entered into the review varied widely from 10 [33] to 8595 [22] with the median sample size being 308. In total, the 23 studies examined 40,908 subjects. Among these 23 papers, Kim et al. [22] reported the prevalence for sensitivity to both *T. urticae* and *P. citri* using separate patient populations. Kim and Lee et al. [25] reported the sensitivity prevalence for both *T. urticae* and *P. ulmi* in the same patient

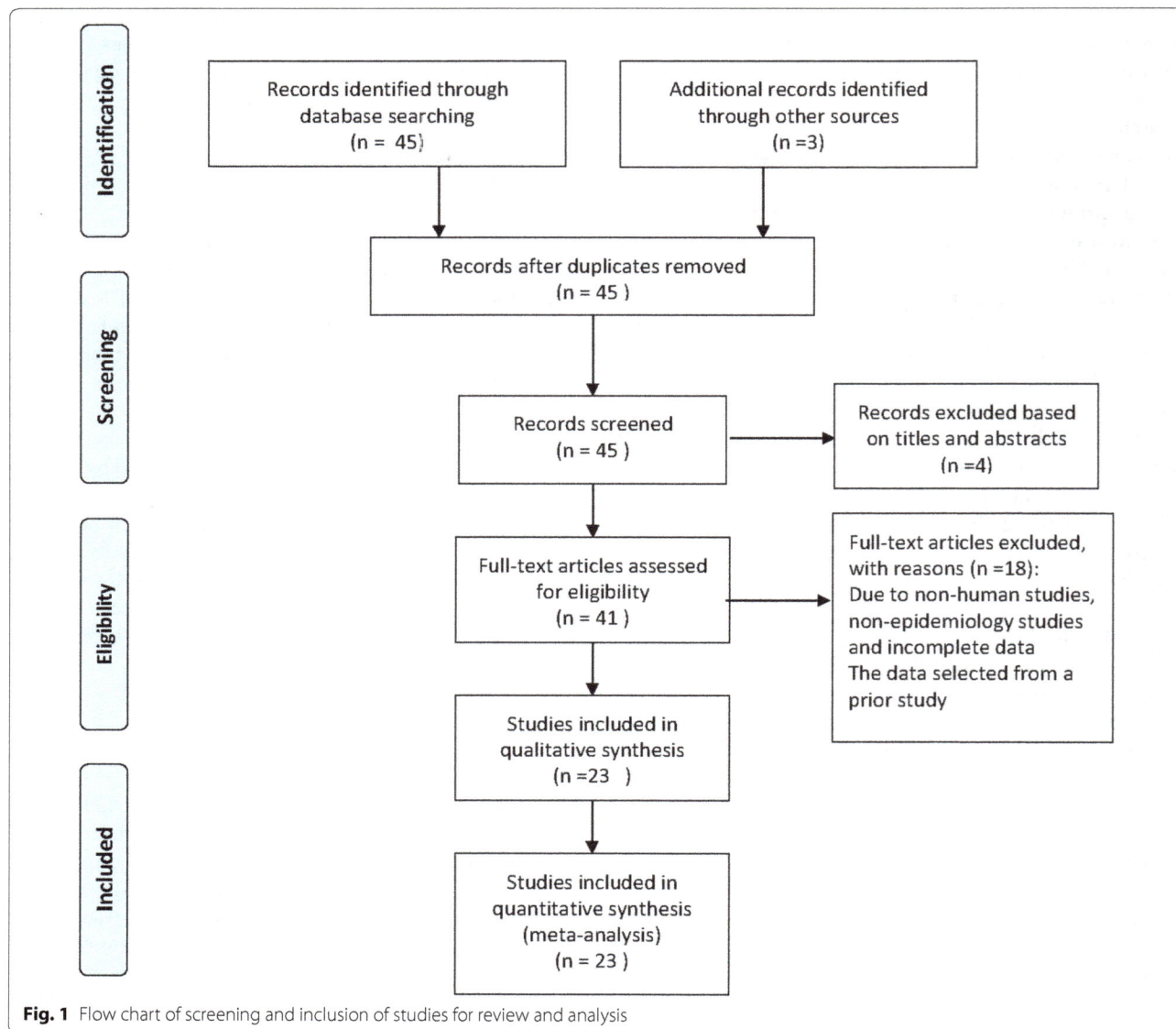

**Fig. 1** Flow chart of screening and inclusion of studies for review and analysis

population. For the purposes of meta-analysis, the different mite species were considered separately. Hence, these two studies contributed to two data points.

### Prevalence of spider mite sensitization

The reported studies included data based on extracts prepared from three spider mite species, i.e., *T. urticae*, *P. citri*, and *P. ulmi* (Table 1). A total of 15 papers reported the prevalence of sensitivity to *T. urticae*, which ranged from 4.3% (95% CI 3.9–4.8%) [22] to 78.3% (95% CI 66.3–90.2%) [34] and reached a global average of 27.0% (95% CI 20.5–33.5%). The heterogeneity found within the studies was high ($I^2 = 99.4\%$, $p < 0.001$, Fig. 2 and Table 2). Nine papers reported the prevalence of sensitivity to *P.*

*citri*, which ranged from 1.3% (95% CI 0.6–2%) [18] to 83.3% (95% CI 62.2–104.4%) [32], reaching a global average of 18.2% (95% CI 12.4–24.0%), and the heterogeneity found within the studies was high ($I^2 = 99.3\%$, $p < 0.001$, Fig. 2 and Table 2). Only one paper reported the prevalence of sensitivity to *P. ulmi*, which was 23.2% (95% CI 19.4–27.1%). The pooled prevalence estimates of spider mite sensitization to any species was 22.9% (95% CI 19–26.8%).

### Publication bias, sensitivity, and meta-regression analysis

Deeks' funnel plot (Fig. 3) was applied to assess publication bias. In Fig. 3, which shows the prevalence among the cases, the prevalence of the analyzed studies

## Table 1  The prevalence of spider mite allergy from included studies

| Study | Prevalence (%) [95% CI] | | | % Weight | Country | Sample Size |
|---|---|---|---|---|---|---|
| *Tetranychus urticae* | | | | | | |
| Astarita et al. [33] | 40.0 | 9.6 | 70.4 | 1.21 | Italy | 10[f,a] |
| Astarita et al. [34] | 78.3 | 66.3 | 90.2 | 3.30 | Italy | 46[f,a] |
| Astarita et al. [35] | 6.0 | 4.5 | 7.5 | 4.77 | Italy | 960[f,a] |
| Delgado et al. [31] | 66.7 | 47.8 | 85.5 | 2.24 | Spain | 24[f,a] |
| Jee et al. [29] | 32.0 | 19.1 | 44.9 | 3.12 | Korea | 50[npo] |
| Jeebhay et al. [28] | 22.1 | 16.2 | 28.0 | 4.32 | South Africa | 190[f,a] |
| Johansson et al. [27] | 25.8 | 10.4 | 41.2 | 2.72 | Sweden | 31[f,a] |
| Kim et al. [8] | 9.9 | 8.7 | 11.1 | 4.78 | Korea | 2467[r,u,a] |
| Kim et al. [22] | 4.3 | 3.9 | 4.8 | 4.80 | Korea | 8595[nao,u,c] |
| Kim et al. [25] | 16.6 | 13.2 | 19.9 | 4.63 | Korea | 465[f,nao,a] |
| Kim et al. [24] | 19.8 | 18.0 | 21.7 | 4.75 | Korea | 1806[u] |
| Kronqvist et al. [21] | 24.0 | 15.4 | 32.5 | 3.89 | Sweden | 96[f,a] |
| Lee et al. [20] | 28.0 | 26.9 | 29.0 | 4.78 | Korea | 7182[c,a] |
| Navarro et al. [16] | 25.3 | 19.8 | 30.8 | 4.38 | Spain | 241[f,a] |
| Seedat et al. [15] | 46.0 | 32.2 | 59.8 | 2.98 | South Africa | 50[u,r,c,a] |
| Sub-total | | | | | | |
| D+L pooled prevalence | 27.0 | 20.5 | 33.5 | 56.67 | | |
| I–V pooled prevalence | 8.7 | 8.4 | 9.1 | | | |
| *Panonychus citri* | | | | | | |
| Ashida et al. [32] | 83.3 | 62.2 | 104.4 | 1.98 | Japan | 12[f,a] |
| Kim et al. [26] | 21.8 | 19.8 | 23.8 | 4.74 | Korea | 1629[nco,c] |
| Kim et al. [22] | 15.6 | 14.8 | 16.4 | 4.79 | Korea | 8029[nco,c] |
| Kim et al. [23] | 14.3 | 13.5 | 15.2 | 4.79 | Korea | 6332[r,c] |
| Kim et al. [14] | 23.0 | 14.8 | 31.2 | 3.94 | Korea | 100[nco,c] |
| Kim et al. [9] | 16.6 | 11.2 | 22.0 | 4.39 | Korea | 181[f,a] |
| Lee et al. [19] | 14.2 | 12.1 | 16.3 | 4.73 | Korea | 1037[nco,c] |
| Lee et al. [18] | 1.3 | 0.60 | 2.00 | 4.79 | Korea | 1000[u,nco,c] |
| Min et al. [17] | 14.9 | 11.3 | 18.5 | 4.61 | Korea | 375[nco,c] |
| Sub-total | | | | | | |
| D+L pooled prevalence | 18.2 | 12.4 | 24.0 | 38.76 | | |
| I–V pooled prevalence | 10.3 | 9.9 | 10.8 | | | |
| *Panonychus ulmi* | | | | | | |
| Kim et al. [25] | 23.2 | 19.4 | 27.1 | 4.58 | Korea | 465[f,naf,a] |
| Sub-total | | | | | | |
| D+L pooled prevalence | 23.2 | 19.4 | 27.1 | 4.58 | | |
| I–V pooled prevalence | 23.2 | 19.4 | 27.1 | | | |
| *Overall* | | | | | | |
| D+L pooled prevalence | 22.9 | 19.0 | 26.8 | 100.00 | | |
| I–V pooled prevalence | 9.5 | 9.2 | 9.7 | | | |

Populations considered in these studies: f, farmers (either outdoor or greenhouse workers); naf, living near apple farms; nco, living near citrus orchards; npo, living near pear orchards; r, rural (unspecified adjacency to specific crop types); u, urban; c, children; a, adults

is presented on the x-axis and the standard error of each study is shown on the y-axis. Visual evaluation revealed that the plot was an asymmetric funnel shape, indicating that publication bias was likely present. Figure 4 shows the random effects estimate, with the line representing the calculated median of all samples (0.23) in the middle and lines representing the lower (0.19) and upper (0.27) 95% confidence values to the left and right, respectively. Each circle represents the new mean obtained when the indicated study is removed from the pool. These means all fell within the 95% confidence interval of the total data set, indicating that no

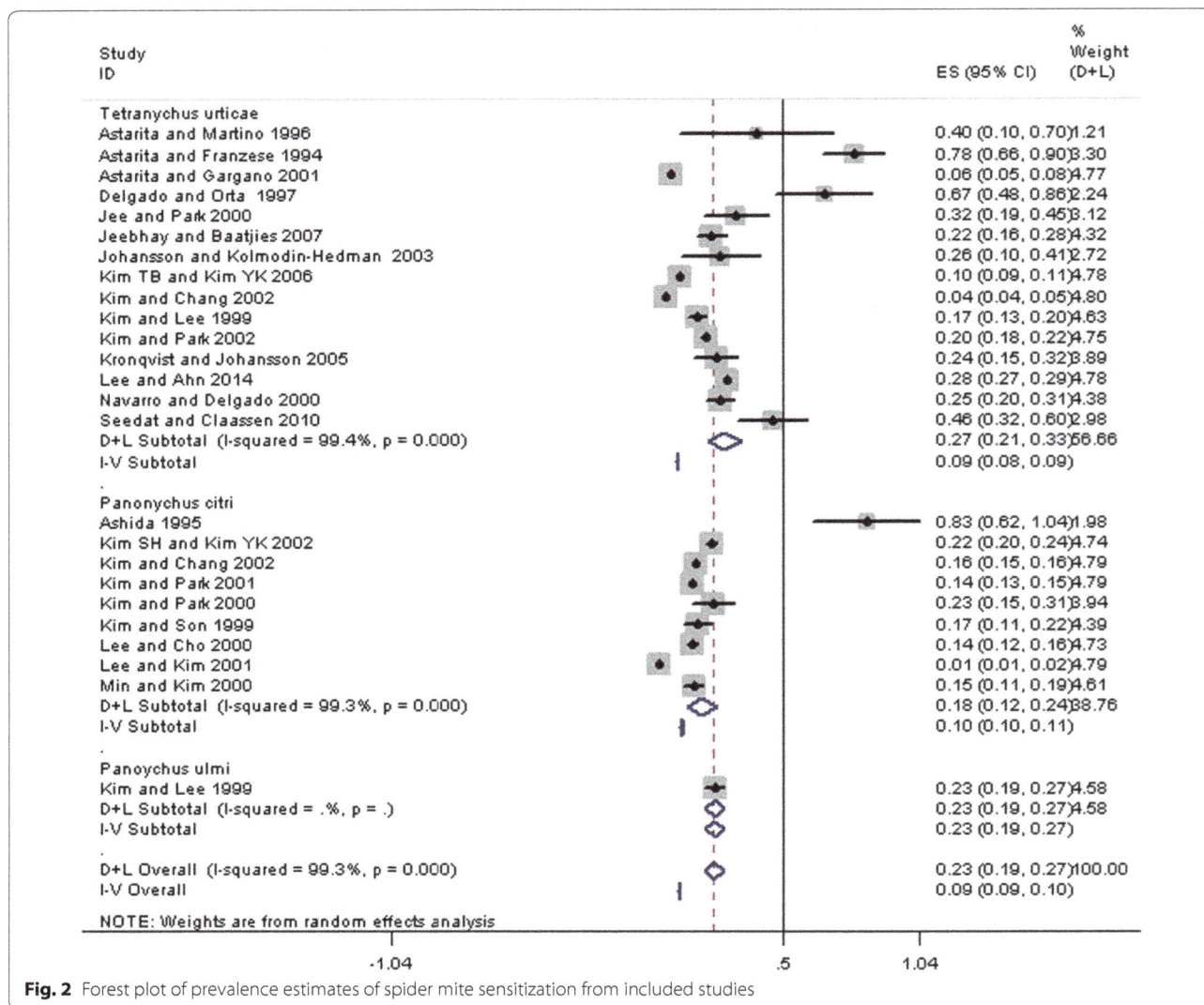

| Study ID | | ES (95% CI) | % Weight (D+L) |
|---|---|---|---|
| **Tetranychus urticae** | | | |
| Astarita and Martino 1996 | | 0.40 (0.10, 0.70) | 1.21 |
| Astarita and Franzese 1994 | | 0.78 (0.66, 0.90) | 3.30 |
| Astarita and Gargano 2001 | | 0.06 (0.05, 0.08) | 4.77 |
| Delgado and Orta 1997 | | 0.67 (0.48, 0.86) | 2.24 |
| Jee and Park 2000 | | 0.32 (0.19, 0.45) | 3.12 |
| Jeebhay and Baatjies 2007 | | 0.22 (0.16, 0.28) | 4.32 |
| Johansson and Kolmodin-Hedman 2003 | | 0.26 (0.10, 0.41) | 2.72 |
| Kim TB and Kim YK 2006 | | 0.10 (0.09, 0.11) | 4.78 |
| Kim and Chang 2002 | | 0.04 (0.04, 0.05) | 4.80 |
| Kim and Lee 1999 | | 0.17 (0.13, 0.20) | 4.63 |
| Kim and Park 2002 | | 0.20 (0.18, 0.22) | 4.75 |
| Kronqvist and Johansson 2005 | | 0.24 (0.15, 0.32) | 3.89 |
| Lee and Ahn 2014 | | 0.28 (0.27, 0.29) | 4.78 |
| Navarro and Delgado 2000 | | 0.25 (0.20, 0.31) | 4.38 |
| Seedat and Claassen 2010 | | 0.46 (0.32, 0.60) | 2.98 |
| D+L Subtotal (I-squared = 99.4%, p = 0.000) | | 0.27 (0.21, 0.33) | 56.66 |
| I-V Subtotal | | 0.09 (0.08, 0.09) | |
| | | | |
| **Panonychus citri** | | | |
| Ashida 1995 | | 0.83 (0.62, 1.04) | 1.98 |
| Kim SH and Kim YK 2002 | | 0.22 (0.20, 0.24) | 4.74 |
| Kim and Chang 2002 | | 0.16 (0.15, 0.16) | 4.79 |
| Kim and Park 2001 | | 0.14 (0.13, 0.15) | 4.79 |
| Kim and Park 2000 | | 0.23 (0.15, 0.31) | 3.94 |
| Kim and Son 1999 | | 0.17 (0.11, 0.22) | 4.39 |
| Lee and Cho 2000 | | 0.14 (0.12, 0.16) | 4.73 |
| Lee and Kim 2001 | | 0.01 (0.01, 0.02) | 4.79 |
| Min and Kim 2000 | | 0.15 (0.11, 0.19) | 4.61 |
| D+L Subtotal (I-squared = 99.3%, p = 0.000) | | 0.18 (0.12, 0.24) | 38.76 |
| I-V Subtotal | | 0.10 (0.10, 0.11) | |
| | | | |
| **Panoychus ulmi** | | | |
| Kim and Lee 1999 | | 0.23 (0.19, 0.27) | 4.58 |
| D+L Subtotal (I-squared = .%, p = .) | | 0.23 (0.19, 0.27) | 4.58 |
| I-V Subtotal | | 0.23 (0.19, 0.27) | |
| | | | |
| D+L Overall (I-squared = 99.3%, p = 0.000) | | 0.23 (0.19, 0.27) | 100.00 |
| I-V Overall | | 0.09 (0.09, 0.10) | |

NOTE: Weights are from random effects analysis

-1.04                    .5          1.04

**Fig. 2** Forest plot of prevalence estimates of spider mite sensitization from included studies

## Table 2 Heterogeneity analysis of the involved studies

| | Heterogeneity statistic | Degrees of freedom | p | I-squared** (%) | Tau-squared |
|---|---|---|---|---|---|
| *Tetranychus urticae* | 2177.04 | 14 | <0.001 | 99.4 | 0.0137 |
| *Panonychus citri* | 1092.73 | 8 | <0.001 | 99.3 | 0.0070 |
| *Panonychus ulmi* | 0.00 | 0 | | | 0.0000 |
| Overall | 3351.78 | 24 | <0.001 | 99.3 | 0.0081 |

Significance test(s) of prevalence = 0

*Tetranychus urticae* z = 8.20, p < 0.001

*Panonychus citri* z = 6.14, p < 0.001

individual study had a disproportionate effect on the mean.

As displayed by the forest plot in Fig. 2 and in Table 2, the heterogeneity was significant for *T. urticae* ($I^2 = 99.4\%$) and *P. citri* ($I^2 = 99.3\%$). One possible source

of heterogeneity was the study population. Eight studies [15, 20, 24, 29, 31–34] enrolled only symptomatic patients (i.e., patients with airway allergy symptoms including asthma and rhinitis or patients with dermatitis) whereas the remaining studies enrolled a mixture of

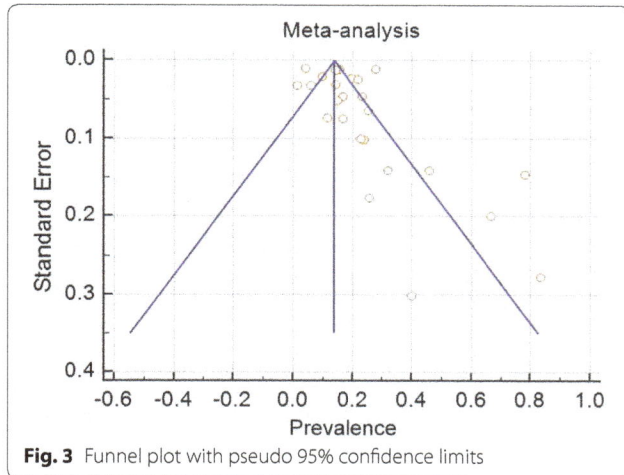

**Fig. 3** Funnel plot with pseudo 95% confidence limits

symptomatic and asymptomatic patients. If all symptom-only studies are removed from the sensitivity analysis, the estimated prevalence dropped to 15.43% outside the 95% confidence interval for the total data set (data not shown). From this, we conclude that these studies inflated the mean. However, it is difficult to conclude whether this is due to the patient populations or some

other factor. The symptomatic studies typically enrolled fewer patients, so study size might have had an influence. Additionally, when subgroup analysis was performed, the heterogeneity of both the symptomatic and mixed studies was still extremely high (Table 3), indicating that patient populations alone did not contribute much to the overall heterogeneity of the included studies. To examine other sources of heterogeneity, a meta-regression analysis considering the publication year, country, number of study subjects, methods, and mite species analysis was performed, and the results showed that no single analyzed factor could account for the large variability in the reported prevalences. It is likely that a combination of factors makes these studies extremely diverse.

**Monosensitization to spider mites**
Of the 15 papers reporting the prevalence of sensitivity to *T. urticae* (Table 4), 9 also reported monosensitization rates ranging from 1% (95% CI 0–1%) to 74% (95% CI 61–87%) and reaching a global average of 7% (95% CI 5–10%). The heterogeneity found within the studies was high ($I^2 = 97.7\%$, p < 0.001). Three papers reported the prevalence of monosensitization to *P. citri*, which was 2% (95% CI 1–3%), 9% (95% CI 7–10%), and 10% (95% CI 6–14%), reaching a global average of 7% (95% CI

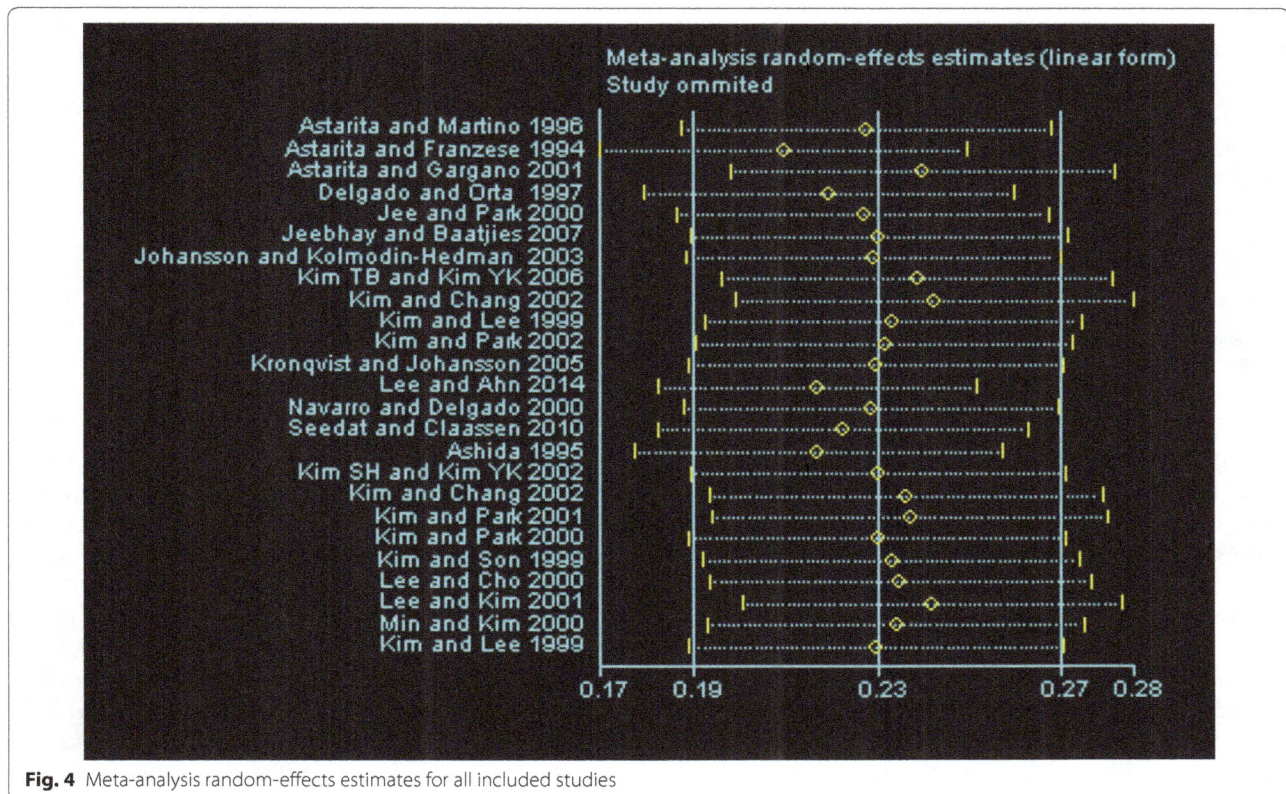

**Fig. 4** Meta-analysis random-effects estimates for all included studies

**Table 3  Effect of population on prevalence of spider mite sensitivity**

|  | N | Number of studies | Prevalence (%) | 95% CI | Heterogeneity statistic (Q) | Degrees of freedom | $I^2$ (%) |
|---|---|---|---|---|---|---|---|
| *All studies* | | | | | | | |
| Overall | 40,908 | 25 | 23.0 | 19.0–27.0 | 2242.56 | 24 | 98.8 |
| *Patient population* | | | | | | | |
| Symptomatic | 9180 | 8 | 44.0 | 35.0–53.0 | 151 | 7 | 95.4 |
| Mixed | 31,728 | 17 | 15.0 | 12.0–20.0 | 1354 | 16 | 98.82 |

**Table 4  Studies reporting monosensitization**

| Study | Monosensitized prevalence (%) [95% CI] | | | % Weight | Country | Sample size |
|---|---|---|---|---|---|---|
| *Tetranychus urticae* | | | | | | |
| Astarita et al. [34] | 74.0 | 61.0 | 87.0 | 2.26 | Italy | 46[f,a] |
| Astarita et al. [35] | 2.1 | 1.0 | 3.0 | 10.23 | Italy | 960[f,a] |
| Jee et al. [29] | 2.0 | − 2.0 | 6.0 | 7.79 | Korea | 50[npo] |
| Jeebhay et al. [28] | 6.0 | 2.0 | 9.0 | 8.35 | South Africa | 190[f,a] |
| Kim et al. [25] | 8.6 | 6.0 | 11.0 | 9.10 | Korea | 465[f,nao,a] |
| Kim et al. [24] | 0.7 | 0.0 | 1.0 | 10.39 | Korea | 1806[u] |
| Kronqvist et al. [21] | 11.0 | 5.0 | 18.0 | 5.45 | Sweden | 96[f,a] |
| Lee et al. [20] | 5.0 | 5.0 | 6.0 | 10.36 | Korea | 7182[c,a] |
| Navarro et al. [16] | 7.0 | 3.0 | 10.0 | 8.53 | Spain | 241[f,a] |
| Sub-total | | | | | | |
|   D + L pooled prevalence | 7.0 | 5.0 | 10.0 | 72.6 | | 11,036 |
|   I–V pooled prevalence | 2.0 | 2.0 | 3.0 | | | |
| *Panonychus citri* | | | | | | |
| Kim et al. [8] | 8.8 | 7.0 | 10.0 | 10.00 | Korea | 1629[nco,c] |
| Kim et al. [9] | 9.9 | 6.0 | 14.0 | 7.31 | Korea | 181[f,a] |
| Lee et al. [19] | 2.2 | 1.0 | 3.0 | 10.24 | Korea | 1037[nco,c] |
| Sub-total | | | | | | |
|   D + L pooled prevalence | 7.0 | 1.0 | 12.0 | 27.54 | | 2847 |
|   I–V pooled prevalence | 4.0 | 4.0 | 5.0 | | | |
| *Overall* | | | | | | |
| D + L pooled prevalence | 7.0 | 5.0 | 9.0 | 100 | | 13,883 |
| I–V pooled prevalence | 3.0 | 2.0 | 3.0 | | | |

Populations considered in these studies: f, farmers (either outdoor or greenhouse workers); naf, living near apple farms; nco, living near citrus orchards; npo, living near pear orchards; r, rural (unspecified adjacency to specific crop types); u, urban; c, children; a, adults

1–12.0%), and the heterogeneity within the studies was high ($I^2 = 97.1\%$, p < 0.001). The pooled prevalence estimate of monosensitization to spider mite sensitization was 7% (95% CI 5–9%) (Fig. 5).

## Discussion

This review provides the first comprehensive search and synthesis of the international literature on the prevalence of spider mite sensitization. The result of our synthesis of all prevalence estimates was 22.9% (95% CI 19.0–26.8%) but may be higher when only symptomatic patients are considered [43.9% (95% CI 35.1–52.9%)]. Our pooled estimate indicates that spider mite sensitivity is moderately common in farming populations. Mite subgroup prevalence estimates were 27% (95% CI 20.5–33.5%) for *T. urticae* sensitivity and 18.2% (95% CI 12.4–24.0%) for *P. citri* sensitivity. Only one paper reported the prevalence of *P. ulmi* sensitivity. Therefore, agricultural workers dealing with fruit trees or working in greenhouses as well as in the surrounding rural population are at risk for developing sensitivity to *T. urticae* and *P. citri*. Further studies are needed to confirm the prevalence of *P. ulmi*

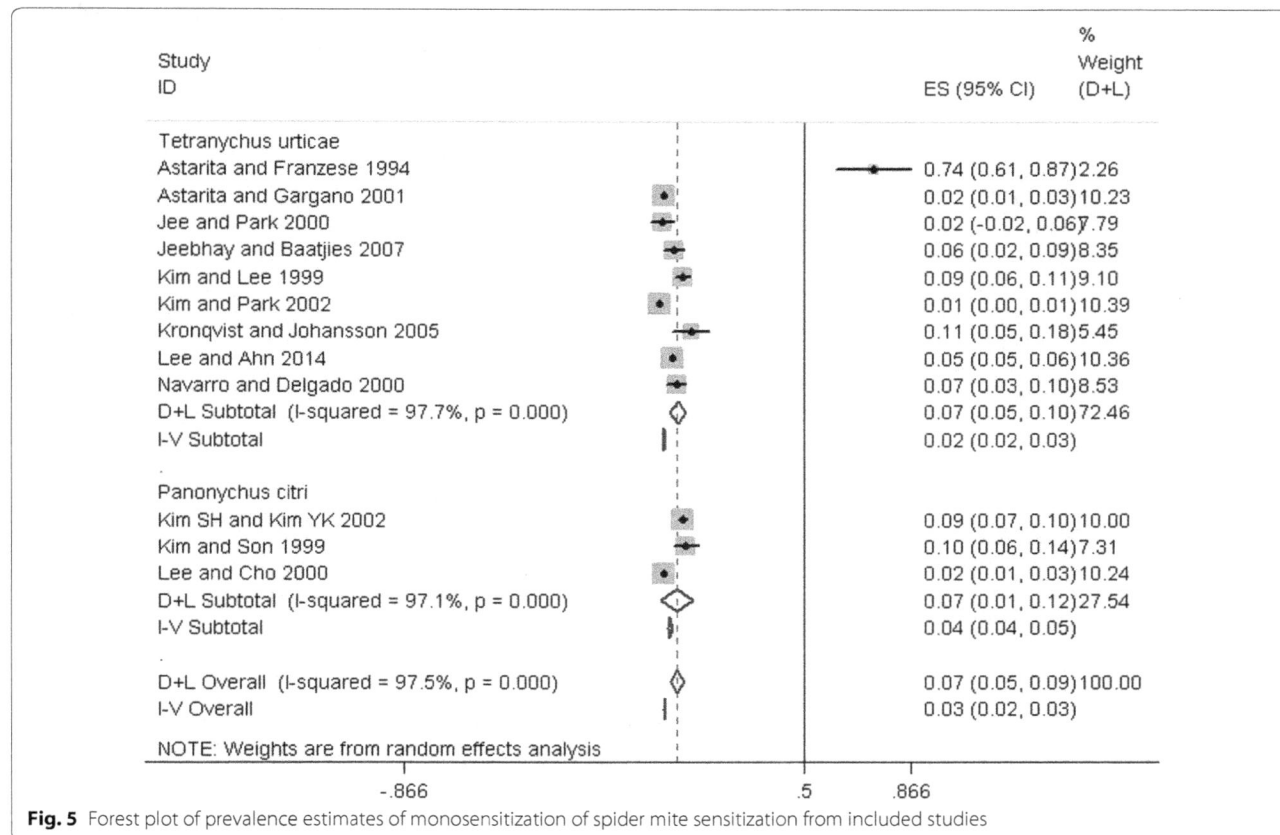

**Fig. 5** Forest plot of prevalence estimates of monosensitization of spider mite sensitization from included studies

sensitivity and to examine if sensitivity to spider mites is a cause of occupational allergies and/or general allergies in rural populations.

The overall sensitivity estimates include patients reactive to spider mite species who may also be sensitized to other environmental allergens. For such polysensitized individuals, a positive skin reaction to spider mites could indicate a primary allergic response or cross-reactivity. To address this, some studies reported the rates of monosensitization (defined as reactivity to spider mites but no other tested allergen). Our pooled prevalence estimate for monosensitization to spider mites was 7% (95% CI 5–9.0%), and subgroup prevalence estimates were 7% (95% CI 5–10%) for *T. urticae* sensitivity and 7% (95% CI 1–12.0%) for *P. citri* sensitivity. This indicates that spider mites are the primary sensitizing agent for a moderate number of individuals living primarily in rural settings. Jee et al. used competitive ELISAs and found that *D. pteronyssinus* extracts could not compete with IgE binding to *T. urticae* proteins in serum from a mono-sensitized patient but could compete in serum from polysensitized patients. Unfortunately, little progress has been made in identifying spider mite-specific antigens. Studies have used SDS-PAGE and IgE-immunoblotting to identify 20

[31], 24 [27] and 10 [36] IgE-reactive bands in spider mite extracts, but which of these components are species specific has yet to be determined. Additionally, it should be noted that patients sensitized to other allergens (including domestic mites and/or non-taxonomically related species) are more likely to also be reactive to spider mites [9, 16, 19, 25, 35]. This generalized atopy is known to be true for a variety of high molecular weight allergens and is believed to indicate a hyper-reactive IgE response in certain sensitive patients [37].

The authors believe that the searches conducted were comprehensive and the sensitivity analysis demonstrates that the calculated mean was not unduly influenced by a single study, and thus our findings are generally robust. However, publication bias is present based on the asymmetric funnel plot, and the heterogeneity of the studies was quite large. The heterogeneity observed could come from the different study settings and populations. The estimated prevalence of spider mite sensitization in symptomatic patients was 43.9% (95% CI 35.1–52.9%) which was 2.9 times higher than that found in mixed populations [15.4% (95% CI 11.6–19.7%)]. Heterogeneity was, however, still very high within the subgroups, hence these results should be interpreted cautiously.

Some studies reporting data from mixed populations did detect an association between spider mite reactivity and symptoms, but others did not. For example, using patient subgroup information published by Kim and Son et al. [9] revealed that, in this study, the prevalence of spider mite allergies in symptomatic patients was 4 times higher than that in asymptomatic patients. However, in Lee et al. [19], prevalence estimates were similar in symptomatic and non-symptomatic patients. Of note, several studies tested the onset of symptoms in response to a *T. urticae* challenge. Astarita et al. [34] examined the onset of allergic symptoms and tracked the peak expiratory flow rate in spider mite-sensitive patients exposed to an infested green-house environment, and two studies [29, 31] performed a bronchial challenge with *T. urticae* extracts and observed responses in the majority of *T. urticae*-sensitive patients. This indicates that spider mite sensitivity has clinical relevance, but this may vary based on the location and population being considered.

We investigated other possible sources of heterogeneity with meta-regression analyses but could not identify a single factor responsible for the variation. Two factors that may be relevant based on individual studies are patient age and site of residence. Kim et al. [8] reported that the sensitization rate to *T. urticae* increased with age, and Kim et al. [22] reported that the prevalence of spider mite allergies in rural areas was higher than the prevalence in urban settings. In regards to age, few studies of *T. urticae* sensitivity included children (Table 1), whereas the majority of the *P. citri* studies only enrolled children. This could account for the lower prevalence of sensitivity in the *P. citri* studies, or it could indicate that *P. citri* is a weaker sensitizing agent.

## Conclusions

In brief, spider mites are important sensitizing agents particularly in farming populations where contact is the most likely. In some of the reviewed studies, the prevalence of spider mite sensitivity was reported to be higher in patients with allergic symptoms (particularly occupational allergies), and thus exposure may correlate with disease. The moderate prevalence of spider mite monosensitization indicates that these organisms produce unique allergens, and thus specific diagnostic tests and treatment regimens for spider mite sensitization are likely warranted. These conclusions should, however, be interpreted cautiously. Publication bias was present, the heterogeneity of the analyzed studies was extremely high, and the sources contributing to this heterogeneity were unclear. Additional cross-sectional studies using more standardized protocols are needed to assess how specific patient characteristics influence

the acquisition of spider mite sensitization and whether and how this progresses to allergic disease.

### Authors' contributions
This paper was drafted by YZ, and search strategy was developed by YC and JQ. The meta analyses were conducted by YZ, HJ, XZ and JZ. It was initially revised following critical review by YC and then by JQ. All authors read and approved the final manuscript.

### Author details
[1] Department of Pediatrics Laboratory, Wuxi Children's Hospital, Wuxi 214023, People's Republic of China. [2] Department of Clinical Laboratory, Wuxi People's Hospital Affiliated to Nanjing Medical University, No. 299 at Qingyang Road, Wuxi 214023, Jiangsu Province, People's Republic of China. [3] Department of Pediatrics, Wuxi Children's Hospital, Wuxi 214023, People's Republic of China.

### Acknowledgements
We acknowledge the freelance editor Kathleen Molyneaux for content and English language editing.

### Competing interests
The authors declare that they have no competing interests.

### Funding
This work was supported by Medical Innovation Team of Jiangsu Province (Grant No. CXTDB2017016) and the National Natural Sciences Foundation of China (NSFC31272369).

### References
1. Voorhorst R, Spieksma FTM, Varekamp H, Leupen MJ, Lyklema AW. The house-dust mite (*Dermatophagoides pteronyssinus*) and the allergens it produces. Identity with the house-dust allergen. J Allergy. 1967;39(6):325–39.
2. Fernández-Caldas E, Puerta L, Caraballo L. Mites and allergy. Chem Immunol Allergy. 2014;100(100):234.
3. Thomas WR. House dust mite allergens: new discoveries and relevance to the allergic patient. Curr Allergy Asthma Rep. 2016;16(9):69.
4. Caraballo L. Mite allergens. Expert Rev Clin Immunol. 2017;13(4):297–9.
5. Calderón MA, Kleine-Tebbe J, Linneberg A, De BF, Hernandez FRD, Virchow JC, Demoly P. House dust mite respiratory allergy: an overview of current therapeutic strategies. J Allergy Clin Immunol Pract. 2015;3(6):843–55.
6. Appel HM, Kunick F, Hoffmann TK, Greve J. Sensitization against domestic mites when perennial nasal symptoms are present. Allergologie. 2016;39:298–301.
7. Manson DCM, Gerson U. Web spinning, wax secretion and liquid secretion by eriophyoid mites. In: Lindquist EE, Sabelis MW, Bruin J, editors. World crop pests, vol. 6. Amsterdam: Elsevier; 1996. p. 251–8.
8. Kim TB, Kim YK, Chang YS, Kim SH, Hong SC, Jee YK, Cho SH, Min KU, Kim YY. Association between sensitization to outdoor spider mites and clinical manifestations of asthma and rhinitis in the general population

of adults. J Korean Med Sci. 2006;21(2):247–52. https://doi.org/10.3346/jkms.2006.21.2.247.

9. Kim YK, Son JW, Kim HY, Park HS, Lee MH, Cho SH, Min KU, Kim YY. Citrus red mite (Panonychus citri) is the most common sensitizing allergen of asthma and rhinitis in citrus farmers. Clin Exp Allergy. 1999;29(8):1102–9.

10. Moher D, Liberati A, Tetzlaff J, Altman DG, PRISMA Group. Preferred reporting items for systematic reviews and meta-analyses: the PRISMA statement. PLoS Med. 2009;6(7):e1000097. https://doi.org/10.1371/journal.pmed.1000097.

11. Higgins JP, Thompson SG, Deeks JJ, Altman DG. Measuring inconsistency in meta-analyses. BMJ. 2003;327(7414):557–60.

12. Devillé WL, Buntinx F, Bouter LM, Montori VM, de Vet HC, Da VDW, Bezemer PD. Conducting systematic reviews of diagnostic studies: didactic guidelines. BMC Med Res Methodol. 2002;2(1):9.

13. Deeks JJ, Macaskill P, Irwig L. The performance of tests of publication bias and other sample size effects in systematic reviews of diagnostic test accuracy was assessed. J Clin Epidemiol. 2005;58(9):882–93.

14. Kim YK, Park HW, Park HS, Kim HY, Kim SH, Bai JM, Cho SH, Kim YY, Min KU. Sensitivity to citrus red mite and the development of asthma. Ann Allergy Asthma Immunol. 2000;85(6 Pt 1):483–8. https://doi.org/10.1016/S1081-1206(10)62576-8.

15. Seedat RY, Claassen J, Claassen AJ, Joubert G. Mite and cockroach sensitisation in patients with allergic rhinitis in the Free State. S Afr Med J. 2010;100(3):160–3.

16. Navarro AM, Delgado J, Sanchez MC, Orta JC, Martinez A, Palacios R, Martinez J, Conde J. Prevalence of sensitization to Tetranychus urticae in greenhouse workers. Clin Exp Allergy. 2000;30(6):863–6.

17. Min KU, Kim YK, Park HS, Lee MH, Lee BJ, Son JW, Kim YY, Cho SH. Bronchial responsiveness to methacholine is increased in citrus red mite (Panonychus citri)-sensitive children without asthmatic symptoms. Clin Exp Allergy. 2000;30(8):1129–34.

18. Lee MH, Kim YK, Min KU, Lee BJ, Bahn JW, Son JW, Cho SH, Park HS, Koh YY, Kim YY. Differences in sensitization rates to outdoor aeroallergens, especially citrus red mite (Panonychus citri), between urban and rural children. Ann Allergy Asthma Immunol. 2001;86(6):691–5. https://doi.org/10.1016/S1081-1206(10)62300-9.

19. Lee MH, Cho SH, Park HS, Bahn JW, Lee BJ, Son JW, Kim YK, Koh YY, Min KU, Kim YY. Citrus red mite (Panonychus citri) is a common sensitizing allergen among children living around citrus orchards. Ann Allergy Asthma Immunol. 2000;85(3):200–4. https://doi.org/10.1016/S1081-1206(10)62467-2.

20. Lee JE, Ahn JC, Han DH, Kim DY, Kim JW, Cho SH, Park HW, Rhee CS. Variability of offending allergens of allergic rhinitis according to age: optimization of skin prick test allergens. Allergy Asthma Immunol Res. 2014;6(1):47–54. https://doi.org/10.4168/aair.2014.6.1.47.

21. Kronqvist M, Johansson E, Kolmodin-Hedman B, Oman H, Svartengren M, van Hage-Hamsten M. IgE-sensitization to predatory mites and respiratory symptoms in Swedish greenhouse workers. Allergy. 2005;60(4):521–6. https://doi.org/10.1111/j.1398-9995.2004.00687.x.

22. Kim YK, Chang YS, Lee MH, Hong SC, Bae JM, Jee YK, Chun BR, Cho SH, Min KU, Kim YY. Role of environmental exposure to spider mites in the sensitization and the clinical manifestation of asthma and rhinitis in children and adolescents living in rural and urban areas. Clin Exp Allergy. 2002;32(9):1305–9.

23. Kim YK, Park HS, Kim HY, Jee YK, Son JW, Bae JM, Lee MH, Cho SH, Min KU, Kim YY. Citrus red mite (Panonychus citri) may be an important allergen in the development of asthma among exposed children. Clin Exp Allergy. 2001;31(4):582–9.

24. Kim YK, Park HS, Kim HA, Lee MH, Choi JH, Kim SS, Lee SK, Nahm DH, Cho SH, Min KU, Kim YY. Two-spotted spider mite allergy: immunoglobulin E sensitization and characterization of allergenic components. Ann Allergy Asthma Immunol. 2002;89(5):517–22. https://doi.org/10.1016/S1081-1206(10)62091-1.

25. Kim YK, Lee MH, Jee YK, Hong SC, Bae JM, Chang YS, Jung JW, Lee BJ, Son JW, Cho SH. Spider mite allergy in apple-cultivating farmers: European red mite (Panonychus ulmi) and two-spotted spider mite (Tetranychus urticae) may be important allergens in the development of work-related asthma and rhinitis symptoms. J Allergy Clin Immunol. 1999;104(6):1285.

26. Kim SH, Kim YK, Lee MH, Hong SC, Bae JM, Min KU, Kim YY, Cho SH. Relationship between sensitization to citrus red mite (Panonychus citri) and the prevalence of atopic diseases in adolescents living near citrus orchards. Clin Exp Allergy. 2002;32(7):1054–8.

27. Johansson E, Kolmodin-Hedman B, Kallstrom E, Kaiser L, van Hage-Hamsten M. IgE-mediated sensitization to predatory mites in Swedish greenhouse workers. Allergy. 2003;58(4):337–41.

28. Jeebhay MF, Baatjies R, Chang YS, Kim YK, Kim YY, Major V, Lopata AL. Risk factors for allergy due to the two-spotted spider mite (Tetranychus urticae) among table grape farm workers. Int Arch Allergy Immunol. 2007;144(2):143–9. https://doi.org/10.1159/000103226.

29. Jee YK, Park HS, Kim HY, Park JS, Lee KY, Kim KY, Kim YK, Cho SH, Min KU, Kim YY. Two-spotted spider mite (Tetranychus urticae): an important allergen in asthmatic non-farmers symtomatic in summer and fall months. Ann Allergy Asthma Immunol. 2000;84(5):543–8.

30. Gargano D, Romano C, Manguso F, Cutajar M, Altucci P, Astarita C. Relationship between total and allergen-specific IgE serum levels and presence of symptoms in farm workers sensitized to Tetranychus urticae. Allergy. 2002;57(11):1044–7.

31. Delgado J, Orta JC, Navarro AM, Conde J, Martinez A, Martinez J, Palacios R. Occupational allergy in greenhouse workers: sensitization to Tetranychus urticae. Clin Exp Allergy. 1997;27(6):640–5.

32. Ashida T, Ide T, Tabata S, Kunimatsu M, Etoh Y, Yoshikawa T, Matsunaga T. IgE-mediated allergy to spider mite, Panonychus citri in occupationally exposed individuals. Arerugi. 1995;44(11):1290–6.

33. Astarita C, Di Martino P, Scala G, Franzese A, Sproviero S. Contact allergy: another occupational risk to Tetranychus urticae. J Allergy Clin Immunol. 1996;98(4):732–8.

34. Astarita C, Franzese A, Scala G, Sproviero S, Raucci G. Farm workers' occupational allergy to Tetranychus urticae: clinical and immunologic aspects. Allergy. 1994;49(6):466–71.

35. Astarita C, Gargano D, Manguso F, Romano C, Montanaro D, Pezzuto F, Bonini S, Altucci P, Abbate G. Epidemiology of allergic occupational diseases induced by Tetranychus urticae in greenhouse and open-field farmers living in a temperate climate area. Allergy. 2001;56(12):1157–63.

36. Kim YK, Oh SY, Jung JW, Min KU, Kim YY, Cho SH. IgE binding components in Tetranychus urticae and Panonychus ulmi-derived crude extracts and their cross-reactivity with domestic mites. Clin Exp Allergy. 2001;31(9):1457–63.

37. Osterman K, Zetterstrom O, Johansson SG. Coffee worker's allergy. Allergy. 1982;37(5):313–22.

# 18

# Visual analogue scale for sino-nasal symptoms severity correlates with sino-nasal outcome test 22: paving the way for a simple outcome tool of CRS burden

Maria Doulaptsi[1,2]* ⬥, Emmanuel Prokopakis[2], Sven Seys[1], Benoit Pugin[1], Brecht Steelant[1] and Peter Hellings[1,3]

**Abstract**

**Background:** A visual analogue scale (VAS) is a psychometric instrument widely used in the Rhinology field to subjectively quantify patient's symptoms severity. In allergic rhinitis, VAS has been found to correlate well with the allergic rhinitis and its impact on asthma severity classification, as well as with rhinoconjunctivitis quality of life questionnaire. In chronic rhinosinusitis (CRS), total VAS score are often used to classify disease burden into mild, moderate, and severe, with few studies correlating VAS scores with more complex and validated instruments assessing disease-specific burden like Sino-Nasal Outcome Test (SNOT)-22.

**Methods:** We correlated VAS scores for total and individual sino-nasal symptom with SNOT-22 scores in a randomly selected group of 180 CRS patients. Pearson's rho was selected as a correlation coefficient for analysis.

**Results:** VAS scores for total nasal symptom score and individual symptoms correlated significantly with SNOT-22, irrespective of VAS based subclasses for sino-nasal, ocular, and bronchial symptoms.

**Conclusions:** VAS for total sino-nasal symptom severity might be used for assessing disease severity, monitoring the course of the disease, and can be used for treatment decisions and disease burden.

**Keywords:** Chronic rhinosinusitis, Patient reported outcome measures, Quality of life, SNOT-22, VAS

## Background

Chronic rhinosinusitis (CRS), with or without nasal polyps, is defined as an inflammation of nose and paranasal sinuses lasting for at least 12 weeks [1]. It is characterized by two or more symptoms, one of which should be either nasal blockage/obstruction or nasal secretions (anterior/posterior nasal drip). Other symptoms might be facial pain/pressure and hyposmia/anosmia. The prevalence of CRS in the European adult population is estimated by GA(2)LEN study to be around 11.9%, while in the USA it is considered even higher [2, 3]. The burden of disease and the impact on patients' every day activity, work

productivity, and overall Quality of Life (QoL) cannot be underestimated, especially in difficult-to-treat cases [4]. The direct cost of CRS in the United States is estimated at $8.6 billion/year, while societal indirect costs from productivity loss are approximately $10,077 per patient each year [5]. Interestingly, general health of CRS patients was worse compared to patients with congestive heart failure, Chronic Obstructive Pulmonary Disease (COPD), and Parkinson disease, using generic health-state utility scores [6].

To accurately assess the burden of disease in CRS patients, multiple disease-specific QoL questionnaires were designed and validated over the past years [7–10]. These questionnaires focus on symptoms and how they affect patients' daily life, emotional condition, and overall QoL. These instruments are designed to have a strong association with principal disease characteristics and the

*Correspondence: mdoulaptsi@gmail.com
[1] Laboratory of Clinical Immunology, Department of Microbiology and Immunology, KU Leuven, Kapucijnenvoer 33, 3000 Louvain, Belgium
Full list of author information is available at the end of the article

ability to reflect response to treatment. Among different disease-specific outcome measurements in CRS, the Sino-Nasal Outcome Test (SNOT)-22 is widely accepted and has been used in several studies even before its validation by Hopkins et al., in 2009. SNOT-22 is a reliable questionnaire, can be used to facilitate clinical practice, and validated in multiple languages [8].

Visual analogue scale (VAS) is a psychometric measurement instrument widely used in the Rhinology field and beyond to subjectively quantify patients' symptoms severity. Originally designed to evaluate workers productivity by senior personnel, VAS gained more attention in the sixties in medicine, social science, and market research [11]. It represents a horizontal line of 10 cm with word anchors at each end representing the extreme feelings. Patients are instructed to indicate the point on the line that best corresponds to their status for the particular characteristic being evaluated. In addition to its high sensitivity, reliability and reproducibility, VAS is easy and simple to use by patients and health care providers [11]. It also does not require training, making VAS a highly valuable tool not only for everyday clinical practice, but also for real-life studies [11].

In allergic disease, VAS was found to correlate well with the Allergic Rhinitis and its Impact on Asthma (ARIA) severity classification system and QoL measurement instruments such as Rhinoconjunctivitis Quality of Life Questionnaire (RQLQ) [12]. Additionally, VAS is utilized to monitor the course of the disease, to assess treatment outcomes, to obtain self-assessments, and to define the level of control in allergic patients by MACVIA-ARIA project [13]. Lately, VAS has been incorporated into the MASK Allergy Diary mobile app, a clinical decision support system assessing allergic rhinitis (AR) severity for feedback to the patient and the doctor on level of disease control [14].

In CRS, VAS for total nasal symptom score (TNSS) is part of routine clinical practice to classify disease as mild, moderate, and severe. In research, VAS for TNSS and individual symptoms are frequently incorporated into studies as an instrument for estimating symptoms severity and burden of disease [15]. In contrast to allergy, correlations between VAS scores with more complex instruments assessing disease-specific burden like SNOT-22 in CRS are scarce [16, 17]. Toma and Hopkins, demonstrated a strong correlation between VAS and SNOT-22 in 65 CRS patients and they further attempted to stratify SNOT-22 score based on disease severity [17]. Here, we aim to study VAS scores for TNSS and individual sino-nasal symptoms in relation to SNOT-22 scores in a larger randomly selected group of CRS patients. In addition, correlation between VAS and SNOT-22 scores is explored in different CRS phenotypes (with/without nasal polyps, controlled/partly controlled/uncontrolled disease).

## Methods

### Study population

A postal questionnaire survey was conducted at the Department of Otorhinolaryngology, Head and Neck Surgery of the University Hospitals of Leuven in Belgium. Subjects who visited the outpatient clinic and coded as CRS between January and May of 2016 were isolated from the clinical workstation. Evaluation of full medical records was performed by an ENT specialist to confirm the coded diagnosis based on EPOS defining criteria for CRS (symptoms, compatible endoscopic findings and/or computed tomography abnormalities when imaging was available). Patients younger than 16 years, those with primary immunodeficiency, ciliary dyskinesia, cystic fibrosis, malignant tumors, and/or surgery for CRS within 6 months were excluded from the study. Patients with a diagnosis of psychiatric disorder were also excluded from the study as their ability to give reliable information regarding their nasal disease could be disputed. Concomitant AR or bronchial asthma was not considered to be a limitation for participation in the study.

After evaluation, a questionnaire was sent to 325 consecutive subjects who met the above criteria. Patients received a postal questionnaire together with the study rationale, and an informed consent. Patients were asked to fill out the questionnaire after signing the informed consent and return all forms by post. In order to reach a response rate of 60%, some of the non-responders to our questionnaire were contacted by phone to communicate the importance of the study and encourage them to participate. This study has been approved by the institutional Medical Ethics Committee.

### Questionnaires

Subjects were asked to give information about their nasal disease, current and past medication for CRS, medical and surgical history, and to provide answers in general items such as profession and smoking habits. In another part of the questionnaire, patients had to give information regarding their allergic status, and their current medication for this condition. The same was asked in case of asthma comorbidity.

A special part of the questionnaire was dedicated to assessing patients' QoL and severity of symptoms by using the SNOT-22 questionnaire and VAS scores. Patients had to draw a vertical line on a 10 cm scale from 0 to 10, according to "how bothersome your total nasal-sinus symptoms were within the last month" (see Additional file 1). Zero represented "not at all" and 10 represented "more than I can imagine" for TNSS. The same was asked for individual symptoms such as nasal blockage, headache/pain on the face, loss of smell, postnasal drip, runny nose, itchy nose, sneezing, itchy eyes, tearing, cough, tightness on the chest, shortness of breath and wheezing.

Level of control was assessed by using the following cut-off points for TNSS: well controlled (VAS $\leq 2$), partly controlled (VAS $> 2$ and $\leq 5$), uncontrolled (VAS $> 5$). In order to exclude a possible responder bias from the written questionnaires, 20 randomly selected non-responders, who met the inclusion criteria, were contacted by phone to repeat the questionnaire. Telephone interviews were performed by a clinical trial assistant with the original questionnaire. As VAS scores are not designed for telephone interview, a verbal instruction was given to obtain a score of 0–100 for studied symptoms to best replicate the effect of the scale.

### Statistical analysis

Discrete data were analysed and presented as frequencies and % frequencies, while continuous variables were mainly presented as mean with standard deviations. Pearson's rho was selected as a correlation coefficient as VAS and SNOT-22 scores are following the normal distribution. VAS bronchial, VAS ocular and VAS sino-nasal were calculated as means of the corresponding category symptoms. Specifically, VAS bronchial score represented means of cough, tightness on the chest, shortness of breath and wheezing. VAS ocular score was obtained from itchy eyes and tearing, whereas VAS sino-nasal score from nasal blockage, headache/pressure on the face, loss of smell, postnasal drip, runny nose, itchy nose, and sneezing. IBM SPSS Statistics 23.0 (IBM Corporation, New York, NY, USA) was used for statistical analysis and a $p < 0.05$ was considered significant.

### Results

Of over 400 patients who met the inclusion criteria, a postal questionnaire was sent to 325 individuals of which 202 returned a filled questionnaire (response rate 62.15%). Twenty-two patients were excluded due to incomplete filling of the questionnaire and/or missing informed consent. A total of 180 patients completed the VAS symptom severity scores and the SNOT-22 questionnaire and were eligible for analysis. Of the 180 subjects analysed, 60% were male and 40% were female. The mean age of the studied population was $51.7 \pm 16.6$, ranged from 16 to 88. About 35.8% had known allergy, 28.7% had asthma, and 12.4% were current smokers. Among patients, 53.9% had CRSwNP, 46.1% had CRSsNP. Using the above mentioned VAS cut-off points for defining the level of control in CRS, 10% were classified as well controlled, 28.3% partly controlled, and 61.7% as uncontrolled (Table 1).

**Table 1 Patients basic demographics, clinical characteristics, co morbidities, and level of control**

| *Demographics* | | |
|---|---|---|
| Gender, n (%) | | |
| Female | 72 | 40.0% |
| Male | 108 | 60.0% |
| Age, years (mean ± SD\|min–max) | | |
| Female | 51.4 ± 17.4 | 18–88 |
| Male | 51.9 ± 16.2 | 16–88 |
| Total | 51.7 ± 16.6 | 16–88 |
| Surgery, n (%) | | |
| Yes | 149 | 83.2% |
| Number of FESS (mean ± SD\|min–max) | 1.8 ± 1.0 | 1–5 |
| Smoking, n (%) | | |
| No | 122 | 68.5% |
| Current | 22 | 12.4% |
| Ex-smoker | 34 | 19.1% |
| Smoking duration, years (mean ± SD\|min–max) | 15.7 ± 10.2 | 1–37 |
| *Clinical characteristics* | | |
| CRSsNP, n (%) | 84 | 46.1% |
| CRSwNP, n (%) | 96 | 53.9% |
| *Co-morbidities* | | |
| Asthma, n (%) | 51 | 28.7% |
| Allergy, n (%) | 63 | 35.8% |
| *Level of control* | | |
| Controlled, n (%) | 18 | 10.0% |
| Partially controlled, n (%) | 51 | 28.3% |
| Uncontrolled, n (%) | 111 | 61.7% |

A significant correlation between SNOT-22 and VAS scores for TNSS (Fig. 1a) and individual symptoms was found, with VAS-TNSS showing the strongest correlation, followed by headache/pressure on the face, postnasal drip, and obstruction (Table 2). The maximum value of Pearson's rho test was estimated at r = 0.655, ($p < 0.001$) for VAS-TNSS, and the minimum value was r = 0.301, ($p < 0.001$) for VAS-Loss of smell score. Correlation between VAS scores and SNOT-22 remained statistically significant, irrespective of the distribution of VAS individual scores into subclasses based on symptoms origin (sino-nasal, ocular, bronchial). In this case, VAS for sino-nasal symptoms showed the strongest correlation with SNOT-22 (r = 0.738; $p < 0.001$), followed by bronchial (r = 0.683; $p < 0.001$), and ocular symptoms (r = 0.559; $p < 0.001$) (Table 2). Furthermore, we found VAS for TNSS to correlate significantly with SNOT-22 in both CRSsNP (r = 0.697; $p < 0.001$), and CRSwNP (r = 0.608; $p < 0.001$) phenotypes (Fig. 1b).

Subsequently, we intended to evaluate the association between VAS and SNOT-22 in different levels of disease control. A significant association was found for SNOT-22 and VAS-TNSS in well controlled (r = 0.337; $p = 0.031$)

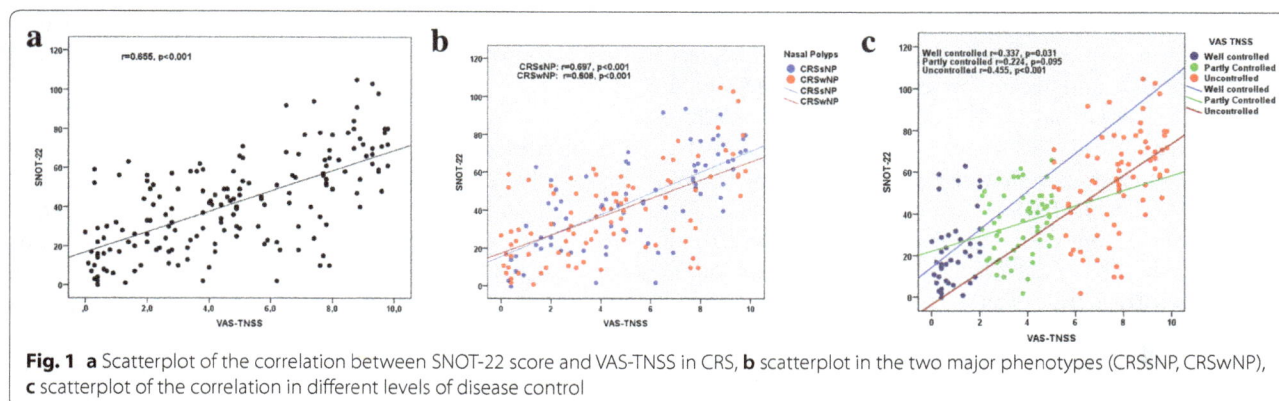

**Fig. 1** **a** Scatterplot of the correlation between SNOT-22 score and VAS-TNSS in CRS, **b** scatterplot in the two major phenotypes (CRSsNP, CRSwNP), **c** scatterplot of the correlation in different levels of disease control

**Table 2** Pearson's correlation of SNOT-22 score with VAS scores in CRS patients

| | SNOT-22 | |
|---|---|---|
| | Pearson's R | P |
| VAS-TNSS | 0.655 | <0.001 |
| VAS-blockage | 0.499 | <0.001 |
| VAS-headache/facial pressure | 0.607 | <0.001 |
| VAS-Loss of smell | 0.301 | <0.001 |
| VAS-postnasal | 0.579 | <0.001 |
| VAS-runny nose | 0.472 | <0.001 |
| VAS-itchy nose | 0.353 | <0.001 |
| VAS-sneezing | 0.460 | <0.001 |
| VAS sino-nasal | 0.738 | <0.001 |
| VAS-itchy eyes | 0.470 | <0.001 |
| VAS-tearing | 0.552 | <0.001 |
| VAS-ocular | 0.559 | <0.001 |
| VAS-cough | 0.549 | <0.001 |
| VAS-tightness of chest | 0.578 | <0.001 |
| VAS-shortness of breathe | 0.579 | <0.001 |
| VAS-wheezing | 0.459 | <0.001 |
| VAS-bronchial | 0.683 | <0.001 |

The maximum value of Pearson's rho test was estimated at $r = 0.655$, ($p < 0.001$) for VAS-TNSS, and the minimum value was $r = 0.301$, ($p < 0.001$) for VAS-Loss of smell and SNOT-22 score

and uncontrolled ($r = 0.455$; $p < 0.001$) but not in partly-controlled ($r = 0.224$; $p = 0.095$) CRS patients (Fig. 1c). No significant differences were found in outcomes of the 20 non-responders to our questionnaire compared to those who responded.

## Discussion

To date, SNOT-22 is used in different research fields and in clinical practice to determine the burden of disease, the outcome of medical or surgical intervention, and to improve candidate selection for surgery [8, 9]. However,

a large number of CRS patients primarily visit their pharmacist or general practitioner to seek advice for their disease or they self-medicate. It is of vital importance to use a simple and reliable tool that can be used by all healthcare providers and patients for self-assessment [16, 18]. As such, VAS has been incorporated into different mHealth tools. Emerging technologies could increase patient participation in treatment decision-making [19]. Consequently, these new tools might improve compliance to treatment, increase level of control, and facilitate doctor-patient communication [19]. Recently, VAS was validated to assess allergic disease control on smartphone screens for the MASK-rhinitis project [14].

We found a significant association between SNOT-22 and VAS for all symptoms ($p < 0.001$), with VAS for TNSS showing the best correlation ($r = 0.655$). Interestingly, nasal obstruction which is considered to have the highest average severity among patients with CRS, did correlate with SNOT-22 but headache/facial pressure, and postnasal drip showed stronger association. Although the importance of headache/facial pressure as a cardinal symptom in CRS has been questioned, it appears to have the second strongest association ($r = 0.607$). VAS for loss of smell was found to have the minimum value of Pearson's rho test ($r = 0.301$). These findings, yet atypical, suggest that patients' perspective of symptoms severity is the result of an interaction between many factors. Age, gender, socio-economic status, psychological profile, and other comorbidities may modify patients' perception of symptoms burden appraisal. In line with this hypothesis, several studies in the literature demonstrated lack of correlation between subjective and objective measures assessing symptoms severity [20, 21].

The strong association observed between VAS for bronchial symptoms and SNOT-22 ($r = 0.683$; $p < 0.001$) is justified on the basis of current knowledge on upper and lower airways interaction [5, 22]. CRS and asthma are common manifestations of an inflammatory process within the contiguous upper and lower airways. Furthermore, it is well established that asthma and CRS frequently coexist, and treatment of one condition could alleviate the coexisting one [5]. Concerning association between allergy and CRS, there is conflicting data in the literature. Nonetheless, allergy testing and treatment remain an option in CRS [5]. Herein, we show a significant correlation between VAS for ocular and bronchial symptoms and SNOT-22. Our results could be explained as patients with allergic, non-allergic rhinitis, and asthma patients were not excluded from the study, and may further support the link between upper and lower airways as stated in the "concept of united airway disease" [1, 5, 22].

Interestingly, a significant association was found for SNOT-22 and VAS-TNSS in well controlled (r = 0.337; p = 0.031) and uncontrolled (r = 0.455; p < 0.001), but not in partly-controlled (r = 0.224; p = 0.095) CRS patients. As this was a postal questionnaire survey, applying the current EPOS criteria for defining the level of control was not feasible [1]. Utilization of specific VAS–TNSS cutoffs for level of control assessment was based on a previous real-life study, where VAS scores of CRS symptoms were compared for different levels of control according to EPOS criteria in 389 patients [15]. Recently, the same cut-off points were used in mySinusitisCoach, an app for patients with CRS developed by medical experts in the field, to assess the level of disease control [23]. The weak correlation observed in the intermediate intervals (VAS > 2 and ≤ 5) could be explained by the halo effect, which may be noticed when several items are to be evaluated with different types of scales [11].

In line with our hypothesis, VAS scores for TNSS and for individual symptoms correlate well with SNOT-22. Among different aspects, mean VAS scores for sinonasal symptoms showed stronger association with SNOT-22 than with ocular and bronchial symptoms. Overall, VAS-TNSS can accurately predict disease severity, level of control, and burden of disease which is in accordance with the revised EPOS statement [1]. Our data confirmed that VAS for TNSS can be used as a first and easy system to evaluate the burden of CRS followed by the more extensive SNOT-22 questionnaire if more detailed analysis is required. The high response rate (62.1%) that was achieved and the fact that data obtained from telephonic interviews were fully in line with the written questionnaires, could allow us to overcome speculation for bias deriving from the nature of the study. Despite the selection of CRS patients being treated in a tertiary referral center, and the relatively small sample size, our data underline the value of a simple tool like VAS for TNSS. As VAS scores are nowadays being used in the novel digital Apps for allergic

rhinitis but also CRS [24], our data support the use of VAS for evaluation of the disease burden in daily life.

## Conclusions

In conclusion, we here show that VAS scores can be used in CRS to evaluate the burden of disease. Undoubtedly, our data are paving the way for a simple evaluation of CRS disease burden. Taking into account that VAS can be easily digitized, it can play a key role not only in everyday clinical practice but also in mHealth tools designed to monitor disease activity in CRS patients.

### Abbreviations
CRS: chronic rhinosinusitis; QoL: quality of life; COPD: chronic obstructive pulmonary disease; SNOT-22: sino-nasal outcome test-22; VAS: visual analogue scale; ARIA: allergic rhinitis and its impact on asthma; RQLQ: rhinoconjunctivitis quality of life questionnaire; TNSS: total nasal symptom score; VAS-TNSS: visual analogue scale for total nasal symptom score; CRSsNP: chronic rhinosinusitis without nasal polyps; CRSwNP: chronic rhinosinusitis with nasal polyps.

### Authors' contributions
The authors verify that they have met all the criteria for authorship and are qualified to be listed as authors of this work by their substantive contribution to the conception and design of the project or analysis of the data, their drafting or critical revision of the content of this manuscript, and their approval of the final version to be published. PH designed the study, revised it critically, and he approved the final version to be published. MD analyzed the data, drafted the manuscript and approved its final version. EP, BS, BP, and SS have all contributed to data interpretation, revised the manuscript. All authors read and approved the final manuscript.

### Author details
[1] Laboratory of Clinical Immunology, Department of Microbiology and Immunology, KU Leuven, Kapucijnenvoer 33, 3000 Louvain, Belgium. [2] Department of Otorhinolaryngology, Head and Neck Surgery, University of Crete School of Medicine, Heraklion, Crete, Greece. [3] Clinical Division of Otorhinolaryngology, Head and Neck Surgery, University Hospitals Leuven, Louvain, Belgium.

### Acknowledgements
Not applicable.

### Competing interests
The authors declare that they have no competing interests.

### Funding
Not applicable.

## References

1.  Fokkens WJ, Lund VJ, Mullol J, Bachert C, Alobid I, Baroody F, et al. EPOS 2012: European position paper on rhinosinusitis and nasal polyps 2012. A summary for otorhinolaryngologists. Rhinology. 2012;50(1):1–12.

2.  Hastan D, Fokkens WJ, Bachert C, Newson RB, Bislimovska J, Bockelbrink A, et al. Chronic rhinosinusitis in Europe–an underestimated disease. A GA$^2$LEN study. Allergy. 2011;66(9):1216–23.

3.  Hamilos DL. Chronic rhinosinusitis: epidemiology and medical management. J Allergy Clin Immunol. 2011;128(4):693–707 **(quiz 708–9)**.

4.  Prokopakis EP, Vlastos IM, Ferguson BJ, Scadding G, Kawauchi H, Georgalas C, et al. SCUAD and chronic rhinosinusitis. Reinforcing hypothesis driven research in difficult cases. Rhinology. 2014;52(1):3–8.

5.  Orlandi RR, Kingdom TT, Hwang PH, Smith TL, Alt JA, Baroody FM, et al. International consensus statement on allergy and rhinology: rhinosinusitis. Int Forum Allergy Rhinol. 2016;6(Suppl 1):S22–209.

6.  Soler ZM, Wittenberg E, Schlosser RJ, Mace JC, Smith TL. Health state utility values in patients undergoing endoscopic sinus surgery. Laryngoscope. 2011;121(12):2672–8.

7.  Piccirillo JF, Edwards D, Haiduk A, Yonan C, Thawley SE. Psychometric and clinimetric validity of the 31-Item Rhinosinusitis Outcome Measure (RSOM-31), vol. 9; 1995.

8.  Hopkins C, Gillett S, Slack R, Lund VJ, Browne JP. Psychometric validity of the 22-item Sinonasal Outcome Test. Clin Otolaryngol Off J ENT-UK Off J Neth Soc Oto-Rhino-Laryngol Cervico-Facial Surg. 2009;34(5):447–54.

9.  Piccirillo JF, Merritt MG, Richards ML. Psychometric and clinimetric validity of the 20-Item Sino-Nasal Outcome Test (SNOT-20). Otolaryngol-Head Neck Surg Off J Am Acad Otolaryngol-Head Neck Surg. 2002;126(1):41–7.

10. Benninger MS, Senior BA. The development of the Rhinosinusitis Disability Index. Arch Otolaryngol Head Neck Surg. 1997;123(11):1175–9.

11. Klimek L, Bergmann K-C, Biedermann T, Bousquet J, Hellings P, Jung K, et al. Visual analogue scales (VAS): measuring instruments for the documentation of symptoms and therapy monitoring in cases of allergic rhinitis in everyday health care: Position Paper of the German Society of Allergology (AeDA) and the German Society of Allergy and Clinical Immunology (DGAKI), ENT Section, in collaboration with the working group on Clinical Immunology, Allergology and Environmental Medicine of the German Society of Otorhinolaryngology, Head and Neck Surgery (DGHNOKHC). Allergo J Int. 2017;26(1):16–24.

12. Brożek JL, Bousquet J, Agache I, Agarwal A, Bachert C, Bosnic-Anticevich S, et al. Allergic Rhinitis and its Impact on Asthma (ARIA) guidelines-2016 revision. J Allergy Clin Immunol. 2017;140(4):950–8.

13. Bousquet J, Schunemann HJ, Fonseca J, Samolinski B, Bachert C, Canonica GW, et al. MACVIA-ARIA Sentinel NetworK for allergic rhinitis (MASK-rhinitis): the new generation guideline implementation. Allergy. 2015;70(11):1372–92.

14. Caimmi D, BaizN, TannoLK, DemolyP, ArnavielheS, Murray R, et al. Validation of the MASK-rhinitis visual analogue scale on smartphone screens to assess allergic rhinitis control. Clin Exp Allergy. 2017;47(12):1526–33.

15. van der Veen J, Seys SF, Timmermans M, Levie P, Jorissen M, Fokkens WJ, et al. Real-life study showing uncontrolled rhinosinusitis after sinus surgery in a tertiary referral centre. Allergy. 2017;72(2):282–90.

16. Hellings PW, Akdis CA, Bachert C, Bousquet J, Pugin B, Adriaensen G, et al. EUFOREA Rhinology Research Forum 2016: report of the brainstorming sessions on needs and priorities in rhinitis and rhinosinusitis. Rhinology. 2017;55(3):202–10.

17. Toma S, Hopkins C. Stratification of SNOT-22 scores into mild, moderate or severe and relationship with other subjective instruments. Rhinology. 2016;54(2):129–33.

18. Hellings PW, Fokkens WJ, Bachert C, Akdis CA, Bieber T, Agache I, et al. Positioning the principles of precision medicine in care pathways for allergic rhinitis and chronic rhinosinusitis: A EUFOREA-ARIA-EPOS-AIRWAYS ICP statement. Allergy. 2017;72(9):1297–305.

19. Bousquet J, Caimmi DP, Bedbrook A, Bewick M, Hellings PW, Devillier P, et al. Pilot study of mobile phone technology in allergic rhinitis in European countries: the MASK-rhinitis study. Allergy. 2017;72(6):857–65.

20. Wabnitz DAM, Nair S, Wormald PJ. Correlation between preoperative symptom scores, quality-of-life questionnaires, and staging with computed tomography in patients with chronic rhinosinusitis. Am J Rhinol Allergy. 2005;19(1):91–6.

21. Hopkins C, Browne JP, Slack R, Lund V, Brown P. The Lund-Mackay staging system for chronic rhinosinusitis: how is it used and what does it predict? Otolaryngol Neck Surg. 2007;137(4):555–61.

22. Bousquet J, Arnavielhe S, Bedbrook A, Fonseca J, Morais Almeida M, Todo Bom A, et al. The allergic rhinitis and its impact on asthma (ARIA) score of allergic rhinitis using mobile technology correlates with quality of life: the MASK study. Allergy. 2017;73(2):505–10.

23. Bousquet J, Schunemann HJ, Fonseca J, Samolinski B, Bachert C, Canonica GW, et al. MACVIA-ARIA Sentinel NetworK for allergic rhinitis (MASK-rhinitis): the new generation guideline implementation. Allergy. 2015;70(11):1372–92.

24. Seys SF, Bousquet J, Bachert C, Fokkens WJ, Agache I, Bernal-Sprekelsen M, et al. mySinusitisCoach: patient empowerment in chronic rhinosinusitis using mobile technology. Rhinology. 2018. https://doi.org/10.4193/Rhin17.253.

# 19

# Severity of allergic rhinitis impacts sleep and anxiety: results from a large Spanish cohort

R. Muñoz-Cano[1,2]* iD, P. Ribó[1,3], G. Araujo[1,2], E. Giralt[4], J. Sanchez-Lopez[5] and A. Valero[1,3]

## Abstract

**Background:** Allergic rhinitis (AR) is a highly prevalent disease that generates high social and health care costs and also has a significant effect on quality of life and quality of sleep. It has also been related to some psychological disorders like anxiety or depression.

**Objective:** To evaluate anxiety, depression, and quality of sleep and life alteration in a group of patients with perennial AR compared to a group of seasonal AR patients.

**Methods:** Six-hundred seventy adults (> 18 years) with perennial and seasonal AR were recruited consecutively in 47 centers in Spain. Individuals were grouped in "Perennial" and "Seasonal" according to the seasonality of their symptoms. Anxiety, depression, sleep quality and health related quality of life were evaluated using the Hospital Anxiety and Depression Scale, Medical Outcomes Study Sleep Scale (MOS Sleep Scale) and the Health-related quality of life questionnaire ESPRINT-15, respectively. Both groups of patients were evaluated in and out of the pollen season.

**Results:** AR symptoms are related to worse quality of life and more anxiety and depression symptoms. Indeed, symptom severity also correlates with worse outcomes (quality of life, sleep and depression/anxiety) regardless allergen seasonality. Symptoms severity, compared with seasonality and persistence, is the most important factor related with more anxiety and depression and poor sleep. However, symptoms severity, persistence and seasonality are independently affecting the quality of life in patients with AR.

**Conclusions:** Although AR symptoms have a great impact on depression and anxiety symptoms, quality of life and quality of sleep in all AR patients, as expected, individuals with more severe AR seem to suffer more intensely their effects.

**Keywords:** Anxiety, Depression, Allergic rhinitis, Sleep

## Background

Allergic rhinitis (AR) is a highly prevalent disease that generates high social and health care costs [1] and also has a significant effect on quality of life (QoL) [2–4]. AR accounts for 55.5% of all cases in Spanish allergy clinics consultations [5], and it is known to alter patients' social life, nighttime rest and inducing daytime drowsiness [6]. Consequently, its adverse impact upon school and work performance has been described [7, 8]. In addition, AR is associated to several disorders with a strong socioeconomic impact such as asthma and rhinosinusitis [1, 9], with the subsequently added impact upon health-related quality of life (HRQL). Olfactory dysfunction is also a very important symptom in patients with AR, and it has been considered as a key contributor to quality of life; its loss is associated to a decrease in both food/drink enjoyment and a social competence [10].

Sleep quality is also altered in patients with AR, and its severity correlates with a poorer sleep quality [2]. AR can impair nocturnal sleep through a mechanical mechanism related to nasal obstruction, snoring and apnea/hypopnea [11, 12]. Sleep impairment has subsequent effects on daytime performance and HRQL. Moreover, the inflammatory cytokines released during allergic reactions

*Correspondence: rmunoz@clinic.cat
[1] Allergy Unit, Pneumology Department, Hospital Clinic, Universitat de Barcelona, ARADyAL, Barcelona, Spain
Full list of author information is available at the end of the article

have been related to the suppression of both rapid eyes movement (REM) and no-REM phase [13, 14].

A positive association between allergies and psychological disorders has been stablished demonstrated in several studies. Patten et al. [15] provided evidence of AR patients having a higher rate of panic disorder and social phobia (OR 1.7 and 1.3, respectively) than healthy individuals, as well as major depression (OR 1.5). Likewise, Cuffel et al. [16] analyzed 850.000 individuals and found that anxiety symptoms were 1.4 times higher in individuals with AR versus healthy controls. Indeed, depression diagnosis was 1.7 times more frequent. Several hypotheses have been formulated to explain the association between AR and psychological disorders. The effects of both anxiety and rhinitis on immunity, affecting cytokine production/release, may account for this relationship. On the other hand, the impairing effects of nasal obstruction on sleep have a negative effect on psychiatric symptoms. Finally, a possible shared genetic risk between both allergy and depression has been postulated [17].

The duration of allergen exposure (i.e. perennial vs seasonal) may have a differential impact on sleep quality, anxiety and QoL [18]. A perennial exposure, with persistent and perennial symptoms, may affect these parameters more deeply than seasonal exposure. Our objective is to compare anxiety and depression levels, sleep disturbance and quality of life in a group of patients with perennial AR with a group of seasonal AR patients.

## Methods

### Patient selection and study design

Six-hundred seventy adults (>18 years) with perennial and seasonal AR were recruited consecutively in 47 centers in Spain. Individuals were grouped in "Perennial" and "Seasonal" groups according to the seasonality of their symptoms and allergic sensitization. Skin prick test with dust mite, molds, dog and cat dander and pollens (plane tree, olive tree, grass, wall pellitory, cypress) were performed in all patients. Patients in the *"perennial group"* had symptoms all over the year and were sensitized to dust mites, molds and animal dander. Those with symptoms limited to pollen season, sensitized to pollen (cypress, grass, olive tree, plane tree and wall pellitory) and symptomatic at visit 1, were included in the *"seasonal group"*. Both groups were evaluated during the pollen season (visit 1 from February to May) and out of the pollen season (visit 2 from September to December). Pregnant women, individuals with psychiatric disorders, patients treated with antidepressants or anxiolytics, and individuals receiving immunotherapy were excluded (see Fig. 1).

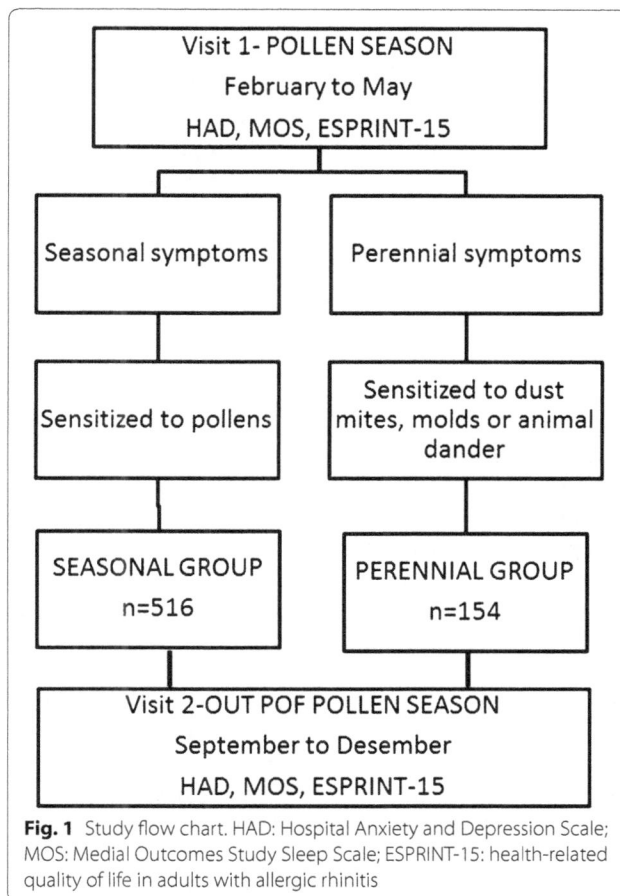

**Fig. 1** Study flow chart. HAD: Hospital Anxiety and Depression Scale; MOS: Medial Outcomes Study Sleep Scale; ESPRINT-15: health-related quality of life in adults with allergic rhinitis

Informed consent was obtained from all participating subjects. The study was approved by the Local Ethics Committee of Hospital Clinic, (Barcelona, Spain).

### Variables

Anxiety, depression, sleep quality and health related quality of life were evaluated using validated questionnaires: the Hospital Anxiety and Depression Scale (HAD) [19, 20], Medical Outcomes Study Sleep Scale (MOS Sleep Scale) [21, 22] and the Health-related quality of life questionnaire ESPRINT-15 [4, 23], respectively.

HAD is a self-administered 14 items questionnaire with a total score from 0 to 42. Seven of these items measure anxiety (score from 0 to 21) and the other seven items measure depression (from 0 to 21). Scores from 11 to 21 indicate a clinical problem, from 8 to 10 the results are not conclusive, and from 0 to 7 are in the range of normality. Participants are asked to work through each question indicating the extent to which they have experienced a particular symptom or state over the past week.

MOS Sleep Scale is a self-administered 12-item questionnaire developed to provide a concise assessment of 6 important dimensions of sleep, including initiation, maintenance, respiratory problems, quantity, perceived adequacy and somnolence. Two sleep problems indexes (sleep index I and II) summarizing information across all these items were also used. Quality of sleep is expressed on a numeric rating scale ranging from 0 ("best possible sleep") to 10 ("worst possible sleep"). Participants are asked to work through each question indicating the extent to which they have experienced a particular symptom or state over the past week.

ESPRINT-15 is a specific and validated instrument to measure health-related quality of life in adult patients with AR, which was first validated for use in Spanish-speaking populations. This questionnaire has shown good reliability, validity, and sensitivity to change. It has also proved easy to use and administer. This self-administered questionnaire contains 15 items distributed within the following dimensions: symptoms (5 items), daily activities (3 items), sleep (3 items), psychological impact (3 items), and general health (1 item). An overall score and a score for each dimension are obtained. The overall score and the dimensional scores range from 0 (no impact on HRQOL) to 6 (maximum impact on HRQOL). Participants are asked to work through each question indicating the extent to which they have experienced a particular symptom or state over the past 2 weeks.

Co-morbidities as rhinitis and asthma and their severity using ARIA and GINA guidelines respectively, were recorded.

### Statistics

Qualitative variables were described using frequencies and quantitative variables by means of centralization and dispersion measures. For comparisons, Fisher's exact test for categorical variables or a Student's $t$ test were used. For comparisons with three or more categories an ANOVA test was implemented. To evaluate the effect of symptoms severity, seasonality and persistence in the variables, a multivariate analysis was performed. Quantitative variables were evaluated using a multiple lineal regression model and post-oc differences were evaluated using Tuckey test. Qualitative variables were evaluated using a logistic regression. A value of $p < 0.05$ was considered significant.

### Results

#### Study population

Among the 670 recruited patients, 516 corresponded to the *seasonal group* and 154 to the *perennial group*. No differences were found between groups, except for conjunctivitis that was more frequently observed in *seasonal*

**Table 1 Demographics, sensitization profile and clinical manifestations**

| | Perennial (n = 154) | Seasonal (n = 516) |
|---|---|---|
| Age (years) (mean ± SD) | 34.2 ± 11.6 | 34.7 ± 10.9 |
| Gender (female %) | 62.5 | 57.8 |
| Rhinitis (%) | | |
|   Persistent | 67.5 | 63.6 |
|   Intermittent | 32.5 | 36.4 |
|   Mild | 20.1 | 19.2 |
|   Moderate | 63 | 56.4 |
|   Severe | 16.9 | 24.4 |
| Co-morbidities (%) | | |
|   Conjunctivitis | 16.2* | 37.8 |
|   Asthma | 40.9 | 41.5 |
|     Intermittent | 58.3 | 49 |
|     Mild persistent | 21.7 | 30 |
|     Moderate persistent | 18.3 | 19 |
|     Severe persistent | 1.7 | 1.9 |
| Sensitization profile (%) | | |
|   Dust mites | 96.1 | 34.8 |
|   Molds | 3.9 | 5.2 |
|   Animal dander | 20.1 | 20.1 |
|   Grass pollen | 0 | 70.7 |
|   Olive tree pollen | 0 | 51 |
|   Cypress pollen | 0 | 20.5 |
|   Plane tree | 0 | 15.9 |
|   Wall pellitory pollen | 0 | 10.8 |

Asthma and rhinitis were classified using GINA and modified-ARIA classification respectively. *$p < 0.01$

*patients* than in *perennial patients* (37.8 vs. 16.2%; $p < 0.001$) (Table 1).

### Effect of allergen exposure in AR patients with perennial symptoms

To assess the effect of allergen exposure on anxiety, depression and quality of sleep and life, results from both *perennial group* and *seasonal group* were compared out of the pollen season. AR patients with seasonal symptoms were asymptomatic out of the pollen season; therefore they were used as a control group. No differences were observed in and out of pollen season in any variable of the study in patients with *perennial symptoms*.

Patients with *perennial symptoms* scored higher for anxiety ($6.4 \pm 3.9$ vs. $5.4 \pm 3.7$; $p = 0.03$) and depression ($4.1 \pm 4.1$ vs. $3.5 \pm 3.3$; $p = 0.17$) compared to asymptomatic individuals (Fig. 2a). However, the total number of patients diagnosed with anxiety (HAD Anxiety > 11; 17.6% perennial vs. 12.1% seasonal; $p = 0.17$) or depression (HAD Depression > 11; 9.9% perennial vs. 5% seasonal; $p = 0.15$) was not different.

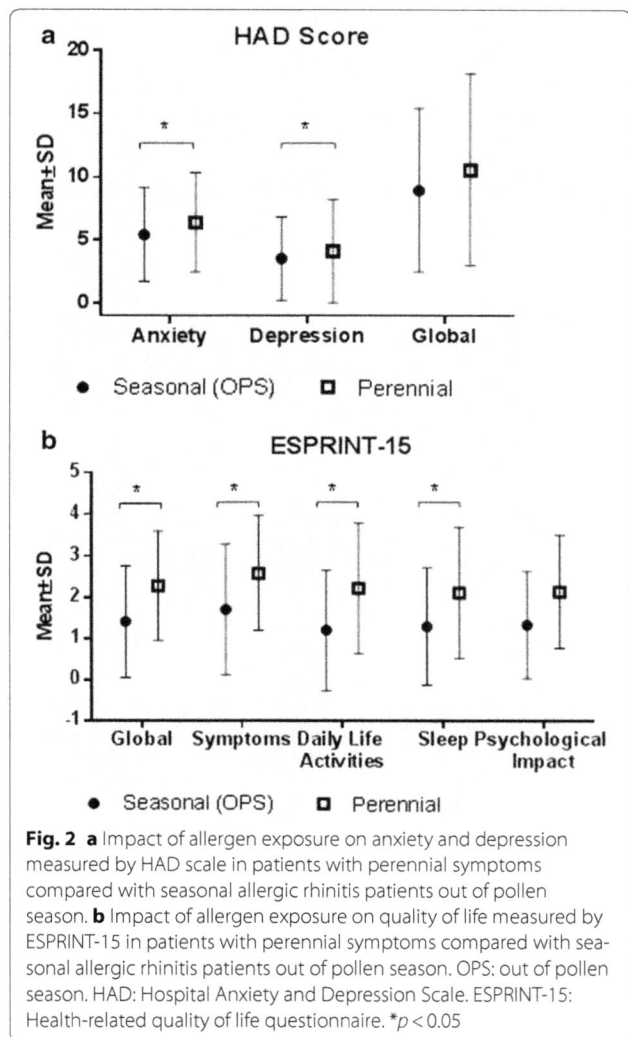

Fig. 2 a Impact of allergen exposure on anxiety and depression measured by HAD scale in patients with perennial symptoms compared with seasonal allergic rhinitis patients out of pollen season. b Impact of allergen exposure on quality of life measured by ESPRINT-15 in patients with perennial symptoms compared with seasonal allergic rhinitis patients out of pollen season. OPS: out of pollen season. HAD: Hospital Anxiety and Depression Scale. ESPRINT-15: Health-related quality of life questionnaire. *$p < 0.05$

Patients in the *perennial group* had a quality of sleep similar to the asymptomatic individuals, and they only scored higher in the dimension "sleep shortness of breath" ($24.2 \pm 26.9$ vs. $15.6 \pm 20.7$; $p = 0.0016$). A similar number of patients had a suboptimal sleep measured by MOS in both groups (36 vs. 29.9%, $p > 0.05$).

Patients with AR in the *perennial group* had a worse quality of life (higher score in all dimensions) measured by ESPRINT-15 questionnaire compared to the asymptomatic control group (Fig. 2b). Global ESPRINT-15 score in *perennial group* was $2.3 \pm 1.3$ and $1.4 \pm 1.3$ in the control group ($p < 0.05$).

Symptoms persistence and severity were related with worse outcomes (anxiety, depression, sleep and quality of life) in perennial AR individuals (Table 2).

### Effect of allergen exposure in AR patients with seasonal symptoms

To assess the effect of allergen exposure on anxiety, depression and quality of sleep, we compared the *seasonal group* patients in and out of pollen season.

Patients with *seasonal symptoms* had higher global HAD scores during pollen season than out of pollen season ($8.9 \pm 6.5$ vs. $10.5 \pm 6.6$; $p < 0.05$). Both anxiety and depression scores were higher during pollen season ($6.3 \pm 3.8$ vs. $5.4 \pm 3.7$; $p < 0.05$; $4.1 \pm 3.4$ vs. $3.5 \pm 3.3$; $p < 0.05$, respectively) (Fig. 3a). However, the number of patients diagnosed with anxiety or depression (HAD > 11) was not different in or out of pollen season (16 vs. 12%; $p > 0.05$; 4.8 vs. 5%; $p > 0.05$ respectively).

Similarly, MOS Sleep indexes were higher during pollen season reflecting a poorer quality of sleep with more somnolence, apneas and snoring (Fig. 3b). Up to 41.5% of patients had a suboptimal sleep during pollen season and 30% out of pollen season ($p = 0.007$).

Quality of life measured using ESPRINT-15 questionnaire was more affected during pollen season in all 5 dimensions, including global score, symptoms, daily life activities, sleep and psychological disturbance. ESPRINT-15 global score was also higher during pollen season, meaning worse quality of life ($2.6 \pm 1.3$ vs. $1.4 \pm 1.3 \; p < 0.05$) (Fig. 3c).

In the seasonal group, symptoms severity but not persistence was related with worse outcomes (anxiety, depression, sleep and quality of life) (Table 2).

### Effect of allergen exposure duration, symptoms seasonality and severity on AR patients

To assess the effect of allergen exposure duration and symptoms seasonality and severity on anxiety, quality of the sleep and quality of life, we compared both groups when symptomatic. That is during pollen season in seasonal group and together in and out of pollen season in perennial group.

When comparing both groups and adjusting for symptoms severity, seasonality and persistence, we found that severity is the most important factor related with worse outcomes in most of the evaluated parameters.

Both symptoms severity and seasonality were independently related with worse HAD scores. Perennial group and patients with more severe symptoms had worse outcomes. In that way, the risk of depression (HAD > 11) was increased 3.3-fold in perennial AR patients compared with seasonal AR, and 2.7-fold in severe AR compared with mild and moderate AR individuals. However, only severity was significantly related with anxiety diagnosis (HAD > 11). Severe AR patients had an increased risk

**Table 2 Anxiety, depression, quality of life and quality of sleep in AR patients with perennial and seasonal symptoms depending on symptoms severity and persistence**

|  | Persistent<br>n = 104 | Intermitent<br>n = 50 | p value | Mild<br>n = 31 | Moderate<br>n = 97 | Severe<br>n = 26 | p value |
|---|---|---|---|---|---|---|---|
| Perennial |  |  |  |  |  |  |  |
| HAD anxiety | 6.4 ± 3.9 | 5.3 ± 3.7 | **c | 4.5 ± 3.8 | 6 ± 3.6 | 7.3 ± 4 | ***a |
| HAD depression | 4.2 ± 3.6 | 3.5 ± 3.4 | *c | 3.4 ± 3.5 | 3.6 ± 3.3 | 5.3 ± 4 | ***a |
| HAD anxiety > 11 | 17.2% | 11% | nsb | 9.4% | 13. % | 23.3% | **a |
| HAD depression > 11 | 31% | 13% | nsb | 6.3% | 4.1% | 13.2% | ***b |
| MOS Sleep index I | 64.8 ± 18.8 | 71.9 ± 17.1 | ***c | 76.4 ± 16.6 | 68.2 ± 17.6 | 57.4 ± 17.8 | ***a |
| MOS Sleep index II | 65.5 ± 18 | 72.6 ± 16.7 | ***c | 77.3 ± 15.9 | 68.7 ± 16.9 | 58.6 ± 17.2 | ***a |
| MOS suboptimal sleep | 40% | 29.7% | *b | 36.4% | 33.5% | 43.4% | nsb |
| ESPRINT global | 2.5 ± 1.4 | 1.3 ± 1.2 | ***c | 0.8 ± 0.9 | 2.2 ± 1.1 | 2.9 ± 1.6 | ***a |
|  | n = 328 | n = 188 |  | n = 99 | n = 291 | n = 126 |  |
| Seasonal |  |  |  |  |  |  |  |
| HAD anxiety | 6.4 ± 3.8 | 6.2 ± 3.8 | ns | 6 ± 4.1 | 5.9 ± 3.5 | 7.3 ± 3.9 | *a |
| HAD depression | 4.3 ± 3.4 | 3.6 ± 3.3 | ns | 4.3 ± 3.9 | 3.4 ± 3 | 5.5 ± 3.6 | ***a |
| HAD anxiety > 11 | 16.1% | 16.1% | ns | 20.8% | 11.4% | 24.1% | nsb |
| HAD depression > 11 | 4.7% | 4.9% | ns | 8.7% | 1.8% | 9.5% | *b |
| MOS Sleep index I | 63.2 ± 19.2 | 67.9 ± 17.3 | ns | 69.2 ± 18.4 | 67.7 ± 18.2 | 56.2 ± 18.1 | ***a |
| MOS Sleep index II | 63.9 ± 18.1 | 67.8 ± 17.4 | ns | 70 ± 17.3 | 67.9 ± 17.4 | 57 ± 18.2 | ***a |
| MOS suboptimal sleep | 43.2% | 35.5% | ns | 41.7% | 37.7% | 48.8% | nsb |
| ESPRINT global | 2.8 ± 1.3 | 1.8 ± 1.1 | ***c | 1.3 ± 0.9 | 2.4 ± 1 | 3.3 ± 1.4 | ***a |

Values expressed as mean ± SD. Comparisons between severity degrees (mild vs. moderate vs. severe) and symptoms persistence (intermittent vs. persistent) in both perennial AR and seasonal AR were made using aANOVA; bFisher's exact test and ct test. p value ≤ *0.01, *0.001, ***0.000001

Rhinitis severity was classified using modified-ARIA (Ref. [30]); HAD: Hospital Anxiety and Depression Scale (Ref. [19]), MOS: Medical Outcomes Study Sleep Scale (ref. [21]); ESPRINT-15: Health-related quality of life questionnaire (Ref. [4, 23])

(2.6-fold) of developing anxiety (HAD > 11) compared to moderate or mild AR individuals, independently of their symptoms seasonality or persistence (Table 3).

Symptoms severity and persistence were independently associated with suboptimal sleep, with patients with moderate and persistent AR symptoms having an increased risk (1.6-fold and twofold respectively) of having trouble sleeping (Table 3).

Finally, all three variables, persistence, severity and seasonality were independently related with worse quality of life measured using ESPRINT. Patients with severe AR, perennial and persistent symptoms had a worse quality of life compared with moderate o mild AR, seasonal and intermittent symptoms respectively (Table 3).

### Effect of the comorbidities on anxiety, depression, quality of sleep and quality of life in patients with AR

The impact of the most common comorbidities in AR, such as asthma and conjunctivitis, on anxiety, depression, quality of sleep and quality of life were evaluated during the symptomatic period of each group.

In *perennial AR patients*, neither asthma nor conjunctivitis were related to worse outcomes: no statistically significant differences were detected in any of the MOS scale domains, HAD depression/anxiety scores or diagnosis or quality of life (data not shown). However, in *seasonal AR patients*, asthma was related with worse sleep quality, mainly in "sleep disturbance" and "sleep shortness of breath". Those patients also scored higher in HAD depression and anxiety, and more patients were diagnosed with anxiety/depression compared to non-asthmatic patients. However, asthmatics' quality of life measured by ESPRINT-15 questionnaire was not statistically different compared to those without asthma (Table 4). On the other hand, conjunctivitis was not related to worse results in any of the measured outcomes (data not shown).

### Correlation between the studied variables

We calculated the correlation between the evaluated variables (anxiety, depression, quality of sleep and quality of life) to study the impact on each other. In both groups, patients with a worse score in quality of sleep had significantly higher scores in HAD depression and anxiety and had significantly worse quality of life measured by ESPRINT-15. No differences in the correlations

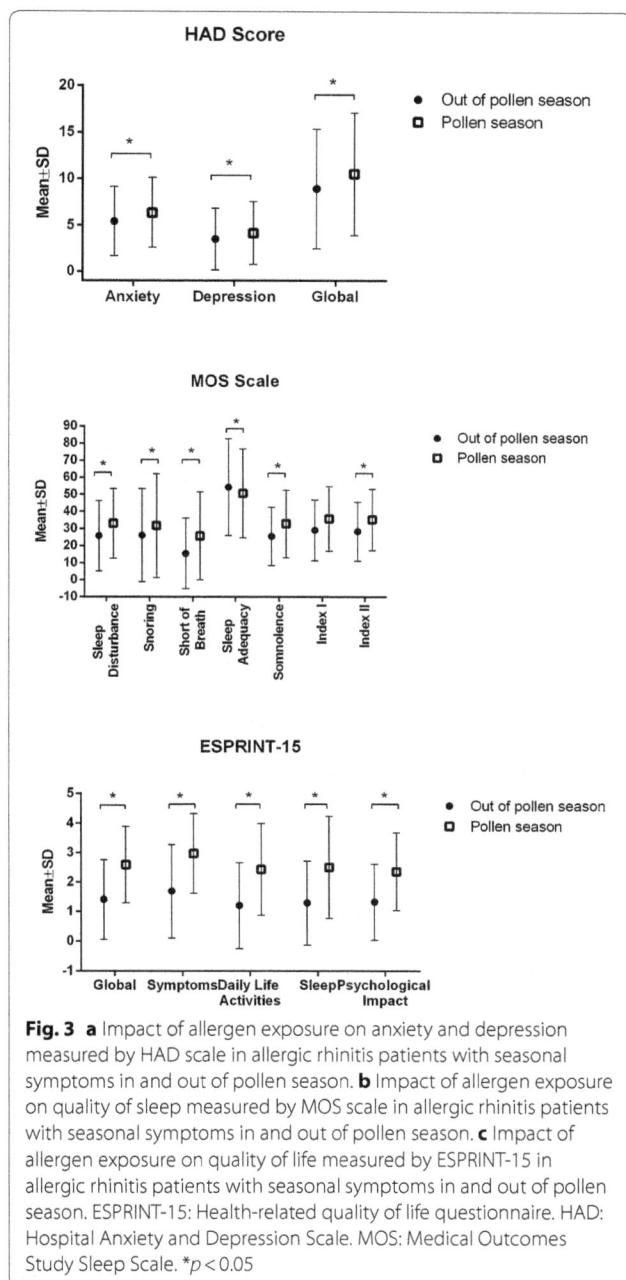

**Fig. 3 a** Impact of allergen exposure on anxiety and depression measured by HAD scale in allergic rhinitis patients with seasonal symptoms in and out of pollen season. **b** Impact of allergen exposure on quality of sleep measured by MOS scale in allergic rhinitis patients with seasonal symptoms in and out of pollen season. **c** Impact of allergen exposure on quality of life measured by ESPRINT-15 in allergic rhinitis patients with seasonal symptoms in and out of pollen season. ESPRINT-15: Health-related quality of life questionnaire. HAD: Hospital Anxiety and Depression Scale. MOS: Medical Outcomes Study Sleep Scale. *$p < 0.05$

were observed when comparing *seasonal* and *perennial patients* (Additional file 1: Suppl Table 1).

## Discussion

This is the first study that has evaluated anxiety and depression, using validated questionnaires, in patients with seasonal and perennial AR. We have found that AR symptoms are related with worse quality of life and more anxiety and depression symptoms. Indeed, symptoms

severity also correlates with worse outcomes (quality of life, sleep and depression/anxiety) regardless allergen seasonality. Interestingly asthma is associated with worse outcomes exclusively in individuals with seasonal symptoms.

In our study, individuals with AR symptoms had worse QoL than asymptomatic ones. Previous studies using different questionnaires (RQLQ, ESPRINT-15) have also revealed the impact of AR on QoL [24]. Indeed, the significant correlation found between QoL and AR severity made possible to differentiate between moderate and severe AR in the modified version of ARIA guideline [3, 4, 25]. We have found that symptomatic AR patients scored higher on anxiety and depression tests than asymptomatic individuals. However, there was no more anxiety/depression diagnosis. Previous works have shown that anxiety symptoms are more frequent in patients with allergies. Cuffel et al. [16] examined the healthcare claims of more than 5000 individuals and found that anxiety symptoms were 1.4 times higher and depression diagnosis was 1.7 times higher in individuals with allergies versus those without allergies. Likewise, in their examination of more than 12,000 individuals, Patten et al. [15] determined that major depression was more frequent in individuals with allergies (OR 1.5). Finally, we found a differential effect of AR symptoms on quality of sleep in perennial AR compared to seasonal AR. Whereas seasonal AR patients had worse quality of sleep when symptomatic, that was not the case of the individuals with perennial AR. Previous studies have shown that patients with AR have an impaired sleep and this correlates with disease severity, either in intermittent or persistent AR [2, 11, 12, 26]. In our study, although no sleep disturbances were found in perennial AR using MOS scale, the ESPRINT-15 domain referring to sleep was significantly affected. The differences between the tests used to evaluate sleep impairment in all those studies may account for the different results. Sleep disturbances make patients more susceptible to psychological consequences, as fatigue, irritability, anxiety and depression, which in the end can result in daytime somnolence and finally contribute to QoL impairment. However, the use of antihistamines to treat AR may also contribute to patient somnolence and cannot be ruled out [27].

We have observed that all three, symptoms persistence, severity and seasonality are affecting independently the quality of life of AR patients. Thus, patients with persistent, severe and perennial AR have worse quality of life measured using ESPRINT. However, other studies did not find differences in the QoL of patients with AR sensitized to perennial and seasonal allergens [28]. A previous study evaluated the psychological status of patients with seasonal and perennial AR [29] and the influence of type,

**Table 3 Effect of symptoms seasonality, persistence and severity on anxiety, sleep and quality of life in AR patients-multivariate analysis**

|  | Perennial versus seasonal p value | Mild versus moderate versus severe p value | Intermittent versus persistent p value |
|---|---|---|---|
| HAD global | 0.02 | <0.0001 | ns |
| HAD anxiety | ns | <0.0001 | ns |
| HAD depression | 0.03 | <0.0001 | ns |
| MOS Sleep index I | ns | <0.0001 | ns |
| ESPRINT | 0.005 | <0.0001 | <0.0001 |

The effect of symptoms severity, seasonality and persistence in each variable was evaluated using a multivariate analysis. Quantitative variables were evaluated using a multiple lineal regression model and post-oc differences were evaluated using Tuckey test. A value of $p < 0.05$ was considered significant

**Table 4 Effect of asthma on anxiety, depression, quality of life and quality of sleep in seasonal allergic rhinitis patients**

|  | Seasonal AR + ASTHMA N = 210 | Seasonal AR without Asthma n = 306 | p value |
|---|---|---|---|
| HAD anxiety | 6.9 ± 3.9 | 5.9 ± 3.6 | *a |
| HAD anxiety > 11 | 20.3% | 12.7% | *b |
| HAD depression | 4.8 ± 3.8 | 3.6 ± 3.1 | **a |
| HAD depression > 11 | 9% | 1.3% | **b |
| ESPRINT Global | 2.6 ± 1.3 | 2.6 ± 1.3 | nsb |
| MOS-Sleep disturbance | 63.4 ± 21 | 69.9 ± 19.4 | **a |
| MOS-Sleep shortness of breath | 70.5 ± 25.6 | 77.5 ± 25.5 | *a |
| MOS Sleep index I | 61.6 ± 19.4 | 66.5 ± 18.3 | *a |
| MOS Sleep index II | 61.9 ± 18.5 | 67.1 ± 17.3 | *a |
| MOS Suboptimal sleep | 46% | 37.7% | nsb |

Values expressed as mean ± SD. Comparison between groups (seasonal AR with vs without asthma) using [a]t test and [b]Fisher's exact test. *$p \leq 0.05$; **$p \leq 0.01$; ns: not significant

duration, and severity of rhinitis on the psychiatric evaluation. Forty-one patients with seasonal and perennial AR and 36 healthy control subjects were enrolled in the study but differences between seasonal and perennial AR patients were not significant. However, severity was positively correlated with anxiety, whereas negatively correlated with the score of satisfaction with the life scale. Actually, a previous study evaluating severity and duration of AR in 3052 patients concluded that the impact that AR severity had on quality of life was more significant than was the duration (intermittent vs persistent) of the disease; 80% of the patients with the severe forms reported impairment in their activities due to the disease, compared with only 40% of those with mild forms [31].

Interestingly, several studies have shown the effect of stress not only in the exacerbation of allergy symptoms but in the development of both asthma and rhinitis. Wright et al. found that, in children predisposed to asthma, increased stress in early childhood was associated with an atopic immune profile [32]. Kilpelainen et al. observed that concomitant parental and personal conflicts increased the risk of asthma (OR 1.72, 95% CI 1.10–2.69) when adjusted by parental asthma, education and passive smoking. However, asthma and atopic dermatitis but not AR, were related to excess of stressful life events [33]. Finally, Rod et al. showed that perceived stress was associated with atopic disorders in a dose-dependent manner. High stress was associated with higher risk of allergic rhinitis (OR 1.64; 95% CI 0.99–2.72), asthma incidence (OR 2.32; 95% CI 1.47–3.65) and first-time asthma hospitalization (HR 2.01; 95% CI 1.41–2.86) among others [34].

Co-morbidities have shown to play a role in AR-related quality of life. However, in our study frequent co-morbidities such as asthma or conjunctivitis had a low impact on the studied outcomes. Conjunctivitis had no effect in any of the tested variables in any group. Asthma was related with higher scores for anxiety/depression and impairment of quality of sleep, but exclusively in seasonal AR. Although the acuteness of asthma symptoms appearance during pollen season may explain their impact only in seasonal AR, whether asthma symptoms were present exclusively during pollen season was not collected. A previous study showed that AR had a more detrimental impact on QoL in patients with comorbid asthma than in patients without asthma, and it was even more important in severe asthma [35]. On the other hand, Colas et al. [2.] found that asthma was related with worse quality of sleep only in moderate AR, but not in mild or severe AR. Another study of 524 patients with intermittent and persistent AR showed that the effect of AR on the psychological profile of patients was independent of age and gender, but it was significantly associated with comorbid asthma [36]. Slattery et al. described that anxiety was associated with asthma and AR, and having both asthma and AR strengthened the association compared to having either disorder alone [37].

However, the relationship between asthma and psychological disorders has been established regardless of AR presence. Mancuso et al. [38] demonstrated that 45% of the 230 asthmatic patients evaluated were positive for depressive symptoms and that these patients reported worse health-related quality of life than asthma patients with similar disease activity but fewer depressive symptoms. Other authors [39] found significant differences in somatization, obsessive–compulsive, depression, and anxiety among patients with a history of eczema or asthma compared with patients who did not have such a history. Collectively, all these findings suggest that asthma may exert an independent effect on the psychological status of patients with AR and show the importance of assessing and treating all AR patients for asthma and for other common chronic comorbid conditions.

This study has some limitations. Patients in the "seasonal group" were recruited at visit 1 (during pollen season) only if they had symptoms (inclusion criteria). Although all patients were symptomatic, at visit 1 some patients may have had symptoms longer than others and this could affect their impact on anxiety, depression, quality of sleep and life. Another limitation is that we did not consider the effect of disease control on the studied variables; uncontrolled AR may have greater impact on anxiety/depression or sleep quality than a well-controlled disease. Finally, we did not use healthy individuals as control group and we used seasonal AR patients out of pollen season instead. Probably, the comparison of seasonal and perennial AR patients with a real control population would be indicative of the real anxious/depressive background of those patients.

In conclusion, AR symptoms have a great impact on quality of life, quality of sleep, and depression and anxiety symptoms in all AR patients. However, individuals with perennial and severe symptoms seem to suffer more intensely their effects.

## Abbreviations
AR: allergic rhinitis; HAD: Hospital Anxiety and Depression Scale; HRQoL: health-related quality of life; MOS: Medical Outcomes Study Sleep Scale; QoL: quality of life.

## Authors' contributions
PR, GA and EG design the study and performed the data analysis. RMC, JSL and AVS also designed the study, developed the methodology and wrote the manuscript. All authors participated in the critical revision of the article and the final approval of the version to be published. All authors read and approved the final manuscript.

## Author details
[1] Allergy Unit, Pneumology Department, Hospital Clinic, Universitat de Barcelona, ARADyAL, Barcelona, Spain. [2] Institut d'Investigacions Biomèdiques August Pi i Sunyer, IDIBAPS, Barcelona, Spain. [3] Allergy Unit, Pneumology Department, Hospital Clinic, Universitat de Barcelona, CIBERES, Barcelona, Spain. [4] Grupo SANED, Barcelona, Spain. [5] Laboratorios LETI SL, Barcelona, Spain.

## Acknowledgements
The study was carried out within the project "ANIMO" thanks to the effort of Cesar Alias Tuduri, Gonzalo Bernaola Hortigüela, Francisco Javier Carballada Gonzalez, Juan Chincoa Gallardo, Jose Antonio Compaired Villa, Nuri Cortes Alvarez, Mari Dias Da Costa, Monica Donado Nortes, Jose Maria Duque San Juan, Susana Duran Macarro, Jose Luis Eseverri Asin, Gaspar Gala Ortiz, Ignacio Garcia Nuñez, Vanesa Gonzalez Nuñez, Miguel Herrerias Peña, Ignacio Jauregui Presa, Joaquin Martin Lazaro, Victoria Moreno Garcia, Pilar Muñoz Garcia, Ramon Nuñez García, Agustin Orovitg Cardona, Rafael Pamies Espinosa, Gustavo Perdomo Gutierrez, Mª Jose Pereira Gonzalez, Celsa Perez Carral, Lucia Rodriguez Ferran, Nuria Rubira Garcia, Maria Rueda Garcia, Noemi Sainz Cordero, Lorena C. Soto Retes, Lucia Valverde Vazquez, Monica Venturini Diaz, Ferran Gomez Tornero, Idoia Gonzalez Mahave, Francisco Alvarez Berciano, Julian Lopez Caballero, German Sanchez Lopez, Eduardo Arcala Campillo, Manuel Alcantara Villar, Lourdes Fernandez Vieira, Iran Sanchez Ramos, Gloria Maria Aloy Pallares, Jose Alberto Martos Velasco, Mª Mercedes Fuentes Cuesta, Mª Dolores Herrero Gil, Elena De Dios Oran, Joaquin Broto Sumalla, Ferran Ballesteros Alonso.

## Competing interests
JSL works for Laboratorios Leti that funded this study. The other authors declare that they have no competing interests.

## Funding
This work was supported by the Laboratorios Leti.

## References
1. Colás C, Brosa M, Antón E, Montoro J, Navarro A, Dordal MT, et al. Estimate of the total costs of allergic rhinitis in specialized care based on real-world data: the FERIN study. Allergy. 2017;6:959–66.
2. Colás C, Galera H, Añibarro B, Soler R, Navarro A, Jáuregui I, et al. Disease severity impairs sleep quality in allergic rhinitis (the SOMNIAAR study). Clin Exp Allergy. 2012;42:1080–7.
3. Valero A, Muñoz-Cano R, Sastre J, Navarro AM, Martí-Guadaño E, Dávila I, et al. The impact of allergic rhinitis on symptoms, and quality of life using the new criterion of ARIA severity classification. Rhinology. 2012;50:33–6.
4. Valero A, Izquierdo I, Sastre J, Navarro AM, Baró E, Martí-Guadaño E, et al. ESPRINT-15 questionnaire (Spanish version): reference values according to disease severity using both the original and the modified ARIA classifications. J Investig Allergol Clin Immunol. 2013;23:14–9.
5. Gamboa PM. The epidemiology of drug allergy-related consultations in Spanish Allergology services: Alergológica-2005. J Investig Allergol Clin Immunol. 2009;19(Suppl 2):45–50.
6. Davies MJ, Fisher LH, Chegini S, Craig TJ. A practical approach to allergic rhinitis and sleep disturbance management. Allergy Asthma Proc. 2006;27:224–30.
7. Jáuregui I, Mullol J, Dávila I, Ferrer M, Bartra J, del Cuvillo A, et al. Allergic rhinitis and school performance. J Investig Allergol Clin Immunol. 2009;19(Suppl 1):32–9.
8. de la Hoz Caballer B, Rodríguez M, Fraj J, Cerecedo I, Antolín-Amérigo D, Colás C. Allergic rhinitis and its impact on work productivity in primary care practice and a comparison with other common diseases: the cross-sectional study to evAluate work Productivity in allergic Rhinitis compared with other common dIseases (CAPRI) study. Am J Rhinol Allergy. 2012;26:390–4.

9. Peroni DG, Piacentini GL, Alfonsi L, Zerman L, Di Blasi P, Visona G, et al. Rhinitis in pre-school children: prevalence, association with allergic diseases and risk factors. Clin Exp Allergy. 2003;33:1349–54.

10. Stuck BA, Hummel T. Olfaction in allergic rhinitis: a systematic review. J. Allergy Clin Immunol. 2015;136:1460–70.

11. González-Núñez V, Valero AL, Mullol J. Impact of sleep as a specific marker of quality of life in allergic rhinitis. Curr Allergy Asthma Rep. 2013;13:131–41.

12. Thompson A, Sardana N, Craig TJ. Sleep impairment and daytime sleepiness in patients with allergic rhinitis: the role of congestion and inflammation. Ann Allergy Asthma Immunol. 2013;111:446–51.

13. Ferguson BJ. Influences of allergic rhinitis on sleep. Ctolaryngol Head Neck Surg. 2004;130:617–29.

14. Berson SR, Klimczak J, Prezio EA, Hu S, Abraham M. Clinical associations between allergies and rapid eye movement sleep disturbances. Int Forum Allergy Rhinol (Published Online First: 20 February 2018). https://doi.org/10.1002/alr.22099.

15. Patten SB, Williams JVA. Self-reported allergies and their relationship to several axis I disorders in a community sample. Int J Psychiatry Med. 2007;37:11–22.

16. Cuffel B, Wamboldt M, Borish L, Kennedy S, Crystal-Peters J. Economic consequences of comorbid depression, anxiety, and allergic rhinitis. Psychosomatics. 1999;40:491–6.

17. Wamboldt MZ, Hewitt JK, Schmitz S, Wamboldt FS, Räsänen M, Koskenvuo M, et al. Familial association between allergic disorders and depression in adult Finnish twins. Am J Med Genet. 2000;96:146–53.

18. Delgado J, Dávila ID, Domínguez-Ortega J, Quirce S, Martí-Guadaño E, Valero A. Quality of life in patients with respiratory allergy is influenced by the causative allergen. J Investig Allergol Clin Immunol. 2013;23:309–14.

19. Zigmond AS, Snaith RP. The Hospital Anxiety and Depression Scale. Acta Psychiatr Scand. 1983;67:361–70.

20. Tejero A, Guimerá EM, Farré JMPJ. Uso clínico del HAD (Hospital Anxiety and Depression Scale) en población psiquiátrica: un estudio de su sensibilidad, fiabilidad y validez. Rev Depto Psiquiatr Fac Med Barna. 1986;13:233–8.

21. Hay R, Stewart A. Measuring functioning and well-being: the Medical Outcomes Study approach. In: Sleep measures. Duke University Press, Durham. 1992: 235–259.

22. Rejas J, Ribera MV, Ruiz MMX. Psychometric properties of the MOS (Medical Outcomes Study) Sleep Scale in patients with neuropathic pain. Eur J Pain. 2007;11:329–40.

23. ESPRINT Study Group and Investigators, Valero A, Alcnso J, Antepara I, Baró E, Colas C, et al. Development and validation of a new Spanish instrument to measure health-related quality of life in patients with allergic rhinitis: the ESPRINT questionnaire. Value Health. 2007;10:466–77.

24. Valero A, Alonso J, Antépara I, Baró E, Colás C, del Cuvillo A, et al. Health-related quality of life in allergic rhinitis: comparing the short form ESPRINT-15 and MiniRQLQ questionnaires. Allergy. 2007;62:1372–8.

25. Valero A, Ferrer M, Sastre J, Navarro AM, Monclús L, Martí-Guadaño E, et al. A new criterion by which to discriminate between patients with moderate allergic rhinitis and patients with severe allergic rhinitis based on the allergic rhinitis and its impact on asthma severity items. J Allergy Clin Immunol. 2007;120:359–65.

26. Leger D, Bonnefoy B, Pigearias B, de La Giclais B, Chartier A. Poor sleep is highly associated with house dust mite allergic rhinitis in adults and children. Allergy Asthma Clin Immunol. 2017;13:36.

27. Hu Y, Sieck DE, Hsu WH. Why are second-generation H1-antihistamines minimally sedating? Eur J Pharmacol. 2015;765:100–6.

28. Valero A, Quirce S, Dávila I, Delgado J, Domínguez-Ortega J. Allergic respiratory disease: different allergens, different symptoms. Allergy. 2017;72:1306–16.

29. Bavbek S, Kumbasar H, Tuğcu H, Misirligil Z. Psychological status of patients with seasonal and perennial allergic rhinitis. J Investig Allergol Clin Immunol. 2002;12:204–10.

30. Valero A, Baró E, Sastre J, Navarro-Pulido AM, Izquierdo I, Martí-Guadaño E, et al. Reference values for facilitating the interpretation of the ESPRINT-15 questionnaire (Spanish version). J Investig Allergol Clin Immunol. 2009;19:396–403.

31. Bousquet J, Neukirch F, Bousquet P, Gehano P, Klossek J, Legal M, et al. Severity and impairment of allergic rhinitis in patients consulting in primary care. J Allergy Clin Immunol. 2006;117:158–62.

32. Wright RJ, Finn P, Contreras JP, Cohen S, Wright RO, Staudenmayer J, et al. Chronic caregiver stress and IgE expression, allergen-induced proliferation, and cytokine profiles in a birth cohort predisposed to atopy. J Allergy Clin Immunol. 2004;113:1051–7.

33. Kilpeläinen M, Koskenvuo M, Helenius H, Terho EO. Stressful life events promote the manifestation of asthma and atopic diseases. Clin Exp Allergy. 2002;32:256–63.

34. Rod NH, Kristensen TS, Lange P, Prescott E, Diderichsen F. Perceived stress and risk of adult-onset asthma and other atopic disorders: a longitudinal cohort study. Allergy. 2012;67:1408–14.

35. Mullol J. A survey of the burden of allergic rhinitis in Spain. J Investig Allergol Clin Immunol. 2009;19:27–34.

36. Xi L, Zhang Y, Han D, Zhang L. Effect of asthma, aeroallergen category, and gender on the psychological status of patients with allergic rhinitis. J Investig Allergol Clin Immunol. 2012;22:264–9.

37. Slattery MJ, Essex MJ. Specificity in the association of anxiety, depression, and atopic disorders in a community sample of adolescents. J Psychiatr Res. 2011;45:788–95.

38. Mancuso CA, Peterson MG, Charlson ME. Effects of depressive symptoms on health-related quality of life in asthma patients. J Gen Intern Med. 2000;15:301–10.

39. Lv X, Xi L, Han D, Zhang L. Evaluation of the psychological status in seasonal allergic rhinitis patients. ORL. 2010;72:84–90.

# 20

# Anti-IgE therapy for IgE-mediated allergic diseases: from neutralizing IgE antibodies to eliminating IgE⁺ B cells

Jiayun Hu[1,2†], Jiajie Chen[1†], Lanlan Ye[1], Zelang Cai[1], Jinlu Sun[2*] and Kunmei Ji[1*]

**Abstract**

Allergic diseases are inflammatory disorders that involve many types of cells and factors, including allergens, immunoglobulin (Ig)E, mast cells, basophils, cytokines and soluble mediators. Among them, IgE plays a vital role in the development of acute allergic reactions and chronic inflammatory allergic diseases, making its control particularly important in the treatment of IgE-mediated allergic diseases. This review provides an overview of the current state of IgE targeted therapy development, focusing on three areas of translational research: IgE neutralization in blood; IgE-effector cell elimination; and IgE⁺ B cell reduction. IgE-targeted medicines such as FDA approved drug Xolair (Omalizumab) represent a promising avenue for treating IgE-mediated allergic diseases given the pernicious role of IgE in disease progression. Additionally, targeted therapy for IgE-mediated allergic diseases may be advanced through cellular treatments, including the modification of effector cells.

**Keywords:** Anti-IgE therapy, Allergic diseases, IgE⁺ B cells, IgE neutralization

## Background

The incidence of allergic diseases has been rising with increasing industrialization and the accompanying changes to the environment and people's lifestyles. According to a 30-nation/region epidemiological investigation conducted by the World Allergy Organization (WAO) Specialty and Training Council, approximately 250 million (22%) of the 1.2 billion people in those regions suffered from allergic diseases, such as allergic rhinitis, allergic asthma, allergic conjunctivitis, eczema, food allergies and drug allergies etc. [1]. Meanwhile, according to the World Health Organization (WHO), the international incidence of asthma specifically has increased from 150 million people in 2005 to 300 million by 2012 [2]. In their White Book on Allergy, the WAO projects the asthma incidence number to reach

400 million by 2025 and estimates that asthma is lethal in about 250 thousand patients per year [3]. Because of their high prevalence and high recurrence rate, allergic diseases pose a serious financial burden for affected households and consume substantial resources in socialized healthcare systems. Thus, the WHO has designated allergic diseases as one of the top disease classes requiring major research and prevention measures in the 21st century [4].

## IgE is a key molecular in the development of IgE-mediated allergic diseases

The mechanism of allergic diseases is complex. In clinical practice, allergic diseases could be divided into two categories: IgE mediated and non-IgE mediated. Allergic disorders are characterized by inflammatory responses involving many types of cells, including mast cells and basophils, and various biological molecules, including cytokines (e.g. interleukin 4) and soluble mediators (e.g. histamine) [5]. IgE, an antibody class found only in mammals, has unique properties and plays a central role in IgE-mediated allergic diseases. Typically, it is the least abundant Ig isotype, with a concentration of about

*Correspondence: sunjinlv@pumch.cn; jkm@szu.edu.cn
†Jiayun Hu and Jiajie Chen have contributed equally to this work
¹ Department of Biochemistry and Molecular Biology, School of Medicine of Shenzhen University, Shenzhen 518035, China
² Department of Allergy, Peking Union Medical College Hospital, Peking Union Medical College and Chinese Academy of Medical Sciences, Beijing 100730, China

150 ng/ml, compared with 10 mg/ml for IgG in the circulation of healthy individuals [6]. The half-life of IgE in serum is about 3 days, compared with 20 days for IgG, but its lifespan can be extended to 2 weeks in skin tissue [6]. Specific IgEs are upregulated in response to exposure to specific allergens. There are two types of IgE molecules: free IgE produced by plasma cells and membrane-bound IgE maintained on the surface membranes of B cells through class switching [7].

### IgE structure and properties
IgE shares the same basic molecular structure of other Igs, with two identical heavy chains and two identical light chains. However, the heavy ε-chain of IgE contains one more domain than the heavy γ-chain of IgG. The Cε3 and Cε4 domains of IgE are sequence homologous and structurally similar to the Cγ2 and Cγ3 domains of IgG; two Cε2 domains, which are the most obvious distinguishing feature of IgE, are present in place of the flexible hinge region found in IgG [8–10]. The Cε2 domains fold back and make contact with the Cε3 and Cε4 domains, perhaps acting as a spacer region between the Fab (antigen-binding fragment) arms and Fc (crystallizable fragment) region, and the compact, bent Cε2 domains provide considerable flexibility in the conformation of IgE [7].

IgE is a glycoprotein with a molecular mass of 190 KD and a sedimentation coefficient of 8S [11]. It is non-thermostable, losing its binding ability after 4 h at 56 °C [12]. The normal range of serum IgE levels is 50–300 ng/mL, markedly lower than typical IgG levels (~ 10 mg/ml) [13]. Serum IgE concentration can fluctuate dramatically. Patients with an allergic disease may have tenfold higher than normal serum IgE levels, and patients with a parasitic or fungal infection can be 1000-fold higher than normal [14]. The half-life of free IgE in the blood is short of ~ 3 days, which makes neutralizing therapy challenging. However, cell surface-bound IgE on basophils, mast cells, and dendritic cells can extend their activity to several weeks, or even several months [6]. When divalent or polyvalent antigens bind cell-surface IgE, they can induce the release of intracellular bioactive substances in the presence of $Ca^{2+}$, thereby triggering an allergic reaction [15].

### IgE plays a critical role in the development of allergic diseases
IgE plays a key role in mediating the initiation and development of allergic diseases. The IgE molecule performs its biological function by binding its receptors on target cells, activating the induction immunomodulatory and protecting against parasitic worms (helminths) and the expulsion of environmental substances that include

toxins, venoms, irritants and xenobiotics [12]. When the body encounters an allergen for the first time, IgM molecules in B cells are converted by class switching to IgE molecules [5]. Then, specific B cells initiate an IgE response, during which IgE[+] B cells start to secrete free IgE into the blood where it can bind the high-affinity IgE receptor FcεR I on mast cells or basophils [16]. This response sensitizes the organism so that when it re-encounters the allergen, the allergen molecules are bound by specific IgE molecules on the surface of mast cells, causing them to undergo degranulation and to synthesize and release large quantities of allergic mediators (i.e., histamine, leukotriene, and platelet-activating factor), which then produce a local or systemic allergic reaction [17]. Apart from binding FcεRI on mast cells and basophils, IgE can also bind its low-affinity receptor FcεRII, which is expressed by B cells and monocytes [18]. Surface receptors on B cells enable them to take in bound allergens, process them, and present them to T cells, priming subsequent targeted innate immunity responses to the allergen in the future [19]. Anti-IgE therapy can reduce IgE receptor expression on effector cells; because IgE is a positive regulator of both FcεRI and FcεRII, reduced IgE results in reduced IgE receptor expression as well [20, 21]. With co-stimulation of CD79A (Ig-α) and CD79B (Ig-β), membrane-anchored IgE can also trigger the proliferation and differentiation of B cells [22].

## IgE targeted therapy for allergic diseases
There is great interest in the development of new drugs or methods that would alleviate allergic diseases by affecting molecular IgE activities in a manner that is safe, effective, and convenient (Table 1).

### Methods for neutralizing IgE in blood
IgE is an important target for allergic disease therapy. The main method of IgE neutralization being pursued involves achieving specific binding and neutralization of free IgE in serum to prevent it from binding receptors on target cells, thereby inhibiting allergen-induced early/late allergic reactions (Fig. 1).

#### Immunoadsorption
Immunoadsorption (IA), also called immune apheresis, has been adopted as an effective treatment for autoantibody-mediated diseases [23]. IA utilizes plasmapheresis to remove immunoglobulin and immune complexes and in cytapheresis, immune cells from the circulation [23]. Accordingly, IA could be successfully applied in patients with severe atopic dermatitis and high total serum IgE levels [24–27]. An IgE-specific adsorber, called IgEnio, has been developed [28]. The pilot study indicates that

**Table 1  Therapies to treat IgE-mediated allergic diseases**

|  | Therapy | Type | Mechanism | Phase | References |
|---|---|---|---|---|---|
| Serum IgEneutral-izization | Immuno adsorption | Plasma-pheresis | Removal of Ig and immune complex from blood | Marketed | Schmidt [23] |
|  | Omalizumab | Monoclonal antibody | Bind Cε3 domain in heavy chain Fc of free IgE | Marketed | Chang [32] |
|  | CMAB007 | Biosimilar of omalizumab | Bind Cε3 domain in heavy chain Fc of free IgE | Phase III Local license | Bo Zhou [37] |
|  | Ligelizumab | Monoclonal antibody | Target Cε3 domain of IgE | Phase II NCT01703312 | Gauvreau [38] |
|  | MEDI4212 | Monoclonal antibody | Bind Cε3/Cε4 domain of IgE | Phase I NCT01544348 | Sheldon [41] |
|  | Recombinant ScFv | Single-chain antibody | Identify IgE, IgE-bound cells, and IgE-secreting cells | Preclinical | Lupinek [43] |
| IgE-effector cells | Anti-FcεRI Fab-conjugated celastrol-loaded micelles | Polymer | Prevent IgE interaction with mast cells, and kill mast cells | Preclinical | Peng [48] |
|  | CTLA4Fcε | Fusion protein | Bind IgE receptors, FcεRI and FcεRII/CD23 | Preclinical | Perez-Witzke [51] |
| IgE + B cells | Quilizumab | Monoclonal antibody | Target CεmX of IgE⁺ B cells | Phase II NCT01582503 | Harris [59] |
|  | Bsc-IgE/CD3 | Monoclonal antibody | Eliminate IgE⁺ target cells by redirected T cells | Preclinical | Talay [61] |
|  | XmAb7195 | Monoclonal antibody | Form complex with B cell IgE receptors and FcγRII β | Phase I NCT02148744 | Chu [66] |

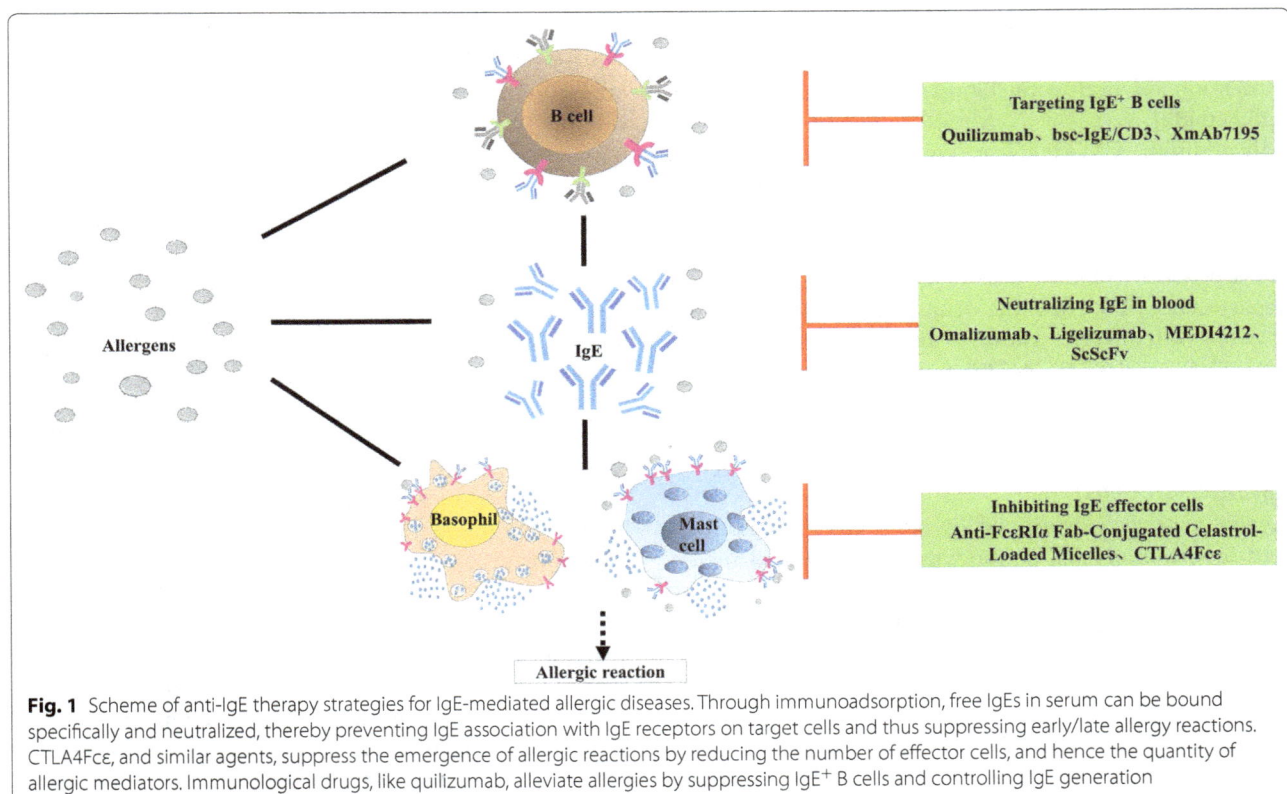

**Fig. 1** Scheme of anti-IgE therapy strategies for IgE-mediated allergic diseases. Through immunoadsorption, free IgEs in serum can be bound specifically and neutralized, thereby preventing IgE association with IgE receptors on target cells and thus suppressing early/late allergy reactions. CTLA4Fcε, and similar agents, suppress the emergence of allergic reactions by reducing the number of effector cells, and hence the quantity of allergic mediators. Immunological drugs, like quilizumab, alleviate allergies by suppressing IgE⁺ B cells and controlling IgE generation

IgEnio may be used to treat pollen-induce allergic asthma [28].

## Omalizumab

Omalizumab, developed by Novartis®, is a recombinant humanized monoclonal antibody against IgE [29]. It binds selectively to the Cε3 domain of the Fc fragment on the heavy chain of free IgE, reducing IgE availability significantly [30]. Because the Cε3 domain mediates IgE binding with the α chain of IgE receptors, omalizumab interferes with IgE-FcεRI interaction, thereby preventing mast cell/basophil degranulation and, ultimately, reducing the activation of inflammatory cells and the release of pro-inflammatory factors [31]. In addition, IgE binding of FcεRII on B cells supports antigen capture and Th2 activation. Thus, omalizumab can block IgE-mediated antigen-presenting processes and inhibit Th2 amplification of inflammatory reactions [32].

However, omalizumab is associated with safety concerns. Because it cannot reduce IgE levels quickly, it requires a long (several weeks), continuous treatment cycle [33]. The US Food and Drug Administration (FDA) warns that long-term use of omalizumab increases the risk of arterial thrombosis slightly and can have negative impacts on cardiac and cerebral circulation [34]. Because the long-term regime is costly, omalizumab is recommended primarily for severe asthma cases [35]. Besides, treatment with omalizumab for patients with chronic spontaneous urticaria resulted in clinical benefits after 12 weeks treatment since the levels of FcεRI and IgE expression on peripheral blood basophils were rapidly reduced [36].

In addition, CMAB007, a biosimilar of omalizumab, was developed by National Engineering Research Center of Antibody Medicine of China. It has the same amino acid sequence as omalizumab and have been finished phase III clinical trial in China approval by local departments [37]. Now, the drug CMAB007 for treating patients with allergic asthma is under large-scale clinical trials (NCT03468790) in China, which is a multi-centre, randomized, double-blind, placebo-controlled phase III study.

## Ligelizumab (QGE031)

Ligelizumab, also developed by Novartis®, is a humanized IgG$_1$ monoclonal antibodytargeting the Cε3 region of IgE [38]. Like omalizumab, ligelizumab inhibits the binding of free IgE to mast cells and basophils, thereby blocking the allergic reaction cascade and yielding clinical benefits to patients suffering from IgE-mediated allergic diseases.

Phase II clinical trials investigating the pharmacokinetics, pharmacodynamics, and safety of ligelizumab showed that it can decrease IgE levels more effectively than omalizumab via inhibition of IgE-FcεRI binding and that it can produce better outcomes, as indicated by skin prick allergen test responses [38, 39]. Hence, ligelizumab has the potential to be a good anti-IgE drug for allergy therapy.

## MEDI4212

MEDI4212, a humanized IgG1λ monoclonal antibody generated by phage display technology, neutralizes free IgE by binding selectively to the Cε3 and Cε4 domains of IgE [40]. The affinity of MEDI4212 to human IgE was demonstrated to be 1.95 pM in vitro, which is one hundred times higher than that of omalizumab [40]. Because the Cε3 region is crucial for IgE interaction with its receptors, MEDI4212 inhibits the binding of IgE with FcεRI/FcεRII.

A phase I clinical trial (NCT01544348) showed that MEDI4212 is more effective than omalizumab in reducing serum IgE levels inpatients with IgE levels $\geq$ 30 IU/ mL and that MEDI4212 treatment reduces FcεRI expression on dendritic cells and basophils [41]. However, pharmacokinetic analysis showed that MEDI4212 is removed rapidly in vivo, making long-term intake likely necessary for maintenance of IgE suppression [41].

The MEDI4121 may be mutagenized to improve the drug's pharmacokinetic properties. A variant of MEDI4121 in which the Fc fragment was altered to enhance affinity for FcγRIIIa, which down-regulates IgE expression by B cells before they have differentiated into IgE secreting plasma cells [42]. Therefore, MEDI4121 variants are new immunotherapeutic candidates for both IgE neutralization and IgE$^+$ B cell elimination.

## Recombinant single-chain variable-fragment (ScFv) antibody

Recombinant ScFv is produced by cDNA encoding the heavy and light Ig chains. Biosensor-based studies have demonstrated that recombinant ScFv binds human IgE rapidly and efficiently (affinity, $1.52 \times 10^{-10}$ M) [43]. It can bind cell-bound IgE (i.e., IgE$^+$ B cells) as well as free IgE in vivo [43]. In vitro experiments showed that recombinant ScFv does not crosslink with IgE$^+$ effector cells or trigger basophil/mast cell degranulation. Recombinant ScFv can also be used to probe IgE activities under both healthy and disease conditions, making it a helpful drug development tool.

## IgE effector cell inhibition

Immune effector cells, including mast cells, basophils, eosinophils, which are critical for the elimination of foreign substances and antigens, are the main sources pro-inflammatory factors. In particular, mast cells are the key cells that induce allergic asthma, and the number of mast cells in asthmatic patients is elevated significantly [44, 45]. After stimulation of allergens, mast cells secrete the autacoid mediators histamine, prostaglandin (PG) D2, and leukotriene (LT) C4, which are capable of inducing bronchoconstriction, mucus secretion, and mucosal edema, all features of asthma [44, 45]. Basophils degranulate for immediate release of histamine, rapidly generate LTC4, and produce Th2 cytokines provides the mechanistic basis whereby basophils can cause immediate hypersensitivity clinical symptoms [46]. The increased number of basophils are common during anaphylactic reaction [46]. Thus, reducing the number of effector cells reduces the material basis of anaphylaxis and can inhibit the fundamental development of allergic reactions.

### Anti-FcεRI Fab-conjugated celastrol-loaded polymeric micelles

Celastrol is bioactive compound extracted from *Tripterygium wilfordii* (Thunder god vine) that can induce T cells apoptosis [47]. Thus, targeting celastrol specifically to mast cells in a manner that also reduces its toxicity is an attractive potential avenue for allergic disease treatment. This approach has been pursued by cross-linking celastrol with anti-FcεRI Fab, which has been shown to induce mast cell apoptosis, eliminating with them their pro-inflammatory factor cargo, and to limit celastrol toxicity [48]. Treatment of allergic asthma model mice with anti-FcεRIα Fab-conjugated polymeric micelles was shown to reduce secretion of inflammatory factors and eosinophil infiltration rapidly and to lead to remission of symptoms of ovalbumin-induced allergic inflammation symptoms [48]. The ability of anti-FcεRIα Fab-conjugated celastrol-loaded polymeric micelles to both block IgE binding of mast cells and induce mast cell apoptosis makes it a very attractive medicine for type I allergic diseases as well as for other mast cell-related diseases.

Anti-FcεRIα Fab-conjugated polymeric micelles have been shown to reduce allergic reactions more efficiently than omalizumab [48]. The following biochemical factors may underlie this favorable efficacy: (1) extension of pharmacokinetics by polymeric micelles; (2) promotion of drug aggregation in target tissues and target cells; and (3) competitive binding with FcεRI on the surface of mast cells resulting in reduced mast cell degranulation.

### Synthetic cytotoxic T-lymphocyte-associated protein 4 (CTLA4) fused with Fcε

CTLA4 (a.k.a., CD152) is a protein receptor that, functioning as an immune checkpoint, down-regulates immune responses. It is constitutively expressed in CD4+CD25+ Foxp3+regulatory T cells, but is upregulated only in conventional T cellsupon activation. CTLA4 is homologous to the T cell co-stimulatory proteinCD28,

and both molecules bind CD80(B7-1) and CD86(B7-2) on antigen-presenting cells [49]. It binds CD80 and CD86 with greater affinity and avidity than does CD28, thus enabling it to outcompete CD28 for its ligands [50]. CTLA4 transmits an inhibitory signal to T cells, whereas CD28 transmits a stimulatory signal [50].

Researchers have constructed a fusion protein containing the CD80/CD86-binding domain of CTLA-4 and the Fcε receptor-binding domain of the IgE H chain [51]. This recombinant protein binds both FcεRI/FcεRII and CTLA-4 receptors (i.e., CD80 and CD86), thereby suppressing Th2 responses. CTLA4 Fcε and CD23-CD80/CD86 combine to form a multi-molecule polymer, which acts as a spacer to influence production of soluble CD23. In an experiment involving human peripheral blood mononuclear cell samples stimulated in vitro, CTLA4 Fcε reduced the rate of lymphocyte proliferation in the presence of the lectin concanavalin A; in the same experiment, CTLA4 Fcε was also shown to bind IgE receptors on effector cells, thereby influencing soluble CD23 biosynthesis and inhibiting lymphocyte proliferation [51]. Given its demonstrated ability to affect IgE levels and the generation of IgE-secreting cells, the recombinant fusion protein CTLA4Fcε may be an effective medicine for controlling IgE-mediated immunodeficiency and other related diseases [51].

### Targeting IgE+ B cells

IgE+ B cells are critical for controlling IgE production. Both transient IgE secreted by plasma blasts in blood and long-living IgE secreted by plasma cells in bone marrow are influenced by IgE+ B cells [52].

### Quilizumab (h47H4)

Membrane-bound IgE on the surface of B lymphocytes is of great importance for IgE production. It has an extra 52-amino acid-long CεmX-containing fragment between the CH4 domain of IgE and its B-cell membrane-anchoring segment [52, 53]. CεmX is the antigen-binding site of IgE-synthesis committed B cells [54, 55]. CεmX is both target-specific and cell-specific, making it a very suitable drug target.

Quilizumab, developed by Genentech®, is a new artificial monoclonal antibody that targets CεmX on IgE+ B cells. It produces crosslinking of membrane-bound IgE antigen receptors on B cells, which induces IgE+ B cell apoptosis, thereby reducing free IgE levels and inhibiting the generation of IgE+ B cells [56, 57]. Because the half-life of free IgE is quite short, this drug represents an efficient means with which to reduce IgE by eliminating the cells that express membrane IgE [58].

A phase II clinical trial showed that quilizumab is an effective candidate for treating allergic diseases safely and with high specificity [59]. Quilizumab was shown to lower total IgE and specific IgE levels in the serum of patients with asthma, and this effect lasted for 6 months [59]. It is hoped that quilizumab will be useful for the treatment and prevention of some IgE-mediated diseases, especially those for which there are no current medicines available [60]. However, quilizumab treatment did not produce a clinically meaningful benefit in allergic asthma patients inadequately controlled by standard therapy, despite its high ability in reducing serum IgE levels and the good tolerability profile [59].

### Bispecific (bsc) IgE-CD3 antibody

There are several types of IgE+ B cells, including plasma blasts, plasma cells, and IgE+ memory B cells [61]. The earliest experiment aimed at eliminating IgE+ B cells specifically sought to modify T-cell receptors in combination with anti-IgE monoclonal antibody activity [62]. The bsc-IgE/CD3 antibody is an artificially modified targeting antibody specific for both IgE and CD3. It binds specifically to cells that express membrane-bound IgE and can re-direct the cytotoxicity of prestimulated human T cells toward IgE+ B cells, at least in vitro, without causing degranulation of mast cells or release of free IgE. Bsc-IgE/CD3 is an antibody that could eliminate both IgE+ B cells and free IgE in serum [63]. Therefore, bsc-IgE/CD3 is a new class candidate medicine for IgE-mediated allergic diseases.

### XmAb7195

FcγRIIβ is involved in B-cell homeostasis and FcγRIIβ abnormalities lead to autoimmune diseases [64]. A novel antibody known as XmAb7195 was produced by humanization, affinity maturation, and Fc engineering using a murine anti-IgE antibody as template [65]. XmAb7195 can isolate free IgE in serum, forming immune complexes with FcγRIIβ and IgE receptors on B cells that impede the formation of IgE+ B cells and reduce free and total IgE levels without affecting the antigen isotypes of other B cells [66]. Because it has the added ability of binding FcγRIIβ, XmAb7195 can inhibit IgE+ B cell differentiation, thereby reducing the number of IgE secreting plasma cells [65]. This reliable double mechanism can be utilized to reduce total IgE levels, while the remaining free IgE can be targeted continuously and effectively. A phase I clinical trial (NCT02148744) showed that XmAb7195 is more efficient at reducing IgE activity than omalizumab [65].

### Prospective

As so far, Omalizumab is the only FDA-approved recombinant humanized monoclonal antibody that neutralizes IgE to treat allergic diseases [67]. Its use is supported by a large number of clinical trials demonstrating its effectiveness [68]. Other IgE-neutralizing antibodies are being developed with the goal of more effectiveness and less side effects. Medicines that target IgE effector cells and IgE+ B cells are also in development. Apart from targeting medicines, cellular treatments are also being developed. For example, T cells may be modified to bind anti-IgE T cell receptors, thereby reducing the number of IgE+ cells [62].

It is a great progress that another new drug dupilumab (Dupixent ®) was approved by the FDA in April 2017 for the treatment of adult patients with moderate-to-severe atopic dermatitis [69]. Dupilumab is a human monoclonal antibody targeting the interleukin-4 receptor (IL-4R) alpha subunit to block interleukin-4 (IL-4)/IL-13 signaling and to inhibit the inflammatory response that plays a role in the development of atopic dermatitis [70].

IgE-targeting is highly promising for the treatment of allergic diseases. Cellular treatments, including selective modification of effector cells, represent an innovative technology for targeted therapy of allergic diseases [71]. Notwithstanding, there remains a serious concern that reducing patients' IgE response ability can increase their risk of cardiovascular disease [72]. Thus, evaluation of secondary effects of these medications in clinical settings remains vitally important.

### Conclusions

IgE is an important therapeutic target in IgE-mediated allergic diseases. Novel IgE targeted therapies are currently being developed, which focus on IgE neutralization in blood, IgE-effector cell elimination and IgE+ B cell reduction. More IgE-targeted medicines such as FDA approved drug Omalizumab are expected for treating IgE-mediated allergic diseases in the future.

### Authors' contributions
JH wrote the manuscript draft. JC, LY and ZC participated the writing. JS and KJ designed the study and wrote the manuscript. The authors read and approved the final manuscript.

### Acknowledgements
We thank the members of Prof. Ji Lab for his valuable comments on this manuscript.

### Competing interests
The authors declared that they have no competing interests.

**Funding**

This study was supported in part by research funding from the NSFC (No. 81571570), Guangdong Province (Nos. 2014A030313563, 2016A030313039 and 2017A010105014), CAMS Innovation Fund for Medical Sciences (CIFMS: 2016-I2M-1003), Shenzhen City (JCYJ20150626141652681 and 2016 Discipline Construction).

**References**

1. Warner JO, Kaliner MA, Crisci CD, Del Giacco S, Frew AJ, Liu GH, et al. Allergy practice worldwide: a report by the World Allergy Organization Specialty and Training Council. Int Arch Allergy Immunol. 2006;139:166–74.
2. Weinberg EG. The WAO white book on allergy 2011-2012: review article. Curr Allergy Clin Immunol. 2011;24(3):156–7.
3. Pawankar RCG, Holgate ST. Wofld allergy organization (WAO) white book on allergy. Update. 2013;2013:248.
4. Nitin J, Palagani R, Shradha NH, Vaibhav J, Kowshik K, Manoharan R, et al. Prevalence, severity and risk factors of allergic disorders among people in south India. Afr Health Sci. 2016;16:201–9.
5. Navines-Ferrer A, Serrano-Candelas E, Molina-Molina GJ, Martin M. IgE-related chronic diseases and anti-IgE-based treatments. J Immunol Res. 2016;2016:8163803.
6. King CL, Poindexter RW, Ragunathan J, Fleisher TA, Ottesen EA, Nutman TB. Frequency analysis of IgE-secreting B lymphocytes in persons with normal or elevated serum IgE levels. J Immunol. 1991;146:1478–83.
7. McCoy KD, Harris NL, Diener P, Hatak S, Odermatt B, Hangartner L, et al. Natural IgE production in the absence of MHC Class II cognate help. Immunity. 2006;24:329–39.
8. Zheng Y, Shopes B, Holowka D, Baird B. Conformations of IgE bound to its receptor Fc epsilon RI and in solution. Biochemistry. 1991;30:9125–32.
9. Zheng Y, Shopes B, Holowka D, Baird B. Dynamic conformations compared for IgE and IgG1 in solution and bound to receptors. Biochemistry. 1992;31:7446–56.
10. Wan T, Beavil RL, Fabiane SM, Beavil AJ, Sohi MK, Keown M, et al. The crystal structure of IgE Fc reveals an asymmetrically bent conformation. Nat Immunol. 2002;3:681–6.
11. Hnasko RM. The biochemical properties of antibodies and their fragments. Methods Mol Biol. 2015;1318:1–14.
12. Sanjuan MA, Sagar D, Kolbeck R. Role of IgE in autoimmunity. J Allergy Clin Immunol. 2016;137:1651–61.
13. Platts-Mills TA, Snajdr MJ, Ishizaka K, Frankland AW. Measurement of IgE antibody by an antigen-binding assay: correlation with PK activity and IgG and IgA antibodies to allergens. J Immunol. 1978;120:1201–10.
14. Lawrence MG, Woodfolk JA, Schuyler AJ, Stillman LC, Chapman MD, Platts-Mills TA. Half-life of IgE in serum and skin: consequences for anti-IgE therapy in patients with allergic disease. J Allergy Clin Immunol. 2017;139(422–428):e424.
15. Wurzburg BA, Tarchevskaya SS, Jardetzky TS. Structural changes in the lectin domain of CD23, the low-affinity IgE receptor, upon calcium binding. Structure. 2006;14:1049–58.
16. Henault J, Riggs JM, Karnell JL, Liarski VM, Li J, Shirinian L, et al. Self-reactive IgE exacerbates interferon responses associated with autoimmunity. Nat Immunol. 2016;17:196–203.
17. Bang LM, Plosker GL. Spotlight on omalizumab in allergic asthma. BioDrugs. 2004;18(6):415–8.
18. Uermosi C, Zabel F, Manolova V, Bauer M, Beerli RR, Senti G, et al. IgG-mediated down-regulation of IgE bound to mast cells: a potential novel mechanism of allergen-specific desensitization. Allergy. 2014;69:338–47.
19. Greiner AN, Hellings PW, Rotiroti G, Scadding GK. Allergic rhinitis. Lancet. 2011;378:2112–22.
20. MacGlashan DW Jr, Bochner BS, Adelman DC, Jardieu PM, Togias A, McKenzie-White J, et al. Down-regulation of Fc(epsilon)RI expression on human basophils during in vivo treatment of atopic patients with anti-IgE antibody. J Immunol. 1997;158:1438–45.
21. Arock M, Le Goff L, Becherel PA, Dugas B, Debre P, Mossalayi MD. Involvement of Fc epsilon RII/CD23 and L-arginine dependent pathway in IgE-mediated activation of human eosinophils. Biochem Biophys Res Commun. 1994;203:265–71.
22. Davis RE, Ngo VN, Lenz G, Tolar P, Young RM, Romesser PB, et al. Chronic active B-cell-receptor signalling in diffuse large B-cell lymphoma. Nature. 2010;463:88–92.
23. Schmidt E, Zillikens D. Immunoadsorption in dermatology. Arch Dermatol Res. 2010;302:241–53.
24. Meyersburg D, Schmidt E, Kasperkiewicz M, Zillikens D. Immunoadsorption in dermatology. Ther Apheresis Dial. 2012;16:311–20.
25. Bresci G, Romano A, Mazzoni A, Scatena F, Altomare E, Capria A, et al. Feasibility and safety of granulocytapheresis in Crohn's disease: a prospective cohort study. Gastroenterol Clin Biol. 2010;34:682–6.
26. Soerensen H, Schneidewind-Mueller JM, Lange D, Kashiwagi N, Franz M, Yokoyama T, et al. Pilot clinical study of Adacolumn cytapheresis in patients with systemic lupus erythematosus. Rheumatol Int. 2006;26:409–15.
27. Sakai Y, Sakai S, Otsuka T, Ohno D, Murasawa T, Munakata K, et al. Efficacy of high-throughput leukocytapheresis for rheumatoid arthritis with a reduced response to infliximab. Ther Apheresis Dial. 2009;13:179–85.
28. Lupinek C, Derfler K, Lee S, Prikoszovich T, Movadat O, Wollmann E, et al. Extracorporeal IgE immunoadsorption in allergic asthma: safety and efficacy. EBioMedicine. 2017;17:119–33.
29. Presta LG, Lahr SJ, Shields RL, Porter JP, Gorman CM, Fendly BM, et al. Humanization of an antibody directed against IgE. J Immunol. 1993;151:2623–32.
30. Zheng L, Li B, Qian W, Zhao L, Cao Z, Shi S, et al. Fine epitope mapping of humanized anti-IgE monoclonal antibody omalizumab. Biochem Biophys Res Commun. 2008;375:619–22.
31. Eggel A, Baravalle G, Hobi G, Kim B, Buschor P, Forrer P, et al. Accelerated dissociation of IgE-FcepsilonRI complexes by disruptive inhibitors actively desensitizes allergic effector cells. J Allergy Clin Immunol. 2014;133:1709–19 e1708.
32. Chang TW, Wu PC, Hsu CL, Hung AF. Anti-IgE antibodies for the treatment of IgE-mediated allergic diseases. Adv Immunol. 2007;93:63–119.
33. Holgate SBJ, Wenzel S. Efficacy of omalizumab, all anti-immunoglobulin E antibody, in patients with allergic asthma at high risk of serious asthma-related morbidity and mortality. Curt Med Res Opin. 2001;17(4):233–40.
34. USFaDA. FDA Drug Safety Communication: FDAapproves label changes for asthma drug Xolair (omalizumab), including describing slightly higher risk of heart and brain adverse events. http://www.fda.gov/drugs/drugsafety/ucm414911.htm. Accessed Sept 29, 2014.
35. Holgate STCA, Hebeft J. Efficacy and safety of a recombinant anti-immunoglobulin E antibody(omalizumab)in severe allergic asthma. Clin Exp Allergy J Br Soc Allergy Clin Immunol. 2004;34(4):632–8.
36. Metz M, Staubach P, Bauer A, Brehler R, Gericke J, Kangas M, et al. Clinical efficacy of omalizumab in chronic spontaneous urticaria is associated with a reduction of FcepsilonRI-positive cells in the skin. Theranostics. 2017;7:1266–76.
37. Zhou B, Lin B, Li J, Qian W, Hou S, Zhang D, et al. Tolerability, pharmacokinetics and pharmacodynamics of CMAB007, a humanized anti-immunoglobulin E monoclonal antibody, in healthy Chinese subjects. mAbs. 2012;4:110–9.
38. Gauvreau GM, Arm JP, Boulet LP, Leigh R, Cockcroft DW, Davis BE, et al. Efficacy and safety of multiple doses of QGE031 (ligelizumab) versus omalizumab and placebo in inhibiting allergen-induced early asthmatic responses. J Allergy Clin Immunol. 2016;138(4):1051–9.
39. Arm JP, Bottoli I, Skerjanec A, Floch D, Groenewegen A, Maahs S, et al. Pharmacokinetics, pharmacodynamics and safety of QGE031 (ligelizumab), a novel high-affinity anti-IgE antibody, in atopic subjects. Clin Exp Allergy J Br Soc Allergy Clin Immunol. 2014;44:1371–85.
40. Cohen ES, Dobson CL, Kack H, Wang B, Sims DA, Lloyd CO, et al. A novel IgE-neutralizing antibody for the treatment of severe uncontrolled asthma. mAbs. 2014;6:756–64.
41. Sheldon E, Schwickart M, Li J, Kim K, Crouch S, Parveen S, et al. Pharmacokinetics, pharmacodynamics, and safety of MEDI4212, an anti-IgE monoclonal antibody, in subjects with atopy: a phase I study. Adv Therapy. 2016;33:225–51.
42. Nyborg AC, Zacco A, Ettinger R, Jack Borrok M, Zhu J, Martin T, et al. Development of an antibody that neutralizes soluble IgE and eliminates IgE expressing B cells. Cell Mol Immunol. 2016;13:391–400.
43. Lupinek C, Roux KH, Laffer S, Rauter I, Reginald K, Kneidinger M, et al. Trimolecular complex formation of IgE, Fc epsilon RI, and a recombinant

nonanaphylactic single-chain antibody fragment with high affinity for IgE. J Immunol. 2009;182:4817–29.

44. Brown JM, Wilson TM, Metcalfe DD. The mast cell and allergic diseases: role in pathogenesis and implications for therapy. Clin Exp Allergy J Br Soc Allergy Clin Immunol. 2008;38:4–18.

45. Bradding P, Walls AF, Holgate ST. The role of the mast cell in the pathophysiology of asthma. J Allergy Clin Immunol. 2006;117:1277–84.

46. Cromheecke JL, Nguyen KT, Huston DP. Emerging ro e of human basophil biology in health and disease. Curr Allergy Asthma Rep. 2014;14:408.

47. Sethi G, Ahn KS, Pandey MK, Aggarwal BB. Celastrol, a novel triterpene, potentiates TNF-induced apoptosis and suppresses invasion of tumor cells by inhibiting NF-kappaB-regulated gene products and TAK1-mediated NF-kappaB activation. Blood. 2007;109:2727–35.

48. Peng X, Wang J, Li X, Lin L, Xie G, Cui Z, et al. Targeting mast cells and basophils with anti-FcεRIα Fab-conjugated celastrol-loaded micelles suppresses allergic inflammatio. J Biomed Nanotechnol. 2015;11:2286–99.

49. Takahashi T, Tagami T, Yamazaki S, Uede T, Shimizu J, Sakaguchi N, et al. Immunologic self-tolerance maintained by CD25(+)CD4(+) regulatory T cells constitutively expressing cytotoxic T lymphocyte-associated antigen 4. J Exp Med. 2000;192:303–9.

50. Krummel MF, Allison JP. CD28 and CTLA-4 have opposing effects on the response of T cells to stimulation. J Exp Med. 1995;182:459–65.

51. Perez-Witzke D, Miranda-Garcia MA, Suarez N, Becerra R, Duque K, Porras V, et al. CTLA4Fcepsilon, a novel soluble fusion protein that binds B7 molecules and the IgE receptors, and reduces human in vitro soluble CD23 production and lymphocyte proliferation. Immunology. 2016;148:40–55.

52. Chen JB, Wu PC, Hung AF, Chu CY, Tsai TF, Yu HM, et al. Unique epitopes on C epsilon mX in IgE-B cell receptors are potential y applicable for targeting IgE-committed B cells. J Immunol. 2010;184:1748–56.

53. Chen HY, Liu FT, Hou CM, Huang JS, Sharma BB, Chang TW. Monoclonal antibodies against the C(epsilon)mX domain of human membrane-bound IgE and their potential use for targeting IgE-expressing B cells. Int Arch Allergy Immunol. 2002;128:315–24.

54. Batista FD, Anand S, Presani G, Efremov DG, Burrone OR. The two membrane isoforms of human IgE assemble into functionally distinct B cell antigen receptors. J Exp Med. 1996;184:2197–205.

55. Peng C, Davis FM, Sun LK, Liou RS, Kim YW, Chang TW. A new isoform of human membrane-bound Ige. J Immunol. 1992;148:129–36.

56. Gauvreau GM, Harris JM, Boulet LP, Scheerens H, Fitzgerald JM, Putnam WS, et al. Targeting membrane-expressed IgE B cell receptor with an antibody to the M1 prime epitope reduces IgE production. Sci Transl Med. 2014;6:243–85.

57. Scheerens H, Zheng Y, Wang Y, Mosesova S, Maciuca R, Liao XC, Wu LC, Matthews JG, Harris JM. Treatment with Memp 1972a, an anti-M1 prime monoclonal antibody, reduced serum Ige in healthy volunteers and patients with allergic rhinitis. Am J Respir Crit Care Med. 2012;185:A6791.

58. Brightbill HD, Jeet S, Lin Z, Yan D, Zhou M. Antibodies specific for a segment of human membrane IgE deplete IgE-producing B cells in humanized mice. J Clin Investig. 2010;120(6):120.

59. Harris JM, Maciuca R, Bradley MS, Cabanski CR, Scheerens H, Lim J, et al. A randomized trial of the efficacy and safety of quilizumab in adults with inadequately controlled allergic asthma. Respir Res. 2016;17:29.

60. Liour SS, Tom A, Chan YH, Chang TW. Treating IgE-mediated diseases via targeting IgE-expressing B cells using an anti-CepsilonmX antibody. Pediatr Allergy Immunol. 2016;27(5):446–51.

61. Talay O, Yan DH, Brightbill HD, Straney EEM, Zhou MJ, Ladi E, et al. IgE(+) memory B cells and plasma cells generated through a germinal-center pathway. Nat Immunol. 2013;13:1302–4.

62. Lustgarten J, Eshhar Z. Specific elimination of Ige production using T-cell lines expressing chimeric T-cell receptor genes. Eur J Immunol. 1995;25:2985–91.

63. Kirak ORG. A novel, nonanaphylactogenic, bispecific IgE-CD3 antibody eliminates IgE(+) B cells. J Allergy Clin Immunol. 2015;136(3):800–2 e3.

64. Pritchard NR, Cutler AJ, Uribe S, Chadban SJ, Morley BJ, Smith KG. Autoimmune-prone mice share a promoter haplotype associated with reduced expression and function of the Fc receptor FcgammaRII. Curr Biol. 2000;10:227–30.

65. Chu SY, Horton HM, Pong E, Leung IW, Chen H, Nguyen DH, et al. Reduction of total IgE by targeted coengagement of IgE B-cell receptor and FcgammaRIIb with Fc-engineered antibody. J Allergy Clin Immunol. 2012;129:1102–15.

66. Chu SY, Yeter K, Kotha R, Pong E, Miranda Y, Phung S, et al. Suppression of rheumatoid arthritis B cells by XmAb5871, an anti-CD19 antibody that coengages B cell antigen receptor complex and Fcgamma receptor IIb inhibitory receptor. Arthritis Rheumatol. 2014;66:1153–64.

67. Kawakami T, Blank U. From IgE to omalizumab. J Immunol. 2016;197:4187–92.

68. Tonacci A, Billeci L, Pioggia G, Navarra M, Gangemi S. Omalizumab for the treatment of chronic idiopathic urticaria: systematic review of the literature. Pharmacotherapy. 2017;37:464–80.

69. Boozalis E, Semenov YR, Kwatra SG. Food and drug administration approval process for dermatology drugs in the United States. J Dermatol Treat. 2018. https://doi.org/10.1080/09546634.2018.1425361 **(Epub ahead of print)**.

70. Han Y, Chen Y, Liu X, Zhang J, Su H, Wen H, et al. Efficacy and safety of dupilumab for the treatment of adult atopic dermatitis: a meta-analysis of randomized clinical trials. J Allergy Clin Immunol. 2017;140:888–91.

71. Kuo CY, Kohn DB. Gene therapy for the treatment of primary immune deficiencies. Curr Allergy Asthma Rep. 2016;16:39.

72. Magen E, Mishal J, Vardy D. Selective IgE deficiency and cardiovascular diseases. Allergy Asthma Proc. 2015;36:225–9.

# 21

# Assessing severity of anaphylaxis: a data-driven comparison of 23 instruments

Esben Eller[1]* ⓘ, Antonella Muraro[2], Ronald Dahl[1,3], Charlotte Gotthard Mortz[1] and Carsten Bindslev-Jensen[1]

**Abstract**

**Backgroud:** The severity of an allergic reaction can range from mild local symptoms to anaphylactic shock. To score this, a number of instruments have been developed, although heterogeneous in design and purpose. Severity scoring algorithms are therefore difficult to compare, but are frequently used beyond their initial purpose. Our objective was to compare the most used severity scoring instruments by a data-driven approach on both milder reactions and anaphylaxis.

**Methods:** All positive challenges to foods or drugs (n = 2828) including anaphylaxis (n = 616) at Odense University Hospital, Denmark from 1998 to 2016 were included and severity was scored according to Sampson5. Based on recommendations from an expert group, the symptoms and values from Sampson5 were for all reactions and anaphylaxis only translated and compared by kappa statistics with 22 instruments, ranging from 3 to 6 steps.

**Results:** For milder reactions, there was a significant correlation between the number of steps in an instrument and the number of challenges that could be translated, whereas all instruments were good to identify food anaphylaxis. Some instruments scored reactions more severely than Sampson5, other scored them milder and some scored food and drug challenges differently. Instruments for hymenoptera reactions were difficult to apply on food and drug reactions, and thus distributed severity differently. Algorithms hampered the translation between instruments, and 7 instruments were poor concerning drug anaphylaxis, including the only instrument developed specifically for drug reactions.

**Conclusion:** The distributions of severity differed between the 23 instruments in both food and drug allergy, and thus rendering translation especially between scoring systems with 3 and 5 grades difficult. Fine-graded and simple instruments are preferred for comparison especially among milder reactions, and instruments applied to non-intended situations may not reflect a true severity picture.

**Keywords:** Severity assessment, Anaphylaxis, Severity comparison, Kappa statistics

## Background

The severity of an allergic reaction can range from subjective local symptoms to lethal anaphylactic shock. Dosage, individual threshold, route of exposure, type of allergen, age, comorbidity and involvement of facilitators can influence the severity, and this combined with the progression of symptoms and the ambiguous definition of anaphylaxis [1], makes severity difficult to capture.

Furthermore, the settings in which the reaction occurs are far from comparable, ranging from accidental exposure in an unknown environment to controlled challenges in a highly specialized clinical setting.

Multiple scoring instruments have been developed to assess the overall severity of an allergic reaction, elicited either by foods [2–9], drugs [10] or hymenoptera stings [11–14]. All instruments cover the whole spectrum of symptoms and signs, and several are using the term anaphylaxis to describe their scoring algorithm, although it is evident that non-anaphylactic milder symptoms neither fulfill the WAO [1, 15] nor the new ICD-11 [16] criteria. Many of these instruments are today applied

*Correspondence: esben.eller@rsyd.dk
[1] Odense Research Center for Anaphylaxis (ORCA), Department of Dermatology and Allergy Center, Odense University Hospital, Odense, Denmark
Full list of author information is available at the end of the article

beyond their initial purpose, whereas others have been adopted to span multiple causes [17–21]. Data-driven instruments are scarce [5, 9, 22] and the majority of tools are designed empirically for data collection in emergency rooms (ER) or intensive care units (ICU) [10, 13, 14, 17–20], in clinical trials (CT) [4, 6, 7, 12], or based on consensus reports, theoretical reviews, position papers, or national guidelines [8, 21, 23–27]. All instruments have organ-specific outcomes, dividing symptoms according to their anatomical origin, i.e. skin, respiratory, gastro-intestinal (GI), cardio-vascular (CV) or neurological symptoms. Some use a detailed predefined "symptom list, ranging from a binary form of "present/not present" to detailed grading of specific symptoms, e.g. urticaria, into mild/local or severe/generalized. Others use more general 'catch-all' symptoms from a specific organ, e.g. all symptoms related to the "GI tract". All operate with an ordinal scale spanning over 3–6 incomparable steps, where the overall severity either is defined by the highest numerical value, i.e. most severe symptoms [7, 8, 10, 11, 14, 17, 21, 23–25], relative allergen exposure [6, 18], milder symptoms obligate for severity progressing [4], fulfillment of "2-or-more" [13], summation of symptoms to get severity [12, 28] or related to number of organs involved [2, 5, 9, 27, 29].

The ideal severity assessing instrument should span all ages (children/adolescents/adults), all allergens (foods, insects, drugs), all exposure circumstances (exercise and other co-factors, injection, inhalation, oral intake etc.) and cope with the whole spectrum of symptoms. This instrument should work as a measuring tool for patients and clinicians, applicable in primary care, ER/ICU, research projects, and combining existing instruments, i.e. being retrograde compatible. A prospective comparison between existing instruments, applied in situ at the same exposure or on the same patient, would be ideal, but this is time consuming, raises ethical dilemmas on when to treat with adrenalin due to ambiguous stop-criteria and does not solve the issue of precise definition of existing tools. Knowing that titrated challenges are not ideal for addressing severity of anaphylaxis, a retrospective data-driven validation, comparing instruments based on robust clinical challenge-verified data could be the second best option to compare the translatability and distribution of severity between instruments, and could form basis for development of a common standardized instrument.

Our aim was retrospectively to compare the distribution of severity in existing grading instruments, by applying each of them to a well-characterized clinical database covering both anaphylactic and milder reactions, based on the definition of an expert-group within the fields of dermato-allergology, respiratory-allergology and pediatric allergology. Ideally, we would provide a platform for subsequent development of a universal scoring instrument for anaphylactic reactions. This study is neither testing the efficacy of intruments to identify anaphylaxis, nor should it be seen as a literature overview of existing severity assessing instruments, but instead as a comparison of the, to our knowledge, most used instruments.

## Methods

Data, i.e. recorded objective signs and/or subjective symptoms, from all positive food (n = 2382) or drug challenges (n = 466) at the Odense Research Center for Anaphylaxis (ORCA) from January 2001 to January 2016 were consecutively entered into a database and included. Anaphylaxis according to WAO criteria [15] was seen in 22% (535/2382) of the food challenges and 19% (84/446) of the drug challenges. Egg (n = 720), peanut (n = 579), hazelnut (n = 264) and milk (n = 230) were the most frequent food allergens, whereas penicillin accounted for $2/3$ and non-steroidal, anti-inflammatory, drug (NSAID) for $1/3$ of the drug challenges (see Table 1).

The most frequently recorded symptoms after food challenges were urticaria (47%), oral allergy syndrome (OAS) (35%), abdominal pain (32%), conjunctivitis (24%), vomiting (24%) and rhinorrhea (22%). For drug

**Table 1  Characteristics of included challenges and severity distribution of Sampson5 for foods and drugs challenges**

|  | n | # Allergens | Mean age (years [SD]) | Gr. 1 | Gr. 2 | Gr. 3 | Gr. 4 | Gr. 5 |
|---|---|---|---|---|---|---|---|---|
| Total | 2848 | 114 | 17.6 [18.4] | 296 (10%) | 1253 (44%) | 843 (30%) | 416 (14%) | 20 (1%) |
| Foods (anaphylaxis[a]) | 2382 (535) | 86 | 11.6 [4.0] | 198 (0) | 1026 (0) | 800 (177) | 347 (347) | 11 (11) |
| 0–3 years | 859 | 22 | 2.3 [1.0] | 33 (4%) | 422 (49%) | 285 (33%) | 118 (14%) | 1 (0%) |
| 4–15 years | 990 | 43 | 7.8 [3.0] | 59 (6%) | 384 (39%) | 408 (41%) | 136 (14%) | 3 (0%) |
| 15+ years | 533 | 73 | 33.9 [14.0] | 106 (20%) | 220 (41%) | 107 (20%) | 93 (17%) | 7 (1%) |
| Drugs (anaphylaxis[a]) | 446 (84) | 28 | 43.8 [17.3] | 98 (0) | 227 (0) | 43 (6) | 69 (69) | 9 (9) |
| Antibiotics | 285 | 21 | 44.6 [17.7] | 79 (28%) | 154 (54%) | 24 (8%) | 21 (7%) | 7 (2%) |
| NSAID | 143 | 7 | 41.1 [16.8] | 15 (10%) | 69 (48%) | 16 (11%) | 41 (29%) | 2 (1%) |

[a] According to WAO [15]

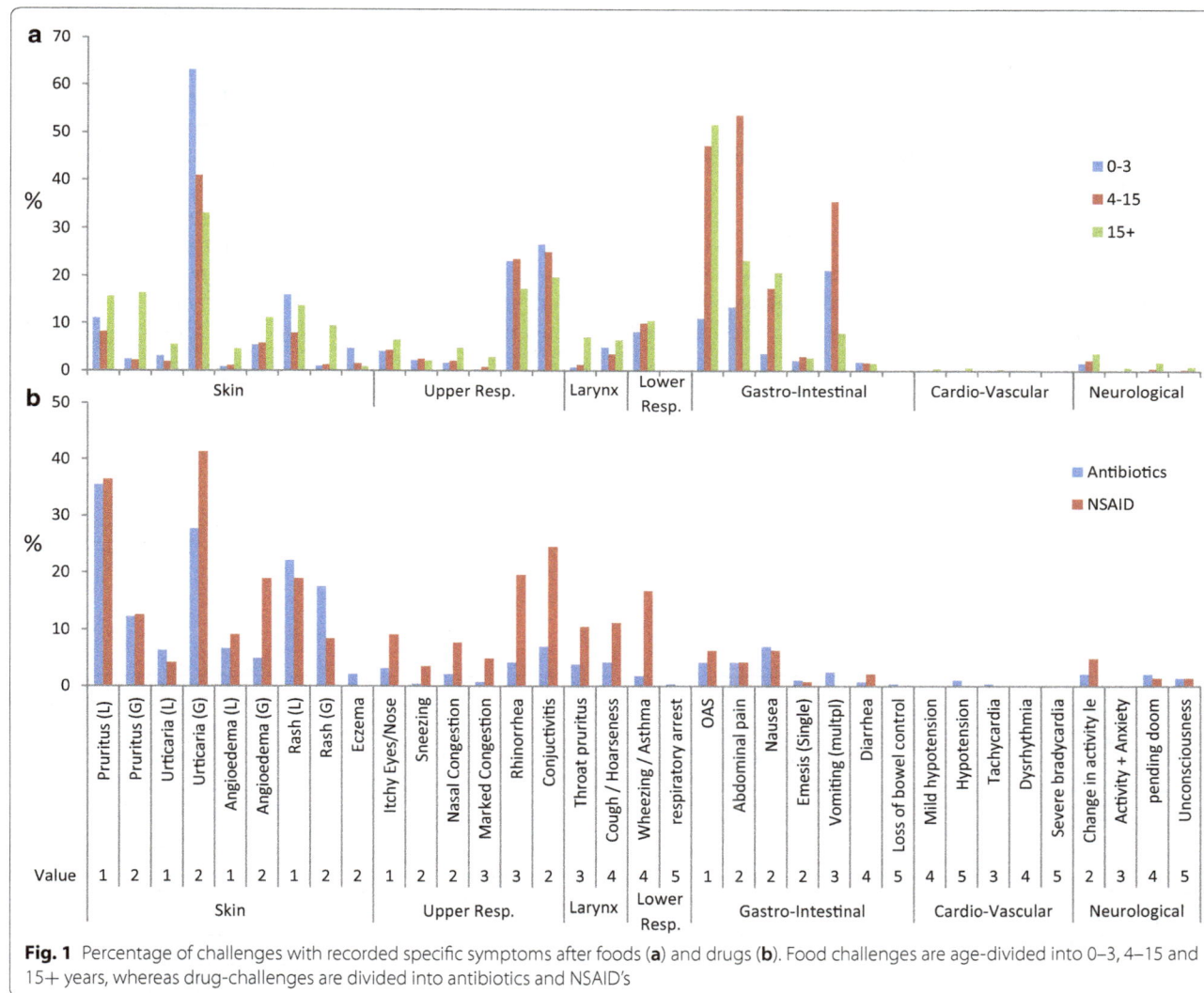

**Fig. 1** Percentage of challenges with recorded specific symptoms after foods (**a**) and drugs (**b**). Food challenges are age-divided into 0–3, 4–15 and 15+ years, whereas drug-challenges are divided into antibiotics and NSAID's

challenges, skin symptoms were predominant; either localized or generalized pruritus (47%), urticaria (36%), rash (35%) or angioedema (17%) (Fig. 1).

The overall severity (Table 1) was based on Sampson5 [8] with an addition of 3 milder symptoms including upper airways and/or eyes (itchy eyes/nose, conjunctivitis) and abdominal pain. Patients challenged to food were significantly younger than patients challenged to drugs (p < 0.001), and food-challenges were therefore subdivided into 3 age-categories (0–3, 4–15, and +15 years). There was a significant difference between the distribution of severity grading between the 3 age-classes (p < 0.001). Children in the 0–3 years group rarely had subjective symptoms, such as OAS, abdominal pain or nausea, whereas 63% of them had urticaria and/or rhino-conjunctivitis, resulting in often having their challenge stopped after

a grade 2 reaction (p < 0.001), compared to older age groups (4–15 years/+15 years). Group +15 years was even more polarized in its severity grading, i.e. often significantly (p < 0.001) milder (gr. 1) symptoms, characterized by a generally higher level in subjective skin symptoms and abdominal pain, but also more frequent severe reactions (gr. 4–5) (p < 0.001). This effect disappeared after adjustment for specific allergens (i.e. milk, egg, peanut, hazelnut) and was entirely driven by more severe objective reactions after a challenge with peanuts [a-OR (95% CI) = 1.77 (1.33–2.35)]. In the +15 years group, food challenges were significantly milder (p = 0.03) than drug challenges. Reactions to NSAID were more severe than antibiotics (p < 0.0001), caused by more frequently respiratory distress, especially laryngeal and lower respiratory symptoms (p < 0.001).

**Translation of symptoms to other instruments**

A direct literature-search identifying severity instruments was not feasible, since the majority of instruments were not published as such, but developed as tools for specific use, e.g. to address severity of reactions in allergen immune therapy trials. Included instruments were therefore identified empirically or in relation to the European Academy of Allergy and Clinical Immunology (EAACI) taskforce initiative on Food Allergy and Anaphylaxis [30]. We identified 22 previously published instruments focusing on severity of allergic reactions [2, 4, 6, 7, 9–14, 17–21, 23–29]; however, 2 were excluded

for not addressing the overall severity but more listing symptoms [19, 26]. Moreover, the new EAACI taskforce guidelines [30] (newEAACI3), a 3-step organ-specific "catch-all" instrument and the new iFAAM oFASS instrument [5], a 5-step observational instrument (iFAAM5) were included. With Sampson5 [8], a total of 23 instruments were compared (Table 2).

Numerical values for symptoms in Sampson5 (e.g. value 2 for generalized urticaria) were then retrospectively translated according to recommendations by the expert group into the corresponding value in the comparing instruments (e.g. value 1 in Mueller4 [13]). As

**Table 2** Overview of the 22 included studies, their origin and exact numerical value (1–6) for each listed symptom ordered by organ and appearance in Sampson5

General discrepancies (Type A–D error) between Sampson5 and the comparing instrument are listed below; symptoms missing in Sampson5 (Type A), symptoms missing in the comparing instrument (Type B), symptoms where comparing instrument contained less information than Sampson5 (Type C—symptoms marked in red), and symptoms with increased information in comparing instrument compared to Sampson5 (Type D—marked in green)

*Pea* peanut, *Ven* venom, *Ped* only pediatric, *Alg* inbuilt algorithm, *Amnt* allergen amount depended, *Org* organ specific, *Rev* review, *Cons* consensus, *CT* clinical trial, *ICU* intensive care unit, *ER* emergency room, *GI* gastro-intestinal, *CV* cardio-vascular, *Neuro* neurological, *Resp* respiratory

*Unspecific "catch-all" symptom

**Added variables to reduced number of Type B error among the most severe cases

[†] Translation depending of number of involved organs

[††] Added variables form Sampson5

[‡] Anaphylaxis according to WAO [15]

illustrated in Table 2, we identified 4 types of systematic translational errors (A–D). Type A errors were symptoms missing in Sampson5, i.e. "incontinence" or "fever", whereas type B were missing variables in the comparing instrument and therefore untranslatable (i.e. localized urticaria in Mueller4 [13]). Sampson5 includes a total of 23 symptoms from 7 "organs" with a total of 34 possible outcomes. Zee3 [9] was, due to its unspecific "catch-all" structure, the only instrument which embraced all symptoms covered by Sampson5, whereas no other instrument showed complete translatability; the best overlap was 32/34 with ASCI6 [28] and poorest overlap was 8/34 with Golden3 [11]. Type B errors reduced the translatability, i.e. the percentage symptoms translated compared to Sampson5 (Table 2) and additionally led to a systematic discrepancy in those cases, where the most severe symptoms were missing, and thereby determining the overall severity by less severe symptoms; half of the recorded grade 5 reactions were caused by fainting, a symptom missing in 5 instruments [2, 6, 10, 21, 29], resulting either in downgrading to other less severe symptoms or being completely lost in translation. "Unconsciousness" was therefore added to these 5 instruments (marked ** in Table 1), corresponding to the highest numerical value for each system. Other errors were type C, where information was lost, because the comparing instrument contained fewer variables than Sampson5, i.e. "local urticaria" or "generalized urticaria" reduced to "urticaria" (marked in red in Table 1). Finally type D, where the comparing instrument incorporated more information than Sampson5, resulting in a translation based on expert interpretation, i.e. whether "wheeze, asthma, dyspnea, cyanosis" should be translated into "mild wheeze" or "pronounced dyspnea" (green in Table 1). "Catch-all" symptoms, e.g. "all symptoms from GI" were encountered to embrace all possible symptoms for that specific organ. Sampson5 included the lower respiratory symptom "wheeze/asthma/dyspnea/cyanosis", which was translated into "asthma" in cases with multiple unambiguous translation possibilities, e.g. "wheeze", "asthma", or "cyanosis". Shock and hypotension was defined as systolic blood pressure < 90 mm Hg.

The majority of instruments applied a simple "most severe" symptom to define the overall anaphylaxis severity [7, 10, 11, 14, 17, 18, 21, 23–25, 30], however 11 of the included instruments instead had a built-in algorithm (marked Alg. in Table 2); Ewans5 [4] mandates at least one symptom from grade 1 (localized skin) or grade 2 (generalized skin) plus symptoms from GI/eyes/nose to accomplish gr. 3. For Niggemann6 [29], Astier5 [2], iFAAM5 [5], and Cox4 [27], grade 2 or grade 3 was directly linked to the number of included organs (one vs. multiple organs). Zee3 [9] calculates a none-linear

severity index in tertiles, based on involved organs regardless of number of observed symptoms. Mueller4 [13] mandates at least 2 milder symptoms plus the defining symptom to qualify for anaphylaxis > grade 1, whereas Pomphrey4 [20], Lockley3 [12] and ASCA6 [28] included different numerical severity indexes, from which specific symptoms were recalculated to give an overall score. Due to absence of specific symptoms (type B error) for the latter 4 instruments, there was a marked reduction in the number of translatable challenges; e.g. for Mueller4 < 50% fulfilled the 2-or-more criteria. The simple "highest" possible symptom was therefore applied to these four instruments.

### Statistics and translational algorithms
Comparison of severity, age, specific symptoms and type of allergen in Sampson5 was performed with ordinal logistic regression. To compare the distribution of severity between instruments with 3 steps, Sampson5 was reduced into three theoretical grade 3 scales; a scale milder than the original Sampson5 was obtained by merging grade $1+2$ into 1, grade $3+4$ into 2 and maintaining grade 5 as a new grade 3 (i.e. grade 1, 2, 3, 4, 5 become $1+2$, $3+4$, 5), a scale with similar severity distribution ($1+2$, 3, $4+5$) and a scale with more severe severity distribution (1, $2+3$, $4+5$) than the original Sampson5. Using weighted kappa statistics, all 3-step-instruments [6, 7, 9, 11, 12, 14, 17, 18, 24, 25, 30] were stepwise compared toward these 3 theoretical scales and the best agreement was identified, thereby ordering them into milder, similar or more severe than Sampson5. Similar, four theoretical 4-step-scales were constructed from Sampson5 for comparison between all instruments containing 4 steps [10, 13, 20, 21, 23, 27]. Five-step scales [2, 4, 5, 8] were directly compared to Sampson5, whereas the two instruments containing 6 steps [28, 29] were converted into 6 possible 5-step scales, which then were compared to Sampson5 using weighted kappa statistics. The cumulative distribution function (CDF) for all instruments was plotted against the relative percentage severity of each instrument, i.e. as tertiles, quartiles, quintiles, and sextiles. The Area Under each CDF Curve (AUC) was calculated and the translatability was compared with nonparametric Spearman correlation test. *WAO criteria [15] of anaphylaxis were applied to all challenges and 619 challenges fulfilled these (see Table 1). Challenges identified as anaphylactic were then translated according to previous description and statistical analysis repeated for these.* All calculations were performed in STATA14 SE (Stata Corporation, College Station, TX, USA). *The study was approved by the local board of* Danish Data Protection Agency (license no. 2012-58-0018/journal no. 16/31454).

## Results

Based on symptoms from all 2382 positive food challenges and 446 positive drug challenges, the 22 instruments were translated from Sampson5. Translatability for foods and drugs for all instruments are presented in Table 2. Best translatability was found for Zee3, iFAAM5, ASCA6, SFFA4 and the NewEAACI3 [5, 9, 23, 28, 30], were >97.5% of all challenges could be translated, whereas only 56% of all challenges could be translated into Golden3 [11]. Mueller4, DSA3, Muraro3, Brown(A)3 and Brown(B)3 [13, 17, 18, 24, 25] were significantly better to translate food challenges than drug challenges, as opposed to Reismann3 and Hourihane(A)3 [7, 14]. There was a significant correlation between the translatability from Sampson5 and the number of steps in the receiving instruments for both foods ($r_s = 0.57$, $p < 0.01$) and drugs ($r_s = 0.72$ $p < 0.005$), meaning that instruments with 5 steps less frequently had incomplete translation compared to instruments only containing 3 or 4 steps. Only applying anaphylactic challenges increased the translatability >90% for all instruments, except 7 instruments on drug anaphylaxis [2, 6, 7, 10, 14, 18, 27]; Ring/Messmer4 criteria [10] only translated 83% of drug anaphylaxis compared to 91%, when milder reactions were included.

The cumulative distribution function (CDF) for all instruments was plotted against the relative percentage severity of each instrument, i.e. the severity in a grade-3 instruments were presented as tertiles (i.e. 33, 66 and 100%) and a grade 5 instruments as quintiles (i.e. 20, 40, 60, 80, and 100%) (Fig. 2). Based on kappa statistics, we could identify three possible scenarios; instruments with left-skewed CDF and thereby overall milder severity-scoring than Sampson5 (Muraro3, Golden3, DSA3, Mueller4, Ring_Messmer4, SFFA4, Cox4, Astier5 and Niggemann6 [2, 10, 11, 13, 23–25, 27, 29]), similar distribution as Sampson5 (Zee3 and BrownB3 [9, 18]) and instruments with a right-skewed CDF and hence a more severe symptom scoring than Sampson5 (Reismann3, HourihaneB3, NewEAACI3, Pomphrey4, Ring_Behrendt4, and ASCA6 [6, 14, 20, 21, 28, 30]). Five instruments (HourihaneA3, Lockey3, BrownA3, Ewan5, and IFAAM5 [4, 5, 7, 12, 17]) showed different distribution on food than drug challenges compared to Sampson5 (red lines in Fig. 2).

The area under curve (AUC) for CDF was calculated (for Sampson5 marked in grey in Fig. 2). Corresponding values of translatability (% translated symptoms compared to Sampson5) and AUC for foods and drugs are presented in Fig. 3, both for all symptoms and signs (Sampson grade 1 through 5) and for the 535 anaphylactic food and 84 anaphylactic drug challenges. The relative severity compared to Sampson5 were for most instruments unaffected when only anaphylactic reactions were

included; only Reismann3, Pomphrey4, Brown(A)3 and Cox4 [14, 17, 20, 27] distributed food challenges milder, whereas Mueller4 [13] appraise anaphylactic food challenges as more severe. Reismann3 and Pomphrey4 [14, 20] scored drug anaphylaxis milder than non-anaphylactic reactions, indicating that they weighted milder symptoms more, than other instruments.

## Discussion

The aim of this project was to compare existing severity instruments and identifying pros and cons among them, thereby forming a backbone for the development of a future instrument, which ideally should be retrograde compatible. To our knowledge, no study has applied multiple instruments on the same allergic reaction, and this paper is the first data-driven comparison of multiple anaphylaxis severity-scoring instruments, based on challenge-data from more than 12,000 titrated challenges.

The overall heterogeneity between included instruments, i.e. their origin, structure and output was large; some instruments are purposed solely for single allergens, e.g. peanut or bee venom, others developed exclusively for specific populations, i.e. children and some to specific situations, e.g. after immunotherapy trials. The consequent extrapolation of instruments into non-intended situations, lead to discrepancies; instruments developed to cope with hymenoptera reactions [11–14] overall had poor translatability and distributed severity differently compared to Sampson5, but were on the other hand not evaluated in venom anaphylaxis in this study. The only instrument intended on adverse drug reactions (Ring_Messmer4) [10] scored for food challenges milder than Sampson5.

Distributions in severity were different, some instruments overestimated e.g. having more severe reactions than Sampson5 (Ring_Berend4, NewEAACI3 [21, 30]), others underestimated (Muraro3, Mueller4, Ring_Messmer4 [10, 13, 25]), some scored food challenges more severe than drug challenges (Hourihane(A)3, iFAAM5 [5, 7]), and others drug challenges more severe than food challenges (Brown(A)3, Evan5, Luckey3 [4, 12, 17]). Anaphylaxis represents the most 'severe, life-threatening, generalized or systemic hypersensitivity reaction' with multiple organs involved [31, 32], but scoring severity of an anaphylactic reaction in relation to exposure is complex due to the overall nature of anaphylaxis (progression, timing and interaction of symptoms), titrated challenges (terminated after the first clear objective signs) and treatment (immediately thereafter, hampering progression and overall severity). Therefore clear-cut anaphylactic reactions were identified and applied separately. Only 22% of the included challenges could by definition be classified as anaphylaxis [15], however all instruments

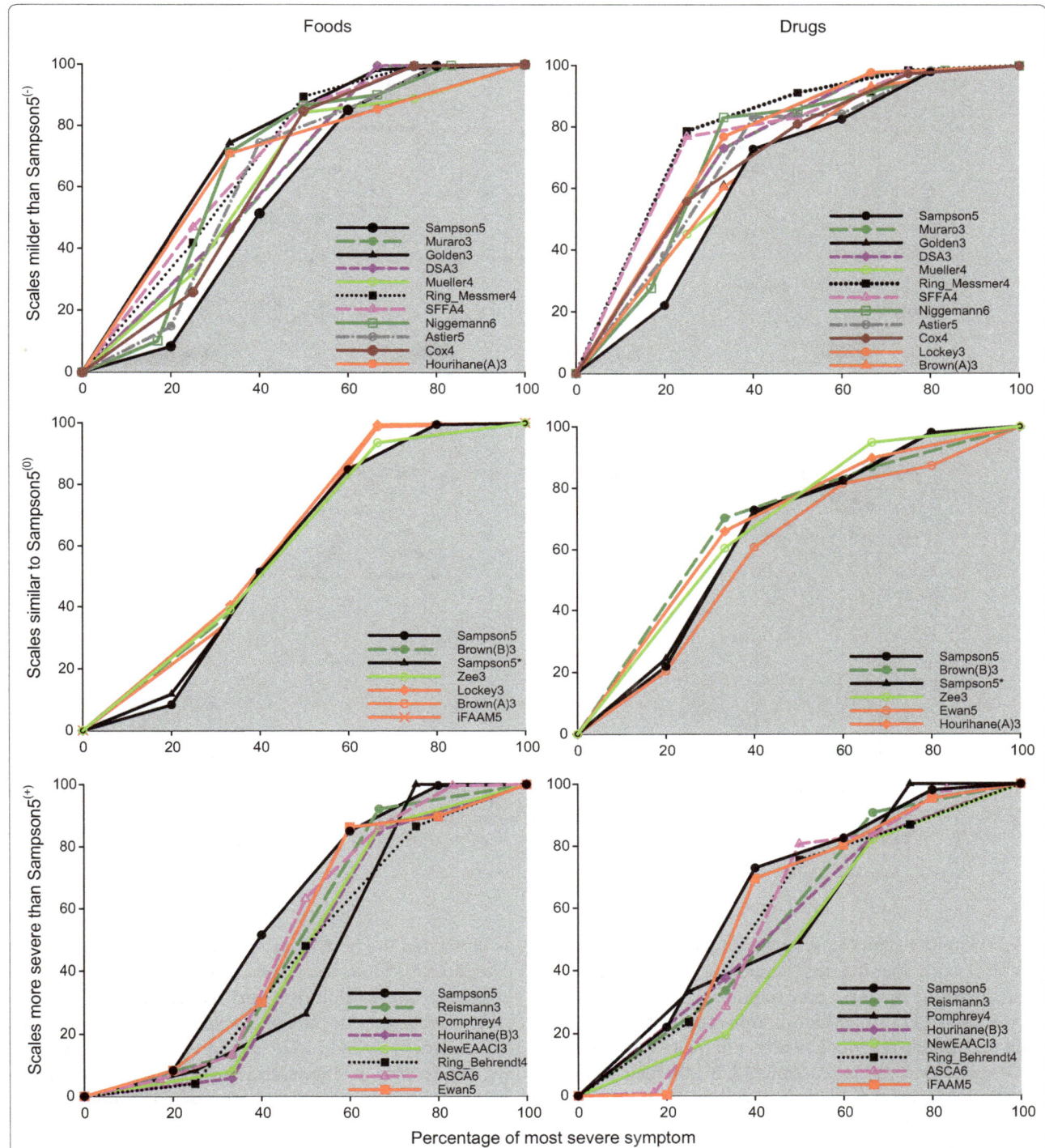

**Fig. 2** Cumulative distribution function (CDF) of all instruments plotted against percentage of most severe value, and presented for food and drug challenges, respectively. Instruments are divided into the relative shift compared to the Sampson5 (black line) based on kappa statistics. Red lines indicate instruments with different distribution between food and drug challenges. [−]3-step scales with best concordance (highest Kappa values) to Sampson5 recalculated as 1 + 2, 3 + 4, 5. 4-step scales with best concordance (highest Kappa values) to Sampson5 recalculated as 1 + 2, 3, 4, 5. Niggemann6 had best concordance to Sampson5 when recalculated into 1, 2, 3, 4 + 5, 6. [0]3-step scales with best concordance (highest Kappa values) to Sampson5 recalculated as 1 + 2, 3, 4 + 5. [+]3-step scales with best concordance (highest Kappa values) to Sampson5 recalculated as 1, 2 + 3, 4 + 5. 4-step scales with best concordance (highest Kappa values) to Sampson5 recalculated as 1, 2, 3, 4 + 5. ASCA6 had best concordance to Sampson5 as when recalculated into 5-step scale = 1 + 2, 3, 4, 5, 6. *Sampson5 unmodified

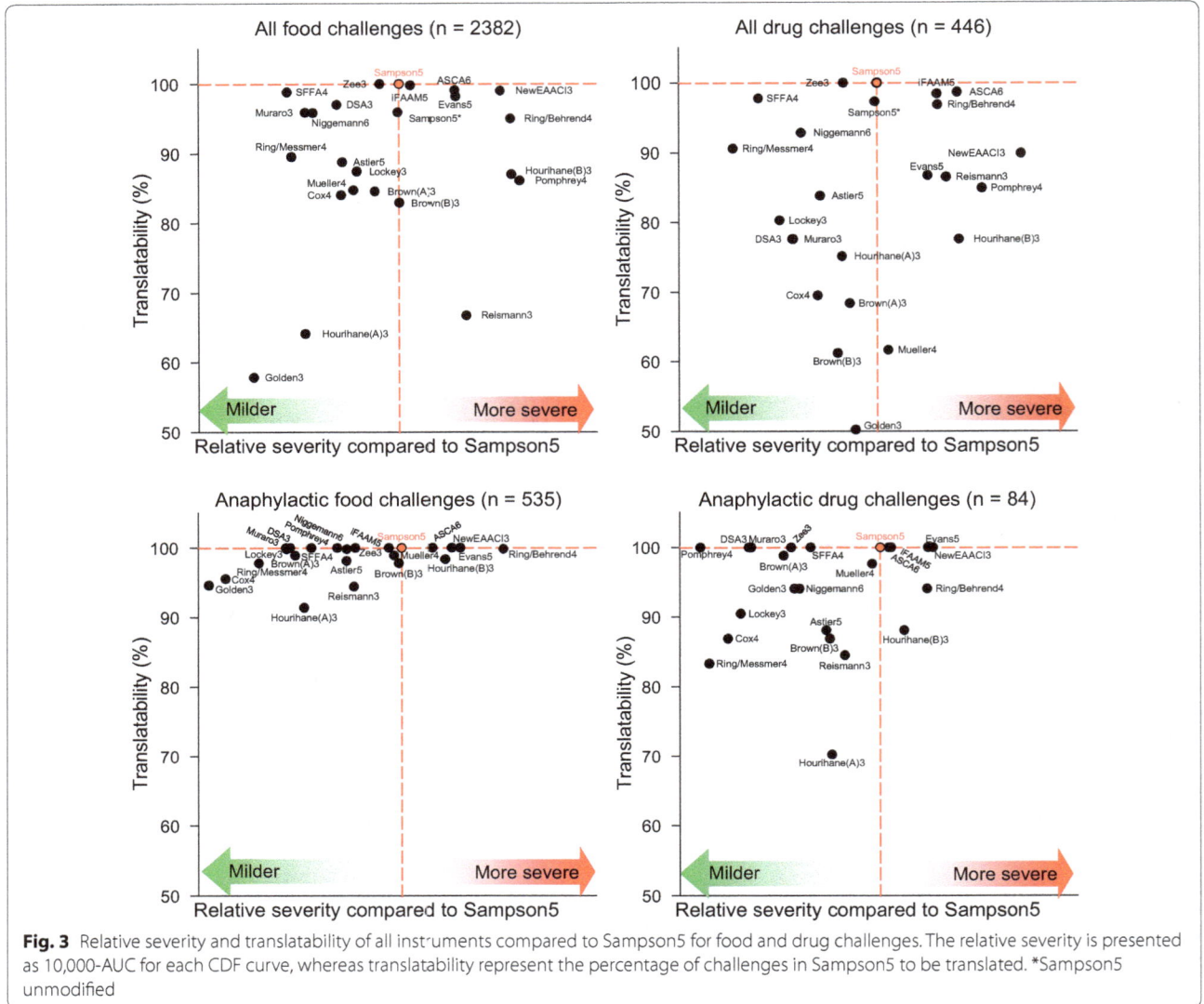

**Fig. 3** Relative severity and translatability of all instruments compared to Sampson5 for food and drug challenges. The relative severity is presented as 10,000-AUC for each CDF curve, whereas translatability represent the percentage of challenges in Sampson5 to be translated. *Sampson5 unmodified

included milder symptoms, such as urticaria (a grade 1–2 reaction) not reflecting life-threatening anaphylaxis [29]. Some instruments only cover the most severe anaphylactic reactions [11, 14], which is reflected in the translatability of milder reactions, while others are designed for the whole spectrum of reactions [5, 8], thereby addressing anaphylaxis and milder reactions similar.

We found a reverse causality between the numbers of steps in instruments and the percentage of all, non-anaphylactic challenges to be translated, meaning that fine-graded instruments were better in agreement with other tools concerning milder symptoms. All instruments could assess >90% of the anaphylactic food challenges, whereas translatability for drug reactions are much more scattered; The explanation for this remains unclear, but

as illustrated in Fig. 1, drug reactions manifest differently compared to food, with overrepresentation of non-anaphylactic skin symptoms. Surprisingly Ring/Messmer4 [10], developed for adverse colloid volume substitution reactions, scored milder than all other instruments applied on drug reactions, and further had reduced translatability on drug anaphylaxis compared to milder reactions. Some instruments entirely [10] or partly [11] focus on cardio-vascular rather than respiratory symptoms and signs, whereas others report that lethality, especially in children, is a result of respiratory compromise [33] or a combination of both [17]. This is mainly interfering with milder reactions and not with anaphylaxis and together with the differences in translatability indicates that fine-graded instruments mainly have their benefits among milder symptoms, whereas all instruments cope with anaphylaxis as "most severe".

All instruments are organ-based, i.e. the skin, respiratory, gastro-intestinal, cardio-vascular, and nervous system, with symptoms classified into ordinal scales from 3 to 6 incomparable steps, ranging from "present" over "mild/moderate/severe" to the 6-step comprehensive Japanese ASCA-system [28]. Anaphylaxis after accidental exposure in non-controlled settings outside a hospital necessitates a relatively simple classification system easy to apply retrospectively. Classifying severity in terms of different grades (mild/moderate/severe) may be more informative for patients and non-allergy specialists, especially if reduced to a limited number of categories. However, for research purposes it may be more useful to have a numerical score of severity with more gradations. The overall/total severity of a reaction is then either based on the highest/most severe symptoms [7, 8, 10, 11, 14, 17, 21, 23–25], or calculated by different algorithms [6, 9, 12, 13, 20, 28–30]. Overall, instruments applying an algorithmic approach were neither superior in translatability nor distribution compared to Sampson5, with Zee3 [9] as only exception. However, a direct comparison of severity between most severe challenges revealed, that only half of grade 5 challenges in Sampson5 were translated into the most severe grade in Zee3, whereas milder reactions from multiple organs were converted into grade 3 in Zee3. Despite algorithms do not seem to add more information, iFAAM5 [5] is currently developing a comprehensive data-driven numerical scoring system (nFASS), which will be interesting to compare among existing instruments in relation to the balance between information gained and simplicity.

The retrospective application of instruments led to translational issues, where comparability and interpretation of known symptoms were critical, and especially type B (symptom missing in comparing instruments) and type D errors (Sampson5 contained less information than comparing instrument) caused discrepancies in the frequency of translation. Missing symptoms were an issue for all but one instrument [9], emphasizing the importance of a stable strategy to cope with these types of errors, which otherwise can lead to misclassification and thereby affect the overall severity of a reaction. In this study, symptoms not available were left untranslated, except for five instruments [2, 6, 10, 21, 29], where none-recorded 'fainting' dramatically would reduce the number of most severe anaphylaxis. One way to overcome missing specific symptoms are "catch-all" definitions [2, 4, 5, 9, 10, 12, 24, 30], i.e. all symptoms related to a specific organ, e.g. the "gastrointestinal tract". Instruments including these have fewer type B arrows and thereby a higher translatability, in contrast to instruments with a predefined "symptom list", which contains more information for research purposes, and avoids the pitfall of overseeing especially milder symptoms.

Skin symptoms usually include pruritus, urticaria, angioedema, flush/rash in 1–2 dichotomous outcomes. GI symptoms consist both of subjective symptoms (OAS, nausea, and abdominal pain) and objective signs (emesis and diarrhea). Brown(A)3 [17] found a direct link between GI symptoms and hypotensive anaphylaxis, whereas Niggemann6 [29] claims that GI symptoms are over-represented, which is reflected in Niggemann6 being milder compared to Samspon5 both after food, where GI symptoms are expectedly predominant, but surprisingly also after drug challenges. Cardio-vascular symptoms are characterized by a change in heart rate (from tachycardia to cardiac arrest) and degrees of hypotension, where only few instruments have an exact definition [11, 17, 18, 25, 28]. Neurological symptoms are less consistent with grades of anxiety and consciousness (from reduced activity level to total loss of consciousness). Niggemann6 [29] claims that subjective symptoms such as anxiety, malaise, weakness or dizziness should not form the basis for grading an allergic reaction, however 70% (77/110) of our challenges with neurological subjective symptoms also have clear-cut objective signs from other organs. Terminating a challenge based on neurological symptoms is therefore rare and can be avoided by strict clinical stop-criteria. The biggest discrepancies are found in respiratory symptoms; some instruments only apply airway obstruction (defined as asthma, cyanosis, or respiratory arrest [8]), symptoms from upper airways, i.e. nose and from eyes are covered by some [8, 20, 25] and are excluded by others [10, 13, 17]. The interpretation of the respiratory system as one system including nose, pharynx, larynx, and bronchial is lacking, and especially symptoms from tongue and pharynx are vaguely mentioned. The compression of 'cough, hoarseness, dysphagia', and 'wheezing, asthma, dyspnea, cyanosis' into two overall 'laryngeal' and 'bronchial' categories, and the lack of 'stridor', a seldom but adrenalin-requiring laryngeal symptom, hamper Sampson5 [8], which have now prompted a change of in our department to facilitate this.

The incomplete translatability and the different number of steps among the instruments make the severity distribution difficult to compare. No standardized or validated method exists to compare multiple heterogeneous scoring systems; some instruments (iFAAM5, Niggemann6, ASCA6, SFFA4, Ring-Behrend4, NewEAACI3 [5, 21, 23, 28–30] have high translatability i.e. percentage translated while others have a similar distribution of severity (Brown(B)3 [18]). The paired kappa comparison probably does not reflect the situation, where two clinical settings intend to compare severity on two different populations, but it is the methodologically correct way to asses this in our retrospective study. By applying the CDF-curve, we assumed that severity obtained under standard challenge conditions was normally (Gaussian) distributed. A linear relationship between the grades, i.e. fixed and equal distance between steps, is also assumed but hypothetical.

The simplified distribution of instruments in reference to Sampson5 place them into 3 categories; milder, similar or more severe than Sampson5. Sampson5 was original applied at our sitting for historical reasons, mainly due to the high numbers of pediatric food challenges performed in our clinic. We do not claim that any of the instruments is better or worse to score severity of anaphylaxis, nor that Sampson5 is the gold standard. This simply identifies the difference between instruments, which reflects their heterogeneous etiology, and should be considered when comparing existing scoring systems for severity in anaphylaxis. This also emphasize, that instruments applied beyond their initial purpose have limitations, especially embracing milder reactions, and might reflect altered distribution of severity.

## Conclusion

We found a reverse causality between the numbers of grades an instrument span and the percentage of non-anaphylactic challenges to be translated, whereas anaphylaxis more easily is translated between instruments. The distributions in severity were different; some over-estimate e.g. having more severe reactions than Sampson5 [21, 30], whereas others under-estimate [10, 13, 25]. There is no consistency between food and drug challenge severity distribution; some scored food challenges more severe than drug challenges [5, 7] and others drug challenges more severe than food [4, 12, 17]. Most instruments appraise milder symptoms identical to anaphylaxis, whereas few weighted them more [14, 17, 20, 27] or less severe [13]. Instruments developed to cope with hymenopteran reactions [11–14] overall had poor translatability and distributed differently compared to Sampson5. Drug challenges are complicated to compare [10], and finally algorithms do not add more information, but compromise comparison of especially milder symptoms.

## Abbreviations

ASCA: Anaphylaxis Scoring Aichi; AUC: area under curve; CDF: cumulative distribution function; CT: clinical trials; CV: cardio-vascular; DSA: Danish Society for Allergology; EAACI: European Academy of Allergy and Clinical Immunology; ER: emergency rooms; GI: gastro-intestinal; ICU: intensive care units; iFAAM: integrated approaches to food allergen and allergy risk management; nFASS: numerical food allergy severity system; NSAID: non-steroidal, anti-inflammatory, drug; OAS: oral allergy syndrome; oFASS: observational food allergy severity system; ORCA: Odense Research Center for Anaphylaxis; SFFA: Svenska Föreningen För Allergologi (Swedish Association for Allergology).

## Authors' contributions

EE performed all quieries, analysis and data stratification preparing and processing the manuscript. All other authors (AM, RD, CGM and CBJ) were enrolled in the expert group, defining, stratifying and ordering symptoms and reviewing the manuscript. All authors read and approved the final manuscript.

## Author details

[1] Odense Research Center for Anaphylaxis (ORCA), Department of Dermatology and Allergy Center, Odense University Hospital, Odense, Denmark. [2] Food Allergy Referral Centre – Veneto Region, Department of Women and Child Health, Padua University Hospital, Padua, Italy. [3] GSK, Brentford, Middlesex, UK.

## Acknowledgements

We would like to acknowledge Kate Crowley, for linguistical support and René Dupont, Biostatistics, Unicersity of Sourthern Denmark for statistical counceling.

## Competing interests

The authors declare that they have no competing interests.

## Funding

The present study was not supported directly, but performed within the the the frame of the Department of Dermatolgy and Allergy Center, Odense University Hospital, Region of Southern Denmark.

## References

1. Sampson HA, et al. Second symposium on the definition and management of anaphylaxis: summary report—second National Institute of Allergy and Infectious Disease/Food Allergy and Anaphylaxis Network symposium. J Allergy Clin Immunol. 2006;117(2):391–7.
2. Astier C, et al. Predictive value of skin prick tests using recombinant allergens for diagnosis of peanut allergy. J Allergy Clin Immunol. 2006;118(1):250–6.
3. Cianferoni A, et al. Predictive values for food challenge-induced severe reactions: development of a simple food challenge score. Isr Med Assoc J. 2012;14(1):24–8.
4. Ewan PW, Clark AT. Long-term prospective observational study of patients with peanut and nut allergy after participation in a management plan. Lancet. 2001;357(9250):111–5.
5. Fernandez-Rivas M. Severity grading of food allergic reactions. In: EAACI. Vienna; 2016.
6. Hourihane JO, et al. Does severity of low-dose, double-blind, placebo-controlled food challenges reflect severity of allergic reactions to peanut in the community? Clin Exp Allergy. 2005;35(9):1227–33.
7. Hourihane JO, et al. Clinical characteristics of peanut allergy. Clin Exp Allergy. 1997;27(6):634–9.
8. Sampson HA. Anaphylaxis and emergency treatment. Pediatrics. 2003;111(6 Pt 3):1601–8.
9. van der Zee T, et al. The eliciting dose of peanut in double-blind, placebo-controlled food challenges decreases with increasing age and specific IgE level in children and young adults. J Allergy Clin Immunol. 2011;128(5):1031–6.
10. Ring J, Messmer K. Incidence and severity of anaphylactoid reactions to colloid volume substitutes. Lancet. 1977;1(8009):466–9.

11. Golden DB, et al. Discontinuing venom immunotherapy: extended observations. J Allergy Clin Immunol. 1998;101(3):298–305.
12. Lockey RF, et al. The Hymenoptera venom study. III: safety of venom immunotherapy. J Allergy Clin Immunol. 1990;86(5):775–80.
13. Mueller HL. Further experiences with severe allergic reactions to insect stings. N Engl J Med. 1959;261:374–7.
14. Reisman RE. Natural history of insect sting allergy: relationship of severity of symptoms of initial sting anaphylaxis to re-sting reactions. J Allergy Clin Immunol. 1992;90(3 Pt 1):335–9.
15. Simons FE, et al. World Allergy Organization anaphylaxis guidelines: summary. J Allergy Clin Immunol. 2011;127(3):587–93 e1-22.
16. Tanno LK, et al. Reaching multidisciplinary consensus on classification of anaphylaxis for the eleventh revision of the World Health Organization's (WHO) International Classification of Diseases (ICD-11). Orphanet J Rare Dis. 2017;12(1):53.
17. Brown SG. Clinical features and severity grading of anaphylaxis. J Allergy Clin Immunol. 2004;114(2):371–6.
18. Brown SG, et al. Anaphylaxis: clinical patterns, mediator release, and severity. J Allergy Clin Immunol. 2013;132(5):1141–1149 e5.
19. Cianferoni A, et al. Clinical features of acute anaphylaxis in patients admitted to a university hospital: an 11-year retrospective review (1985–1996). Ann Allergy Asthma Immunol. 2001;87(1):27–32.
20. Pumphrey RS, Stanworth SJ. The clinical spectrum of anaphylaxis in north-west England. Clin Exp Allergy. 1996;26(12):1364–70.
21. Ring J, Behrendt H. Anaphylaxis and anaphylactoid reactions. Classification and pathophysiology. Clin Rev Allergy Immunol. 1999;17(4):387–99.
22. DunnGalvin A, et al. Highly accurate prediction of food challenge outcome using routinely available clinical data. J Allergy Clin Immunol. 2011;127(3):633–9 e1-3.
23. Gottberg L. Anafylaxi; Rekommendationer för omhändertagande och behandling. In: Swedish National Society of Allergology (Svenska Föreningen För Allergologi—SFFA). SFFA. 2015. http://www.sffa.nu/wp-content/uploads/2015/12/Anafylaxi_sept_2015.pdf.
24. Grinsted P, et al. Akutberedskab ved procedurer med øget risiko for anafylaksi, specielt med henblik på allergen-specifik immunterapi. In: Danish Society for General Medicine, Danish Society of Anesthesiology, Danish Society of Allergology. 2004. http://danskallergi.dk/wp-content/uploads/beredskab_it6.pdf.
25. Muraro A, et al. The management of anaphylaxis in childhood: position paper of the European academy of allergology and clinical immunology. Allergy. 2007;62(8):857–71.
26. Sampson HA, et al. Standardizing double-blind, placebo-controlled oral food challenges: American Academy of Allergy, Asthma & Immunology-European Academy of Allergy and Clinical Immunology PRACTALL consensus report. J Allergy Clin Immunol. 2012;130(6):1260–74.
27. Cox L, et al. Speaking the same language: The World Allergy Organization Subcutaneous Immunotherapy Systemic Reaction Grading System. J Allergy Clin Immunol 2010;125(3): 569–74, 574 e1–574 e7.
28. Hino A, et al. Establishment of "Anaphylaxis Scoring Aichi (ASCA)," a new symptom scoring system to be used in an oral food challenge (OFC). Arerugi. 2013;62(8):968–79.
29. Niggemann B, Beyer K. Time for a new grading system for allergic reactions? Allergy. 2016;71(2):135–6.
30. Muraro A, et al. The urgent need for a harmonized severity scoring system for acute allergic reactions. Allergy. 2018.
31. Johansson SG, et al. A revised nomenclature for allergy. An EAACI position statement from the EAACI nomenclature task force. Allergy. 2001;56(9):813–24.
32. Muraro A, et al. EAACI food allergy and anaphylaxis guidelines: diagnosis and management of food allergy. Allergy. 2014;69(8):1008–25.
33. Hompes S, et al. Provoking allergens and treatment of anaphylaxis in children and adolescents—data from the anaphylaxis registry of German-speaking countries. Pediatr Allergy Immunol. 2011;22(6):568–74.

# Permissions

# List of Contributors

**Alexandra F Santos**
Department of Paediatric Allergy, Division of Asthma, Allergy and Lung Biology, King's College London, London, UK
MRC and Asthma UK Centre in Allergic Mechanisms of Asthma, London, UK
Immunoallergology Department, Coimbra University Hospital, Coimbra, Portugal

**Luis Miguel Borrego**
CUF Descobertas Hospital, Lisbon, Portugal
CEDOC, Nova Medical School, Universidade Nova de Lisboa, Lisbon, Portugal

**Giuseppina Rotiroti and Glenis Scadding**
The Royal National Throat, Nose and Ear Hospital and University College London Hospitals, London, UK

**Graham Roberts**
David Hide Asthma and Allergy Research Centre, St Mary's Hospital, Isle of Wight, UK
Human Development and Health and Clinical Experimental Sciences Academic Subunits, University of Southampton Faculty of Medicine, Southampton, UK
Respiratory Biomedical Research Unit, University Hospital Southampton NHS Foundation Trust, Southampton, UK
Paediatric Allergy and Respiratory Medicine, University Child Health (MP803), University Hospital Southampton NHS Foundation Trust, Southampton, UK

**Liz Tulum, Zoë Deag, Matthew Brown, Annette Furniss, Lynn Meech, Anja Lalljie and Stella Cochrane**
SEAC Unilever Colworth, Colworth Science Park, Sharnbrook, Bedfordshire MK44 1LQ, UK

**Sangeeta Dham**
Evidence-Based Health Care Ltd, Edinburgh, UK

**Aadam Sheikh**
UCL, London, UK

**Antonella Muraro**
Food Allergy Referral Centre Veneto Region, Department of Women and Child
Health, Padua General University Hospital, Padua, Italy

**Graham Roberts**
The David Hide Asthma and Allergy Research Centre, St Mary's Hospital, Newport Isle of Wight, NIHR Respiratory Biomedical Research Unit, University Hospital Southampton NHS Foundation Trust, Southampton, UK
Faculty of Medicine, University of Southampton, Southampton, UK

**Susanne Halken**
Hans Christian Andersen Children's Hospital, Odense University Hospital, Odense, Denmark

**Monserat Fernandez Rivas**
Hospital Clínico San Carlos - Jefe del Servicio de Alergia, Madrid, Spain

**Margitta Worm**
Chartie-Universitatsmedizin, Berlin, Germany

**Aziz Sheikh**
Allergy and Respiratory Research Group, Asthma UK Centre for Applied Research, Usher Institute of Population Health Sciences and Informatics, The University of Edinburgh, Edinburgh, UK

**Georg Boelke, Karl-Christian Bergmann and Torsten Zuberbier**
Charité – Universitätsmedizin Berlin, corporate member of Freie Universität Berlin, Humboldt-Universität zu Berlin, and Berlin Institute of Health, Department of Dermatology and Allergy, Allergy-Center-Charité, Berlin, Germany

**Uwe Berger**
Department of Otorhinolaryngology, Aerobiology and Pollen Information
Research Unit, Medical University of Vienna, Vienna, Austria.

**Carsten Bindslev-Jensen**
Department of Dermatology and Allergy Centre, Odense University Hospital, Odense, Denmark

**Jean Bousquet**
CHRU, Montpellier University Hospital Center, Montpellier, France

**Julia Gildemeister**
Mobile Chamber Experts GmbH, Berlin, Germany

**Marek Jutel**
ALL-MED Medical Research Institute, Wrocław, Poland
Department of Clinical Immunology, Wroclaw Medical University, Wrocław, Poland

**Oliver Pfaar**
Department of Otorhinolaryngology, Head and Neck Surgery, Universitätsmedizin Mannheim, Medical Faculty Mannheim, Heidelberg University, Mannheim, Germany
Center for Rhinology and Allergology, Wiesbaden, Germany

**Torsten Sehlinger**
Bluestone Technology GmbH, Woerrstadt, Germany

**Peter W. Hellings**
Department of Otorhinolaryngology, University Hospitals Leuven, KU Leuven, Louvain, Belgium
Department of Otorhinolaryngology, Academic Medical Center, Amsterdam, The Netherlands

**David Borrelli**
Italian Member of the European Parliament, EFDD Group, Brussels, Belgium

**Sirpa Pietikainen**
Finnish Member of the European Parliament, Brussels, Belgium

**Ioana Agache**
Faculty of Medicine, Transylvania University, Brasov, Romania

**Cezmi Akdis**
Swiss Institute of Allergy and Asthma Research (SIAF), University of Zurich, Davos, Switzerland
Christine Kühne – Center for Allergy Research and Education (CK-CARE), Davos, Switzerland

**Claus Bachert**
Upper Airways Research Laboratory, ENT Department, Ghent University Hospital, Ghent, Belgium.

**Michael Bewick**
Q4U Consultants Ltd, London, UK

**Erna Botjes**
EFA - European Federation of Allergy and Airways Diseases Patients' Associations, Brussels, Belgium

**Jannis Constantinidis**
1st Department of ORL, Head and Neck Surgery, Aristotle University, Thessaloníki, Greece

**Tari Haahtela**
Skin and Allergy Hospital, Helsinki University Hospital, Helsinki, Finland

**Claire Hopkins**
ENT Department, Guy's and St Thomas' Hospitals, London, UK

**Maddalena Illario**
Division for Health Innovation, Campania Region and Federico II University Hospital Naples (R&D and DISMET), Naples, Italy

**Guy Joos**
Department of Respiratory Medicine, Ghent University Hospital, Ghent, Belgium

**Valerie Lund**
Royal National Throat, Nose and Ear Hospital, University College London Hospitals, LondonUK

**Antonella Muraro**
Food Allergy Referral Centre Veneto Region, Department of Women and Child Health, Padua General University Hospital, Padua, Italy

**Benoit Pugin and Sven Seys**
European Forum for Research and Education in Allergy and Airway Diseases (EUFOREA), Brussels, Belgium

**Sven Seys**
Lab of Clinical Immunology, Department of Immunology and Microbiology, KU Leuven, Brussels, Belgium

**David Somekh**
European Health Futures Forum (EHFF), Isle of Wright, UK

**Pär Stjärne**
Rhinology Department of Otorhinolaryngology, Karolinska University Hospital, Stockholm, Sweden

**Arunas Valiulis**
Vilnius University Clinic of Children's Diseases and Public Health Institute, Vilnius, Lithuania
European Academy of Paediatrics (EAP/UEMS-SP), Brussels, Belgium

**Erkka Valovirta**
Department of Lung Diseases and Clinical Allergology, Univ. of Turku, and Allergy Clinic, Terveystalo, Turku, Finland

**Jean Bousquet**
MACVIA-France, Contre les MAladies Chroniques pour un VIeillissement Actif en France European Innovation Partnership on Active and Healthy Ageing Reference Site, Montpellier, France
INSERM U 1168, VIMA: Ageing and Chronic Diseases Epidemiological and Public Health Approaches, UMR-S 1168, Université Versailles St-Quentinen-Yvelines, Villejuif, Montigny le Bretonneux, France

EUFOREA aisbl, 132, Ave. Brand Whitlock, 1200 Brussels, Belgium

**David Price**
University of Aberdeen, Aberdeen, UK

**Glenis Scadding**
The Royal National Throat, Nose and Ear Hospital, London, UK

**Dermot Ryan**
Woodbrook Medical Centre, Loughborough, UK
University of Edinburgh, Edinburgh, UK

**Claus Bachert**
Upper Airways Research Laboratory, Ghent University Hospital, Ghent, Belgium

**G. Walter Canonica**
Allergy and Respiratory Clinic, IRCCS AOU S. Martino, Genoa, Italy

**Joaquim Mullol**
Hospital Clínic, IDIBAPS, CIBERES, Barcelona, Catalonia, Spain

**Ludger Klimek**
Center for Rhinology and Allergology, Wiesbaden, Germany

**Richard Pitman**
ICON, Oxford, UK

**Sarah Acaster**
Acaster Consulting, London, UK

**Ruth Murray**
Medscript Ltd, Dundalk, Ireland

**Jean Bousquets**
University Hospital, Montpellier, France
MACVIA-LR, Contre les Maladies Chronique spour un Vieillissement Actif en Languedoc Roussilon, European Innovation Partnership on Active and Healthy Ageing Reference Site, Montpellier, France
INSERM, VIMA : Ageing and Chronic Diseases, Epidemiological and Public Health Approaches, U1168, Paris, France
UVSQ, UMR-S 1168, Université Versailles St-Quentin-en-Yvelines, Versailles, France

**Yubao Cui, Qiong Wang and Haoyuan Jia**
Department of Clinical Laboratory, Wuxi People's Hospital Affiliated to Nanjing Medical University, No. 299, Qingyang Road, Wuxi 214023, Jiangsu Province, People's Republic of China

**Alberto Alvarez-Perea and María L. Baeza**
Allergy Service, Hospital General Universitario Gregorio Marañón, Doctor Esquerdo, 46, 28007 Madrid, Spain
Gregorio Marañón Health Research Institute, Madrid, Spain

**Luciana Kase Tanno**
Hospital Sírio Libanês, São Paulo, Brazil
Division of Allergy, Department of Pulmonology, University Hospital of Montpellier, Montpellier, France
Pierre and Marie Curie Institute of Epidemiology and Public Health, Sorbonne Universités, Paris, France

**María L. Baeza**
Biomedical Research Network on Rare Diseases (CIBERER)-U761, Madrid, Spain

**Emilia Mikola, Tuomo Puhakka and Lotta Ivaska**
Department of Otorhinolaryngology, Turku University Hospital and Turku University, Turku, Finland

**Varpu Elenius, Maria Saarinen, Riitta Turunen and Tuomas Jartti**
Department of Paediatrics and Adolescent Medicine, Turku University Hospital and Turku University, 20520 Turku Finland

**Oscar Palomares, Beate Rückert, Alar Aab and Mübeccel Akdis**
Swiss Institute of Allergy and Asthma Research, University of Zürich, Davos, Switzerland
Christine Kühne-Center for Allergy Research and Education, Davos, Switzerland

**Oscar Palomares**
Department of Biochemistry and Molecular Biology, School of Chemistry, Complutense University of Madrid, Madrid, Spain

**Matti Waris**
Department of Clinical Virology, Turku University Hospital, Turku, Finland
Department of Virology, University of Turku, Turku, Finland

**Tuomo Puhakka**
Department of Otorhinolaryngology, Satakunta Central Hospital, Pori, Finland

**Tero Vahlberg**
Department of Biostatistics, University of Turku and Turku University Hospital, Turku, Finland

**Tobias Allander**
Department of Clinical Microbiology, Karolinska University Hospital, Stockholm, Sweden

**Carlos A. Camargo Jr.**
Department of Emergency Medicine, Massachusetts General Hospital, Harvard Medical School, Boston, USA
Division of Rheumatology, Allergy and Immunology, Department of Medicine, Massachusetts
General Hospital, Harvard Medical School, Boston, USA

**C. Cingi**
Department of Otorhinolaryngology, Eskisehir Osmangazi University School of Medicine, Eskisehir, Turkey

**P. Gevaert**
Upper Airway Research Laboratory, Ghent University Hospital, Ghent, Belgium

**R. Mösges**
Institute of Medical Statistics, Informatics, and Epidemiology, Medical Faculty, University of Köln, Cologne, Germany

**C. Rondon**
Allergy Unit, IBIMA, Regional University Hospital of Malaga, UMA, Malaga, Spain

**V. Hox**
Clinical division of Otorhinolaryngology, Head and Neck Surgery, University Hospitals Leuven, Louvain, Belgium

**M. Rudenko**
London Allergy and Immunology Centre, London, UK

**N. B. Muluk**
ENT Department, Faculty of Medicine, Kirikkale University, Kirikkale, Turkey

**G. Scadding**
Royal National Throat, Nose and Ear Hospital, London, UK

**F. Manole**
Faculty of Medicine, ENT Department, University of Oradea, Oradea, Romania

**C. Hupin**
Institut de Recherche Expérimentale et Clinique (IREC), Pole de Pneumologie, ORL and Dermatologie, Université catholique de Louvain, Louvain-la-Neuve, Belgium

**W. J. Fokkens**
Department of Otorhinolaryngology, Head and Neck Surgery, Academic Medical Centre (AMC), Amsterdam, The Netherlands

**C. Akdis**
Christine Kuhne-Center for Allergy Research and Education, Swiss Institute of Allergy and Asthma Research, University of Zurich, Davos, Switzerland

**P. Demoly**
Hôpital Arnaud de Villeneuve, University Hospital of Montpellier, Montpellier, France

**J. Mullol**
Unitat de Rinologia i Clinica de l'Olfacte, Servei d'Otorinolaringologia, Hospital Clínic, Barcelona, Catalonia, Spain

**A. Muraro**
The Referral Centre for Food Allergy Diagnosis and Treatment Veneto Region, Department
of Mother and Child Health, University of Padua, Padua, Italy

**N. Papadopoulos**
Allergy Department, 2nd Pediatric Clinic, University of Athens, Athens, Greece

**R. Pawankar**
Nippon Medical School, Tokyo, Japan

**P. Rombaux**
Service d'ORL, Cliniques Universitaires St-Luc, Brussels, Belgium

**E. Toskala**
Department of Otorhinolaryngology-Head and Neck Surgery, Temple University, Philadelphia, PA, USA

**L. Kalogjera**
Department of Otorhinolaryngology and Head and Neck Surgery, University Hospital Sestre milosrdnice, Zagreb, Croatia

**E. Prokopakis**
Department of Otorhinolaryngology, University Hospital of Crete, Crete, Greece

**Peter W. Hellings**
Department of Otorhinolaryngology, University Hospitals Leuven, Leuven, Belgium

**Peter W. Hellings and Wytske Fokkens**
Department of Otorhinolaryngology, Academic Medical Center (AMC), Amsterdam, The Netherlands

**Antonella Muraro**
Department of Women and Child Health, Food Allergy Referral Centre, Padua University Hospital, Veneto Region, Padua, Italy

**Joaquim Mullol**
Hospital Clinic, IDIBAPS, CIBERES, Barcelona, Catalonia, Spain

**Claus Bachert**
Upper Airways Research Laboratory (URL), University Hospital Ghent, Ghent, Belgium

**G. Walter Canonica**
Allergy and Respiratory Diseases, Department of Internal Medicine, IRCCS S Martino, IST, University of Genoa, Genoa, Italy

**David Price**
Centre of Academic Primary Care, University of Aberdeen, Aberdeen, UK

**Nikos Papadopoulos**
Allergy Department, 2nd Pediatric Clinic, University of Athens, Athens, Greece

**Glenis Scadding**
RNTNE Hospital, London, UK

**Gerd Rasp**
Department of Otorhinolaryngology, Paracelsus Medical University, Salzburg, Austria

**Pascal Demoly**
Division of Allergy, Department of Pulmonology, Hôpital Arnaud de Villeneuve, University Hospital of Montpellier, Montpellier, France

**Ruth Murray**
MedScript Ltd, Dundalk, Co. Louth, Ireland

**Jean Bousquet**
University Hospital, Montpellier, France
MACVIA-LR, Contre les Maladies Chronique pour un Vieillissement Actif en Languedoc Roussilon, European Innovation Partnership on Active and Healthy Aging Reference Site, Montpellier, France
INSERM, VIMA: Ageing and Chronic Diseases. Epidemiological and Public Health Approaches, U1168 Paris, France
UVSQ UMR-S1168, Universite Versailles St-Quentin-en-Yvelines, Versailles, France

**Maria D'Amato, Antonio Molino and Giovanna Calabrese**
Respiratory Department, 'Federico II University' – Division of Respiratory Medicine and Allergy, Hospital Dei Colli, Naples, Italy

**Lorenzo Cecchi**
Interdepartmental Center of Bioclimatology, University of Florence, Florence, Italy

**Isabella Annesi-Maesano**
Epidemiology of Allergic and Respiratory DIseases Department, IPLESP, INSERM and Sorbonne Université, Medical School Saint-Antoine, Paris, France

**Gennaro D'Amato**
Department of Respiratory Diseases, High Specialty Hospital 'A. Cardarelli' and University of Naples Federico II, School of Specialization in Respiratory Diseases, Rione Sirignano, 10, 80121 Naples, Italy

**Glynnis De Greve and Peter W. Hellings**
Department of Otorhinolaryngology-Head and Neck Surgery, UZ Leuven, Louvain, Belgium

**Peter W. Hellings and Wytske J. Fokkens**
Department of Otorhinolaryngology, Academic Medical Center, Amsterdam, The Netherlands

**Peter W. Hellings**
Upper Airways Research Laboratory, Department of Otorhinolaryngology-Head and Neck Surgery, Ghent University, Ghent, Belgium

**Benoit Pugin, Brecht Steelant and Sven F. Seys**
Laboratory of Clinical Immunology, Department of Immunology and Microbiology, KU Leuven, Herestraat 49/PB811, 3000 Louvain, Belgium

**J. van Tongeren, K. I. L. Röschmann, S. M. Reinartz, S. Luiten, W. J. Fokkens and C. M. van Drunen**
Department of Otorhinolaryngology, Academic Medical Center (AMC), Amsterdam, The Netherlands

**E. C. de Jong**
Department of Cell Biology and Histology, Academic Medical Center (AMC), Amsterdam, The Netherlands

**Chunquan Zheng**
Department of Otolaryngology-Head and Neck Surgery, Eye Ear Nose and Throat Hospital, Fudan University, 83 Fenyang Road, Xuhui District, Shanghai 200031, People's Republic of China

**Yue Ma and Le Shi**
Shanghai Key Clinical Disciplines of Otorhinolaryngology, Shanghai, People's Republic of China

**M. H. Foss-Skiftesvik and M. S. Opstrup**
Department of Dermato-Allergology, National Allergy Research Centre, Copenhagen University Hospital Gentofte, Kildegårdsvej 28, 2900 Hellerup, Denmark

**M. H. Foss-Skiftesvik, H. Søsted and J. D. Johansen**
Department of Dermato-Allergology, Research Centre for Hairdressers and Beauticians, Copenhagen University Hospital Gentofte, Hellerup, Denmark

**L. Winther, H. F. Mosbech, M. S. Opstrup and C. R. Johnsen**
Allergy Clinic, Department of Dermato-Allergology, Copenhagen University Hospital Gentofte, Hellerup, Denmark

**C. Zachariae**
Department of Dermato-Allergology, Copenhagen University Hospital Gentofte, Hellerup, Denmark

**P. S. Skov**
Reflab ApS, Copenhagen, Denmark

**Ying Zhou**
Department of Pediatrics Laboratory, Wuxi Children's Hospital, Wuxi 214023, People's Republic of China

**Haoyuan Jia, Xuming Zhou and Yubao Cui**
Department of Clinical Laboratory, Wuxi People's Hospital Affiliated to Nanjing Medical University, No. 299 at Qingyang Road, Wuxi 214023, Jiangsu Province, People's Republic of China

**Jun Qian**
Department of Pediatrics, Wuxi Children's Hospital, Wuxi 214023, People's Republic of China

**Sven Seys, Benoit Pugin, Brecht Steelant and Peter Hellings**
Laboratory of Clinical Immunology, Department of Microbiology and Immunology, KU Leuven, Kapucijnenvoer 33, 3000 Louvain, Belgium

**Maria Doulaptsi and Emmanuel Prokopakis**
Department of Otorhinolaryngology, Head and Neck Surgery, University of Crete School of Medicine, Heraklion, Crete, Greece

**Peter Hellings**
Clinical Division of Otorhinolaryngology, Head and Neck Surgery, University Hospitals Leuven, Louvain, Belgium

**R. Munoz-Cano, P. Ribó, G. Araujo and A. Valero**
Allergy Unit, Pneumology Department, Hospital Clinic, Universitat de Barcelona, ARADyAL, Barcelona, Spain

**R. Muñoz-Cano and G. Araujo**
Institut d'Investigacions Biomèdiques August Pi i Sunyer, IDIBAPS, Barcelona, Spain.

**P. Ribó and A. Valero**
Allergy Unit, Pneumology Department, Hospital Clinic, Universitat de Barcelona, CIBERES, Barcelona, Spain

**E. Giralt**
Grupo SANED, Barcelona, Spain

**J. Sanchez-Lopez**
Laboratorios LETI SL, Barcelona, Spain

**Jiayun Hu, Jiajie Chen, Lanlan Ye, Zelang Cai and Kunmei Ji**
Department of Biochemistry and Molecular Biology, School of Medicine of Shenzhen University, Shenzhen 518035, China

**Jiayun Hu and Jinlu Sun**
Department of Allergy, Peking Union Medical College Hospital, Peking Union Medical College and Chinese Academy of Medical Sciences, Beijing 100730, China

**Esben Eller, Ronald Dahl, Charlotte Gotthard Mortz and Carsten Bindslev-Jensen**
Odense Research Center for Anaphylaxis (ORCA), Department of Dermatology and Allergy Center, Odense University Hospital, Odense, Denmark

**Antonella Muraro**
Food Allergy Referral Centre – Veneto Region, Department of Women and Child Health, Padua University Hospital, Padua, Italy

**Ronald Dahl**
GSK, Brentford, Middlesex, UK

# Index